Man in the Trap

This el, OP
7⁵⁰

Current db - 7⁹⁵

Man in the Trap

by

ELSWORTH F. BAKER, M.D.

COLLIER BOOKS
A Division of Macmillan Publishing Co., Inc.
New York
COLLIER MACMILLAN PUBLISHERS
· *London*

Macmillan Publishing Co., Inc.
866 Third Avenue, New York, N.Y. 10022
Collier Macmillan Canada, Ltd.

Library of Congress Cataloging in Publication Data
Baker, Elsworth F.
Man in the trap.
Bibliography: p.
Includes index.
  1. Orgonomy. I. Title.
RZ460.B3   1980   615.5′3   79-26675
ISBN 0-02-083650-3 pbk

First Collier Books Edition 1980

Man in the Trap is also published in a hardcover edition by
Macmillan Publishing Co., Inc.

Printed in the United States of America

Permissions for the use of certain material in this book previously contained in works of Wilhelm Reich, M.D., deceased, have been obtained from the publisher, Farrar, Straus & Giroux, Inc.

This book is dedicated to the memory of Wilhelm Reich and to all those who give his concepts life through natural living.

After thousands of years of concentration upon the riddle of the nature of man, humanity finds itself exactly where it started: with the confession of utter ignorance. The Mother is still helpless in the face of a nightmare which harasses her child. And the physician is still helpless in the face of . . . a running nose. . . . Wherever we turn we find man running around in circles as if trapped and searching for the exit in vain and in desperation. . . . *The trap is man's emotional structure, his character structure.* There is little use in devising systems of thought about the nature of the trap if the only thing to do in order to get out of the trap is to know the trap and to find the exit. . . . The exit is clearly visible to all trapped in the hole. Yet nobody seems to see it. Everybody knows where the exit is, yet nobody seems to make a move toward it. More: whoever moves toward the exit or whoever points toward it is declared crazy or a criminal or a sinner. . . . It turns out that the trouble is not with the trap or even with finding the exit. The trouble is *within the trapped ones.* . . . The keys to the exit are cemented into your own character armor and into the mechanical rigidity of your body and soul.

Wilhelm Reich, The Murder of Christ

Contents

PART III

CHARACTER MANAGEMENT: *The Removal of Armoring*

PART IV

CHARACTER MANAGEMENT: *The Prevention of Armoring*

Preface

IN THIS BOOK I have tried to present in organized form the basic
concepts of Reich's theory of character, a theory growing out of
his discoveries about the movement and blocking of energy in
the body. The purpose of the book is to provide a deeper understanding of "character" structure generally in Reich's sense of the
word, and to aid in recognizing and diagnosing character from a
bioenergic point of view. The material is presented concisely but,
I hope, clearly enough to be understood. Parts I and II will be
more understandable if they are reread after the case histories in
Part III, which should give the reader a view of the theory in
application.

The material is based upon my twenty years' experience as a
medical orgonomist, eleven of which were spent in close association with Reich, attendance at his seminars and personal discussions with him. It is based also upon Reich's discoveries which
are recorded in his published works. The reader's attention is
directed to the selected bibliography for a more extensive treatment by Reich of certain of the subjects contained in this book.

Before going to a more general discussion of these theories, I
wish to express my appreciation to all those who helped both
materially and technically in the production of this volume. Of
those who helped materially I must thank my students, who
kept careful notes on my seminars and offered many helpful suggestions in clarifying the material presented. My thanks also to
Dr. Chester M. Raphael for permission to use his article on
orgonomic treatment in labor; to Dr. Barbara Goldenberg for
permission to include her technique of the use of light in therapy

of the eye segment. This I believe is the most important contribution to treatment since Reich. Also for her help in writing several of the character types. My thanks to Paul Mathews for his valuable help and free use of his paper, "Functional Energetic Thought and Contemporary Social Phenomena" in writing my chapter on the liberal and conservative characters; Dr. Charles Konia for his suggestion on the mechanism of guilt.

For technical advice my especial thanks to Professor Paul Edwards without whose valuable help this book would have suffered immeasurably in the writing. I wish to make it clear that Dr. Edwards' help does not mean that he necessarily agrees with what I have written nor is he responsible for any of the contents. This likewise applies to all others who offered technical advice. My thanks to Virginia Carew for her very reliable advice and aid in preparing the manuscript; Marguerite M. Baker, Patricia R. Greene, and James E. Payne for criticisms and suggestions; Martin Berkon for the drawings; and my wife for her tireless retyping of the manuscript each time I made changes.

Referring to material that is specifically mine, I should particularly mention placing the eye as a major erogenous zone. As far as I know no one has specifically done this before, although Reich emphasized the importance of armoring in the eye segment. The more I have worked with patients the more important the eye has become in therapy, both as a means of maintaining objectivity or, conversely, losing it. The eye is also important as a means of erotic excitation and pleasure. This is quite evident neurotically in voyeurism. There is also little doubt in my mind from my experience that armoring in the eye segment fixes the character structure of schizophrenia, epilepsy, and, I believe, voyeurism just as armoring in the anal zone, for example, produces the compulsive, passive feminine, and the masochist. See "The Ocular Stage," in Chapter 2, "The Ocular Segment" in Chapter 4 and Chapter 12.

In writing the chapter on the liberal and conservative characters I am attacking the problem of the third sacred cow, politics. The other two of course are sex and religion. Psychiatry has discussed these two rather fully and the initial furor has largely subsided. I expect a great deal of controversy about the socio-political chapter.

Over many years of professional experience as a psychiatrist and orgone therapist I have been aware of these two other broad types of character structure which, like the emotional plague character, manifest themselves specifically and prominently in social and political functioning. Reich was aware of these types and made frequent allusions to them both in his writings and in private conversation, especially to the liberal character. He wrote extensively on the extreme types of each, namely: communism and fascism. He did not, however, present an organized analysis dealing with these individuals from the standpoint of the therapist. There is no question but that Reich regarded what I define as the modern, characterological liberal, or more accurately the collectivist, as pathological.

Reich himself was basically conservative in his approach to problems of political and social change. This attitude stemmed from his broad experience with human beings, professionally and socially, and his unmatched insight into the human dilemma, i.e. the contradiction between human longings for freedom and the biophysical incapacity to accept it. It was this knowledge which imbued him with a terrible sense of responsibility and a fear and hatred of the "freedom peddlers" whom he felt would bring the world to ultimate disaster in the name of "peace," "freedom," and "justice." It should be understood that Reich was not a modern liberal nor a leftist—although he was "radical" in his scientific explorations and discoveries—in the root-seeking sense of the word. Only the most "hideous distortions" of orgonomic truth—as Reich put it—could possibly equate his work, thinking, and hopes for mankind with those of present-day liberals, leftists, and beatnik-bohemians who have in one way or another attempted to identify themselves with orgonomy.

I shall be dealing with the liberal and conservative characters in an organized manner—for what, I believe, is the first time in clinical, psychiatric literature. The explosive reactions to the analyses of these types have convinced me that an understanding of them is vital to an effective approach to therapy.

The material in this book is in reality an outline of orgonomic biopsychiatry and has been greatly condensed for presentation in one volume. It is my feeling, however, that if the essential features are understood, the complexities can be handled. The basic theory—that character is based on movement and blocking of energy in the body—effectively removes the dichotomy of mind-body functioning. It is a dynamic energetic point of view which I have found provides tools that are unknown to classical psychiatry for treating emotional disorders, and which greatly enhances the therapist's ability to correct these disorders.

Orgonomy[1] is no panacea; not every case can be helped, and cures are at best difficult and require courage and hard work. But the energic concept strikes at the very roots of disease and mobilizes many patients who could not otherwise be touched. I believe the concept is sound; what is necessary is more knowledge of how to use it. Theoretically, it should be possible to help everyone, but we do not yet know enough. Character structures are usually mixtures of classical types and often quite complex; some cannot be understood at all. At best, therapy is only a personal solution, the final solution lies in *prevention* of neurosis, not in its çure. Here, too, Reich showed the way.

Although some general indications are given here about biopsychiatric techniques, this book is not designed as a manual on therapeutic technique. Use of the technique requires personal restructuring through therapy, a minimum of three years of training in seminars, and laboratory and clinical work. Only a physician should attempt to use these methods of treatment, and even the physician must be adequately trained in both conventional methods and orgonomy. The tools are powerful and disaster can result if they are mishandled.[2]

Therapy is functional, and must be made to fit each case; it does not restrict itself to a rigid technique and it does not ignore conventional methods where they can be helpful. Classical medicine is constantly called upon where it can be of use. The primary

---

[1] "Orgonomy" is here used loosely. Actually, it includes physical, biological, sociological, and the medical sciences generally.

[2] Reich's latest discovery in the treatment of emotional problems by directly drawing energy from the armor is not described. Reich's preliminary studies warrant hopeful expectations, especially in schizophrenia, epilepsy, and the cancer biopathy.

concern is to see and fulfill the needs of the patient in his struggle toward health.

Until comparatively recent years, the cause and the mechanism of neuroses were unknown; we did not know why or how it is possible for man to harbor such disease. Prior to Freud, emotional illness was considered evidence of degeneration.

Man has always pondered the nature of life and tried to understand it. How, for example, does a living cell differ from a dead one, or a living being from a dead one? From ancient times, to explain this mystery, man has postulated a dualism of the soul and the body: when the body dies the soul escapes and lives on. In recent times, this theme has been developed into the cult of spiritualism, while at the opposite pole the mechanists have rejected the idea of soul and tried to explain life purely in terms of chemical processes. Each theory emphasized one side and more or less ignored any contradictory facts from the other. The complete picture remained obscure.

It is logical to assume that life must be a natural process that at some time evolved from non-living processes, but purely mechanical thinking leaves too many gaps to be explained. For example, what is an emotion? Rage? Love? Anxiety? What happens in the body when you thrill to pleasure or shrink from pain? Exactly what is a nerve impulse? A psychic impulse? The spark when you touch a metal doorknob after walking over a woolen rug? These are energy phenomena, yes; but is this an energy that is foreign to the body? What explains your effect on a sensitive television set when you stand near it without touching it?

All of the examples cited seem rather obviously to be energy processes in which free energy in the body affects or is affected by energy from outside it. Popular speech accepts this concept. People say, "You have a lot of energy," or "I've no energy at all today." Yet if you probe to discover exactly what people mean you get no satisfactory answer, and your questions are likely to arouse uneasiness and a desire to change the subject. Aristotle called this energy "hormone." Bergson, the French philosopher, explained it with his idea of *"élan vital."* Freud, in a narrower sense, termed it the "libido." Wilhelm Reich, after a quarter of a century of dealing with emotional problems and conducting research into their causes, identified a specific energy in the body which he called bioenergy or "orgone" (organism) energy, hence "orgonomy." He presented a wealth of experimental confirmation of its natural primordial origin and life-giving properties, its direct linkage with natural functioning. This was too much for the experts to accept all at once, and Reich became one of the most controversial figures of our time.

No one who has any knowledge of Reich's work can be indifferent. People are either violently opposed and accuse him of being insane, a sex maniac, or a fraud; or they are just as violently in favor and work to build up a cult designed to put into practice what they believe he stood for. Unfortunately, neither group has been able to understand him or his teachings, and both do him a great injustice. This is understandable, because his work touched man in his deepest emotions: love, hate, fear, and longing. To defend themselves from such painful self-knowledge, people must either turn away and fight bitterly, or follow blindly and mystically.

It is a great pity for the world that each new scientist who comes to upset old theories and change old concepts must meet the same kind of distortion, falsehood, and persecution, only to be lauded hundreds of years later. Reich will not be properly evaluated in our generation or the next, or perhaps even for generations beyond that. Each of us has a limitation on how far he can follow objectively and with an open mind; classical psychiatry, for example, can accept him as far as *Character Analysis,* but beyond that insists his teachings are unsound.

As one who worked closely with Reich for over ten years and tried very hard to enter neither of the groups mentioned above, but rather to allow Reich to demonstrate and prove his work, I can say categorically that as a therapist and as a teacher he has never been surpassed. His amazing insight and ability to go directly to the root of a problem were a constant revelation to his students. He was always cautious, thorough, and frank to admit it when he did not know.

Reich became a pupil of Freud at a time when psychoanalytic theory was just taking recognizable form. Freud had already determined that the neurotic was not a degenerate as previously believed, but rather was an average person suffering from an illness the cause of which was sexual inhibition. He had worked out the psychic structure of the ego, superego, ego ideal, and id—the unconscious influences on functioning—and a concept of psychic or sexual energy which he termed "libido." Freud's technique enabled him to unravel the chaotic functioning of the neurotic through free association and through the interpretation of dreams. He insisted that material should not be selected, but should be interpreted as it came up from the unconscious and called the process psychoanalysis. He thought that success in therapy depended upon utilizing the positive transference of the patient to enable him to face his anxiety and his problems. Such transference was therefore a vital part of therapy. The average person was considered healthy. His latest theory was that of the death instinct, which he proposed in order to explain the enigma of the masochist and of those others who seemed to prefer suffering or even death to health.

Reich, as Freud's pupil, soon established himself as an innovator. Seeking to find a method of establishing a firmer positive transference, he moved down from behind the couch to sit beside the patient and look at him, and allow the patient to see him. He thus made contact with the individual behind the neurosis he was treating. He repeatedly came up against resistances in the patient. Resistance was not new but handling it was not well understood, especially latent resistance, which was frequently not even recognized. Previously the transference had been utilized to overcome resistance and was thus considered all-important. Reich attacked the resistance directly by pointing out that the patient was resistant and telling him how he was showing it. That is, he described the patient's attitudes and handled each new resistance as it appeared.

Co-workers argued against such tactics, but Reich kept on and found that as resistances were dissolved painful material at the root of the neurosis spontaneously began to appear in logical order until basic conflicts were reached. When these were overcome, the patient showed a great change, both in his attitudes and in his functioning, and eventually was capable of true positive transference.

Reich thus demonstrated that the former "positive transfer-ence" was actually a latent resistance designed to avoid painful material. He finally concluded that there was no such thing as genuine positive transference early in therapy.

When resistances were analyzed the personality structure, or character, began to change. This change showed that not only were symptoms evidence of neurosis, but that *the character itself was neurotic.* Character neurosis was a new concept and Reich called his new method "character analysis." By its means he solved the problem of masochism and proved that the idea of the death instinct was a fallacy. It was not that the masochist did not want to get well because of a biological death instinct, nor was it that he preferred to suffer, but rather it was that his in-tolerance of expansion and movement made response to therapy impossible. Even the masochist is following the pleasure prin-ciple.

A study of patients cured and not cured, regardless of the extent of the analysis, revealed consistently that the former had developed a satisfactory sexual life while the latter had not. This brought into focus the need for regulating the organism's energy; in order to cure a patient, libido stasis had to be overcome. Previously, sexual problems were considered only symptoms, not the core of the neurosis, and erective potency in the male and any kind of pleasurable response in the female were considered evidence of adequate sexual functioning. But now it was clear that in order to cure a patient, the libido stasis had to be over-come. Sexual activity in itself did not guarantee this, but gratifi-cation in the sexual act did. Reich called the capacity for gratifi-cation "orgastic potency."

Some psychiatrists still insist that there are neurotics who lead normal sexual lives. Indeed, I have had several patients who described their sexual lives in terms of typical orgastic potency. Such patients are apt to be schizophrenics. This appearance of perfect sexual health is easily disturbed, and can usually be completely dissipated by telling the patient that it is all an illu-sion. True sexual potency, however, cannot be eliminated in that way. When these apparently sexually healthy patients develop genuine sexual feelings they recognize that earlier feelings had been quite different.

Establishment of orgastic potency brings about very definite changes in the individual—changes which are not properly recognized or understood by most psychiatrists even today. The recognition of orgastic potency was crucial. Such potency includes the ability to discharge excess energy and thus maintain a stabilized energy level. This process of energy metabolism takes place in a four-beat rhythm of:

TENSION ⟶ CHARGE ⟶ DISCHARGE ⟶ RELAXATION

Reich called this the *orgasm formula*.

The orgastic potency concept confronted Reich with another inescapable conclusion. The libido must be more than a psychic concept. *It must be a real energy.* A person who develops truly adequate sexual release cannot maintain a neurosis. Neuroses exist only on repressed excess energy, or stasis. Moreover, as a patient achieves orgastic potency and emerges from his neurotic character, he undergoes certain basic changes. His attitudes toward society change. Many social mores become incomprehensible; for example, living with a mate he does not love merely because the law says he is married, or an insistence on faithfulness out of duty. He has morals, true, but they are concerned with different values: sex is a desire only with one he loves, promiscuity is uninteresting, pornography is distasteful. He is not interested in perversion but feels tolerance toward it and intolerance toward the unbending attitude of society. He becomes *self-regulating*.

Furthermore, certain other changes occur. His face becomes relaxed and expressive. His body loses its stiffness and appears more alive. He is able to give freely and react spontaneously to situations.

What has made this change? His body is relaxed where formerly it was rigid through permanent muscular contraction as a defense against feeling and giving. The neurosis was anchored in this rigidity—the "armor" which produced and maintained the character.

Reich's discovery of the armoring of the musculature was a

major advance, for when the armor is dissolved in therapy it releases the orgasm reflex—the ability of the organism to yield to its normal functioning. But equally important, it led to an unexpected and revolutionary turn in his research. What produces the muscular contraction and holds it? Investigation led to the realm of the vegetative nervous system and the basic antithesis of vegetative functioning. Excitation of the sympathetic nervous system causes *contraction,* which is felt as anxiety. Parasympathetic excitation causes *expansion,* which is felt as pleasure. It is chronic sympatheticatonia, therefore, which causes and maintains the armor, which in turn maintains the neurosis.

With these findings, Reich left the psychic realm of psychoanalysis, entered into biophysics, and found a new concept for health—a concept based on energy metabolism of charge and discharge, which he called *sex economy.* His therapeutic technique improved, for he found that by working on the muscular armor directly as well as working on the character he could release the pent-up emotions more effectively. He called this *character analytic vegetotherapy.* It was faster and more thorough than psychoanalysis or even character analysis, and was effective with a greater number of patients.

As "emotions" more and more came to mean to him the manifestations of a tangible bioenergy, and "character" to mean simply specific blockings of the flow of that energy, he found that it was possible to change character directly by freeing biological energy, rather than indirectly through the use of psychological techniques. His therapy thus came to be called *medical orgone therapy.* Nevertheless, the psychological aspect was not ignored; its importance depended on the individual case. In some cases, character analysis is still the major approach; in others, it is largely unnecessary, and verbal communication consists of education, understanding of goals, and discussions of problems and resistances.

Thus three major steps, whose value cannot be overestimated, had been discovered and had opened a vast opportunity for understanding human functioning: the reality of the libido (it is a flow of energy), the function of the orgasm (it regulates the flow of energy), and the muscular armor (it prevents regulation of energy). Let us examine the three in more detail.

In the first place, the isolation of the function of the orgasm made it necessary to study the distinction between a satisfactory sexual life and an unsatisfactory sexual life and their separate effects on the organism. The difference between satisfaction and mere sexual expression was that the satisified organism could remain healthy even though analytically his therapy had not been complete, while those with thorough analysis remained untouched where they had not accomplished satisfaction in sex. Somehow this satisfaction drained off the neurosis so that ideas or complexes could no longer be considered the important factor. We were literally dealing with physiology, not just concepts. Nor was it just a matter of expression of the sexual substance, since ejaculation occurred in unsatisfactory experiences also. The determining factor in satisfaction was the experiencing of pleasure in the act. Pleasure is felt in the skin, so the next logical step was to investigate skin reactions.

Reich believed that, in pleasure, there was an electrical charge at the skin surface and he set out to investigate. He used a galvanometer and found that there actually was a charge. The greater the pleasure the higher the charge that showed on the galvanometer. Furthermore, in unpleasurable situations the charge disappeared. Here was concrete evidence of a real energy. Reich called it "bioelectric energy." Further research indicated that it was not a type of electric energy, so Reich renamed it "orgone" (organism) energy, or life energy. Later he showed that this energy radiated out beyond the skin surface as an energy field.

Precise clinical studies showed that in satisfactory sexual experiences this energy was somehow concentrated in the genital area and then discharged, relieving stasis in the organism. Where anxiety was present no charge reached the skin and discharge could not occur. The genital could thus be looked upon as a specialized organ of the skin capable of discharging energy.

The function of the sexual act seemed to be primarily to maintain an economic energy level in the organism. That function could not be carried out adequately unless anxiety was absent and the organism could surrender completely to its pleasurable sensations. With surrender, the act ended with the total convulsions of the body and momentary loss of consciousness known as the orgastic convulsion or orgasm. Thus Freud's theory of the libido found startling confirmation.

We pause to ask why such a mechanism should be necessary: why doesn't the body just use up its energy? In the normal course of events, more energy is built up than can be used. Energy is stored in the body like money in a bank for emergency situations. During such emergencies as battle, worry, or exhausting work, this excess energy is used up and the organism is asexual. In ordinary circumstances, however, energy keeps piling up, so that the organism would have to grow continually or would eventually burst unless some mechanism were present to discharge the accumulated energy after it had reached a certain level. This level of energy is known as the "lumination point," and in the healthy individual is experienced as sexual excitement. Where excitation is blocked, it is felt as tension or restlessness, or other discomfort. This discharge is necessary at more or less regular intervals, depending on other mechanisms for handling energy (work, worry, growth, etc). (One recalls, here, Freud's theory of sublimation. It is effective to a very limited extent in preventing stasis.)

Now, what happens if a child is taught that sex is forbidden and this avenue of release is blocked? Energy builds up to the point of sexual excitement, but he finds himself forced to hold back. He pulls back his pelvis, tightens the muscles of his thighs and buttocks, holds his breath or clenches his teeth, and does not allow himself to think of or to look at anything that will disturb his self-control. Eventually he loses the sensation of sexual desire, but finds his body tight from tensed muscles. In other words, he has become armored. This process may continue until all the muscles of his body are involved and still the energy increases. In the end it overflows in the form of neurotic symptoms. This process is started at birth, because of the universal anti-sexual attitude of our society. Few people grow up as nature intended, and the average person is not healthy, even though he may not have reached the stage of having overt symptoms.

Again, Reich asked if all this repression is necessary. Why is it so universal? This question was not easy to answer, but one finding was consistent. Every patient under therapy reacted with terror when he reached the end phase where all armor was dissolved and he was confronted with the necessity of surrendering to his bodily sensations. His body had been so accustomed to holding still that it could not tolerate free movement. Stillness, immobility, unchangingness—they were safe. They were something to cling to, a certainty to save one from destruction.

Functional ideas have been developed in the past, only to be stifled by the application of an absolute, an immobility. Normal urges were killed and themselves became killers because of this great terror, orgastic anxiety. Neurotic man cannot stand natural movement and fights bitterly against it wherever he finds it; his consistent source of error is in this fight against nature which results from armoring and orgasm anxiety. What terror to make contact with the cosmos and feel the pulsating eternity around him! So man has never accepted a continuum of moving, luminating energy in which all atoms, planets, suns, and galaxies are included in the pulsation and react vibrantly to each other's charge.[3] He quiets himself and so egotistically quiets the universe.

Yet stillness is not satisfying and never can be, for deep within man is a stirring always calling for expression. He longs for the freedom he once felt ("heaven lies about us in our infancy") and promises himself he will find it again when he dies. God will give it back to him when the spirit is free of the armored body. Even here on earth he strives for that freedom, but unfortunately he does not know what he seeks.

Christianity and brotherly love will bring it, he says, but instead they brought prejudice. Freedom from tyranny will bring it—but more tyranny came. Monarchy is at fault, he says, but revolution brought new wrongs, Capitalism is to blame—but the workers were more tyrannical. Man cannot be free because he cannot tolerate freedom. His body is rigid and when his soft

[3] Opik, internationally known astronomer, offers a similar concept which he calls, "The Oscillating Universe." Cf. his book by the same name published by The New American Library. Opik, however, does not postulate a primordial all-pervasive cosmic energy as Reich did. Astronomers are now concerned that none of their current theories of the origin of the universe account for the energy manifested.

nature does try to reach out, it backs up at the armor. When there is sufficient push to pass through the armor the energy emerges as something harsh and brutal. Natural strivings, when they pass through armor, change from soft to harsh. Primary drives become secondary drives, and secondary drives are destructive; so the world is filled with destructiveness and man seems bent on destroying himself and his natural environment in spite of all his knowledge and efforts to improve his lot.

He has become the master of the earth but he destroys and wastes its resources with little consistent thought for the future. Everywhere he upsets the fine balance nature has established in effective functioning. He destroys the forests, and the waters rush away and the land dries up and erodes. He plows land that should be left for grazing and winds blow away the topsoil and produce desert. He kills off animals and birds that keep down rodents and insects. He spreads his diseases far and wide. He builds houses and buries his dead on the best land, and lets the bad land remain useless. He pollutes his streams and lakes and even his atmosphere, and now, even worse, fills it with radioactivity, the results of which no one can yet foresee. Not content with all this, he sets about destroying his own kind and even his own self. Peaceful peoples are mercilessly butchered or put into slavery. He prepares for and makes war, destroying resources the people need—and the people themselves. He stifles his children and adolescents and makes it wrong to express emotions nature gave them. He even poisons the very food he eats.[4] Such is incredible man.

Moreover, each organized effort he makes to correct his destructiveness becomes in itself destructive. The brotherly love of Christianity turned into the Inquisition; the effort to escape from religious persecution led to the witch hunts of Salem; the overthrow of the tyranny of the Czar led to the even worse tyranny of communism.

Classical psychiatry accepts this destructiveness as natural and

[4] Preservatives, artificial coloring and flavoring, or antiseptics are added to almost all processed foods; further, hormones and antibiotics fed to meat animals are not always proven harmless to humans, and outright poisons are used to kill insects on growing fruit and vegetables. Cf. *Silent Spring* by Rachel Carson.

believes that the child needs more "civilizing" and "control" instead of sensing that the destructiveness is a result of such "control." This problem of destructiveness cannot be solved by reform or law. It cannot be solved at all as long as we armor ourselves. And we must armor as long as we repress sexuality. And we must repress sexuality as long as our culture exists in its present form. It is a chain of destruction.

Reich did not like this unraveling any more than man does generally, but the world hounded him to death because of his insights. It is easier to accept armoring than to discover and live with nature. If we do not like our situation and seriously wish to save ourselves, we have only one alternative, and that is to bring up children naturally and to accept adolescent sexuality. This cannot be done suddenly or chaos would develop from licentious abandon or paralysis would arise from lack of direction and control of pent-up neurotic pressures. Without self-regulation, there must be regulation, so constructive change must come gradually and from the hearts of enough people to make it work. First we must recognize the goal, then work toward it.

Reich's findings of armor plus orgastic anxiety explain many enigmas of human functioning, such as mysticism and mechanistic thinking. One of the most important of these he termed the *emotional plague*. This is the social or individual structure that consistently blocks all progress toward natural functioning. No one of us is free of it completely, but there are certain persons who function essentially as emotional pests. They are capable, intelligent, and have a high energy level, but they are anti-sexual and prone to seek positions of authority where they can dictate rules of living. They are the bulwark of society—and they cannot tolerate natural functioning. It creates a longing in them which is intolerable, and so their prime purpose in life is to place restrictions on any natural living that might disturb them. At the same time, they rationalize their behavior so successfully that it is accepted as for the common good.

It was the emotional plague that caused persecution of people in order to maintain the belief that the world was flat, that the sun revolved around the earth, that evolution was against the ideas of God, and that children were asexual. Any finding that increases knowledge of natural functioning or man's relation to the cosmos is forbidden and comes to acceptance only after a bitter struggle and much persecution, as with Socrates, Jesus, Galileo, Copernicus, Roger Bacon, Semmelweis, Pasteur, Lister, Darwin, and Freud. And now Reich.

Destructive knowledge is accepted at once. Man has lost his ability to surrender to his nature, a surrender which sends energy streaming through his pelvis, a surrender where love is really felt and oneness with nature exists. Such natural findings cannot be accepted thus because they cannot be felt or tolerated within the organism, and so we fight against them, or do not see them, or explain them away.

Our greatest weapon against such restrictions is knowledge. Our hope must be to know what is really true and what is natural and why man fights against it so fiercely. Reich has told us much that is true about man, if we can listen and remain objective even though we wish to run from it.

Glossary

Anorgonia—The condition of diminished or complete lack of energy charge in the organism.

Anxiety—The emotional perception of the organism as it is constricted by a contraction against expansion. A distressing sense of oppression, or a vague, formless worry.

Armor—The sum total of the muscular attitudes (chronic muscular spasms) which an individual develops as a defense against the breakthrough of emotions and vegetative sensations, especially anxiety, rage, and sexual excitation. Functionally identical with character armor.

Bioenergy—The energy in the living organism which provides the ability for functioning.

Biophysical—The status of charge and movement of energy in the organism.

Biopsychiatry—Psychiatry from the energic point of view.

Block—Contraction in the organism which prevents the free flow of energy or its excitation.

Character armor—The sum total of the character attitudes which an individual develops as a defense against anxiety, resulting in character rigidity, lack of contact, "deadness." Functionally identical with muscular armor.

Contact—The perception of sensation produced by movement of energy above a certain minimal level plus excitation.

Contactlessness—Absence of contact.

Core—The vegetative nervous system from which involuntary stimuli arise to maintain functioning of the organism.

Cosmic feelings—The sensation of being a part of nature and the universe, of belonging to it rather than an isolated entity.

Depersonalization—The loss of self-perception which depends on contact between the excitation and the subjective feeling of the excitation.

DOR energy—The resultant state when primordial orgone energy reacts with an energy which has come out of matter, especially radioactivity. It is black, lusterless, immobile, oxygen and water hungry, and toxic. Reich felt that it was a normal stage of metabolism in the body but when the body fails to metabolize it adequately disease results.

Energy charge—The quantitative estimation of energy present.

Erogenous—Capable of intense pleasure sensations usually felt as sexual excitation.

Fixation—The arrest of emotional development or desire, especially sexual desire, upon some person or object.

Genital character—The un-neurotic character who does not suffer from sexual stasis and is therefore capable of natural self-regulation.

Hook—A block that for some reason, either in its development or in a particular significance to the individual, is particularly difficult if not impossible to overcome.

Libido—The sexual energy. Energy in the organism above a certain level which is felt as sexual excitation.

Neurotic character—The character which, due to chronic sexual stasis, operates according to the principle of compulsive moral regulation.

Orgasm anxiety—Anxiety produced by final and complete surrender of the organism giving in to its involuntary convulsion. Seen in the final stages of therapy. In the final analysis orgasm anxiety is behind all armored manifestations.

Orgasm reflex—The unitary involuntary contraction and expansion of the total organism seen when the organism is at rest and energy flow is uninhibited. Also seen at the acme of the sexual act, suppressed in most humans.

Orgastic impotence—The absence of orgastic potency. By damming up of biological energy in the organism it provides the source of energy for all kinds of psychic and somatic symptoms.

Orgastic potency—The capacity for complete surrender to the involuntary contraction of the organism and complete discharge of sexual excitation in the acme of the sexual act. It is always lacking in neurotic individuals.

Orgone energy—Primordial cosmic energy, universally present and demonstrated visually, thermically, electroscopically, and with the Geiger-Muller counter. In the living organism it is biological energy.

Orgonomy—The natural science of orgone energy and its functions.

Orgonotic charge—The same as energy charge.

Orgonotic pulsation—The pulsation of the energy in the body which can be determined by an oscillograph.

Parasympathetic—That part of the vegetative system where excitation produces expansion in the organism.

Paresthesias—Distorted sensations arising out of blocking of the energy flow through a part. Felt as prickling, tingling, or creeping.

Plasmatic shrinking—The state of gradual lowering of the energy level through depression or disease such as cancer.

Pleasure anxiety—The fear of pleasurable excitation which means expansion, basically the fear of expansion and movement.

Pleasure streamings—The perception of pleasant, wavelike movement of energy in the body much as a soft breeze flowing through. It gives a three-dimensional perception of the body.

Pregenital—Development occurring before genital primacy is attained at approximately five years of age.

Primary drive—The natural expressions of the body which occur when there are no enforced inhibitions.

Secondary drive—Expressions of the body which have to come through armor and are therefore forceful and destructive.

Sex economy—The body of knowledge which deals with the economy of the biological energy in the organism, with its energy household.

Stasis—The damming up of sexual energy in the organism, thus the source of energy for the neuroses.

Substitute contact—An attempt to make contact in the absence of real contact. It is therefore stilted and artificial.

Sympatheticatonia—A continual state of sympathetic excitation due to continuing anxiety.

Vegetative contact—Natural contact—see contact.

Vegetative functioning—Natural unblocked functioning.

Warded off—Prevented from expression.

Notes to the 1980 Printing

On pp. xxvii-xxix, definitions for "Armor," "Character armor," "Genital character," "Neurotic character," "Orgasm reflex," "Orgastic impotence," "Orgastic potency," "Orgone energy," "Orgonomy," "Pleasure anxiety," "Sex economy," and "Stasis" were given by Wilhelm Riech, M.D.

On p. 37, "The solution occurs in three stages." From *Character Analysis, op. cit.,* pp. 147 ff.

On p. 48, *The Ocular Segment*: The description of the segments within this chapter which follow, and related symptoms, are based upon corresponding material contained in *Character Analysis, op. cit.,* pp. 370 ff. and *Function of the Orgasm, op. cit.,* pp. 266 ff.

On p. 67, present footnote references are to pp. 293 ff.

On p. 77, "Reich distinguished three groupings . . . self-gratification in childhood." From Wilhelm Reich, M.D., "About Genital Self-satisfaction in Children," in *Orgone Energy Bulletin,* Vol. 2, No. 2, pp. 64-65.

On p. 93, the following replaces the present footnote: The material which follows is essentially a condensation of material found in *The Sexual Revolution, op. cit.,* pp. 103 ff.

On p. 124, *Characteristics and Symptoms*: Cf. *Character Analysis, op. cit.,* pp. 193 ff.

On p. 130, *The Masochistic Character*: For a more complete discussion, see *Character Analysis, op. cit.,* pp. 208 ff.

On p. 143, "Reich has found . . . the individual's reaction to both." From *Character Analysis, op. cit.,* p. 435.

On p. 210, addition to present footnote: Also *Function of the Orgasm, op. cit.,* pp. 320 ff.

On p. 296, "Careful periodic examination . . . was also made." See "Children of the Future," *Orgone Energy Bulletin,* Vol. 2, No. 4, p. 195, where Reich discussed the Orgonomic Infant Research Center.

PART I

.

CHARACTER FORMATION:

The Factors in Armoring

1 · General Introduction

The Energic Process of Life

MAN IS THE MOST COMPLEX and incredible accomplishment of nature. One of his great problems has been to understand himself. Self study has caused him anxiety so intense that he studied or explored the universe around him before he dared to look inside his own body. This book is concerned with his understanding of emotions, particularly of those emotions he faces when natural functioning is blocked through muscular contraction (armoring). To understand this study better, let us first observe reactions of the simplest animal, a one-celled creature called the amoeba.

The amoeba consists of a nucleus or core, protoplasm, a membrane, and an energy field. The nucleus is the energic center of the organism and contains the highest charge, drawing energy from the protoplasm which ingests the food.[1] From the nucleus, waves of excitation flow through the organism. These waves are intermittent. What happens is probably that energy concentrates until the organism reaches a point of excitation with lumina-

[1] Determined by microscopic study of energy concentration and movement in the amoeba under magnification of 2,000x. The energy itself of course cannot be seen, only its manifestations.

tion.[2] Then discharge occurs and the organism shortly begins to rebuild the charge. The result is an intermittent pulsatory effect and an appearance of alternating expansion and contraction. In the normal course of events the amoeba is never still; waves of excitation continually flow through the protoplasm. Careful observation can determine an energy field surrounding the membrane and pulsating with the organism. It appears much like the corona of the sun.

More energy is ingested through food than is used up, so that energy in the organism gradually increases. When energy builds up toward the lumination point, tension increases in the membrane and the amoeba begins to elongate, eventually narrowing in the center until the opposing sides of the membrane meet. Two amoebas are then formed by division. This division creates a larger surface area, which reduces tension; this is the amoeba's means of handling excess energy and avoiding bursting. Propagation is a corollary phenomenon, we believe, and not the cause of division.

The normal expansion seen in the pulsatory movement is exaggerated when the amoeba reaches out pseudopodia for food and the excited energy flows toward the membrane and pushes it out. The reverse action occurs when the membrane is attacked by the environment. For instance, if it is stuck with a pin, the amoeba contracts. After a single prick the amoeba soon expands as before. After several attacks it becomes "cautious" and expands anxiously and incompletely. After repeated attacks the amoeba remains contracted, and for practical purposes we can say that it is now armored and experiencing a state of anxiety. It has defended itself from its environment by reduction in size, but at the expense of lowered motility and increased inner pressure. If now the attacks continue and it is not allowed to expand, it will cease to build up energy and in fact the energy level will slowly diminish and the amoeba will eventually lose its tonicity, the membrane will wrinkle, the field will narrow

2 Lumination means literally what it says: the energy lights up as does a spark when it bursts into flame. In the human it is identical with thrill or genital excitation. We say the person glows or sparkles.

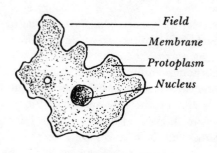

_____ Field
_____ Membrane
_____ Protoplasm
_____ Nucleus

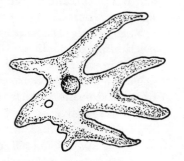

Amoeba
in state of rest

Amoeba
in state of expansion

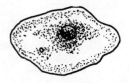

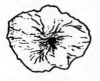

Amoeba
in state of contraction

Amoeba
in process of shrinking

and disappear, and it will gradually shrink and die (like a human depression or cancer case).

These simple demonstrations are comparable to the basic mechanisms of emotional disorders—however complex they may be and in whatever animal they may occur.

The human organism, although infinitely more complex, basically consists of the same structures as the amoeba:[3] the core or vegetative nervous system; the protoplasm consisting of the blood, lymphatic, and tissue fluids; the membrane or skin; and an energy field.[4] Of course, in such a complex organism there has been specialization: the various internal organs which serve specific functions, the skeletal structure which maintains the characteristic form, and the musculature which provides means of locomotion.

The vegetative nervous system consists of two opposing nerve systems: the parasympathetic and the sympathetic. The former produces expansion or "reaching out" from the standpoint of the total organism (although the internal organs actually contract and force their contents toward the skin surface), and the latter causes contraction of the total organism (even though the internal organs actually expand and in so doing keep their contents from going to the surface). It is interesting to note that chemically the parasympathetic is functionally identified with alkalinity and sodium and potassium ions,[5] the sympathetic with acidity and Ca ions. This is important to remember in the

---

[3] Even galaxies have a similar structure. Dr. Jan H. Dort reported to the general assembly of the International Astronomical Union at Hamburg, Germany, that galaxies, including our own, have nuclei which may be the seats of unknown forms of energy and even of an unknown state of matter. It consists of a swiftly spinning disk with a sharp edge. Outside this the material rotates rather slowly. Although the main body of the galaxy seems to be a spinning pinwheel it is enclosed in a spherical halo populated by stars formed before stellar processes had brewed heavy elements. Enveloping this is a corona the extent of which is still unknown. New York *Tmes*, Science Section, September 6, 1964.

[4] The energy field can be demonstrated by a field meter, or by watching the effect of one's body on a television set when standing near it, or by feeling the drawing sensation on the palms of the hands when they are moved toward and away from each other. The field can be seen under certain lighting conditions. Cf. "The Currents of Life," *M.D.* magazine, June, 1959.

[5] This material is covered fully in good neurology or physiology texts.

production of certain conditions and diseases such as the peptic ulcer, calcification of arteries, bones, ligaments, etc.

Both the sympathetic and the parasympathetic systems are composed of ganglia and nerves. The parasympathetic ganglia are largley situated in the brain and pelvis, or at both ends of the organism where the erogenous zones are located and contact with the environment is most important. The parasympathetic expands the organs near these ganglia actually *and* from the standpoint of total expansion (e.g. the genitals in sexual excitement). The sympathetic ganglia are largely in the abdomen and chest, along with the internal organs, and actually expand these organs; but from the standpoint of the total organism, the sympathetic ganglia produce contraction (e.g. the chest during inspiration, which, from a total standpoint, is a contraction.)

The antithetical effects of the expansion of the parasympathetic system and the contraction of the sympathetic system have come to be recognized in popular speech. Hands are "cold as icicles," and people have "chills of terror," or are "cold with disgust." All such phrases refer to the sympathetic contraction of the organism. Conversely, "bursting with enthusiasm" or "swollen with pride" refer to parasympathetic expansion.

Normal Human Body Functioning
(The Orgasm Theory)

Like the amoeba, the human is in a state of constant expansion and contraction. This is present in all the tissues of the body, but is most easily observed in the pulse and respiration. Energy is carried to the surface and the specialized organs chiefly by the blood, but it undoubtedly flows also, to some extent, directly through the tissues. The circulatory system can quickly carry energy to any specific part of the body at need; for example, to the muscles when the organism is attacked. Excitation comes from the vegetative nervous system which sets the direction of the flow of energy by opening some blood channels and closing others. The intensity of the excitation and the amount of energy together determine the strength of the charge or push in any particular flow.

This energy flow is felt as emotion. For example, *rage* results when energy flows into the muscles; *pleasure,* identical with expansion, results when energy flows to the skin surface (the genitals are part of the skin or ectoderm); and *anxiety* follows if the flow is to the internal organs and therefore causes contraction of the organism. These are the three important basic emotions.

There are two subsidiary emotions: longing and sadness. In longing, energy flows chiefly to the chest and arms, but also to the pelvis and mouth (a desire for superimposition), causing a reaching out for something which is not there but is desired. In sadness, which is a reaction to a loss, there is longing with no prospect of fulfillment,[6] and the organism simply contracts.

Withdrawal of energy from a part of the body results in a weakness known as *anorgonia*. Or, the energy can remain in the part and the organism contract on it through the muscular system. *Armoring* is the condition that results when energy is bound in a muscular contraction and does not flow through the body. Of course, armor also appears as a temporary self-protective response to environment and is not a disadvantage to the organism so long as it is abandoned when the occasion for it passes.

Energy is built up in the organism by the intake of food, fluid, and air, and is also absorbed directly through the skin. It is discharged by activity, excretion, emotional expression, the process of thinking, and by conversion into body heat which radiates to the environment. Also, it is used up in growth. In the usual course of events, more energy is built up than is discharged; if this were to continue the organism would either have to grow continually or burst. To maintain a stable, economic energy level, excess energy must be discharged at more or less regular intervals. This economic discharging of energy is the function of the orgasm. (In the female, it is probable that menstruation may help serve this purpose and childbirth certainly does. Before menstruation, blood flows to the pelvis and creates tension which is discharged with menstruation.)

In expansion (breathing out), the impulse seems to move down

---

[6] Sadness is to be distinguished from the secondary emotion depression, which is due to hate turned inward and is a neurotic manifestation, a result of armoring.

from the head to the genital, and a wave of excitation can be seen moving in this direction.[7] In contraction (breathing in), the excitation spreads from the solar plexus both up and down. Thus, in expansion the impulse covers twice the distance necessary in contraction. This may account for the normal pause after expiration while pleasure is felt in the organism.

As energy increases the body regularly builds up tension. At a certain point, known as the lumination point, the tension is felt as sexual excitement in the healthy individual. Energy above the level of the lumination point may be looked upon as sexual energy, or the libido which Freud described. Then, normal expansion, described above, markedly increases. The skin becomes warm and dry, the pulse is full and slow, breathing is deep, vision is sharp, and the genitals fill with blood and become acutely sensitive. The field expands and is highly charged. In full sexual excitement not only must energy reach the skin surface, especially the genitals, but this energy must be excited from the core. For excitation to come from the core, acceptance of the genital feeling and anticipation of the genital embrace are necessary.

Excitation is further increased through the field and membrane of the sexual object until closer contact and union of the genitals become imperative. Rhythmic friction rapidly produces a maximum peak of energy concentration and excitation in the genital. Discharge occurs through total convulsions of the body —the orgasm—and the economic energy level is reestablished. The whole occurs in the four beat stages (tension, charge, discharge, relaxation) discovered by Reich and which he called the orgasm formula.

Normal contraction is exaggerated in anxiety states.[8] The skin

[7] Cf. Wilhelm Reich, *Character Analysis*, 3rd ed. (New York, Orgone Institute Press, 1949), p. 388. Reich states in reference to the orgasm reflex: "These convulsions go with deep *expiration* and a wave of excitation from the diaphragmatic region to the head on the one hand and the genitals on the other." I do not believe this is in contradiction to the statement above. The convulsion occurs at the end of full expiration and is a muscular contraction discharging energy after total expansion. The stimulus for this contraction may well originate in the solar plexus, comparable to an "extra systole."

[8] Anxiety actually is a contraction against expansion. Contraction alone does not produce anxiety, e.g., contraction from cold.

becomes cold and moist, blood leaves the surface of the body, the pulse is rapid and shallow, breathing is inspiratory in type (that is, there is full inspiration but incomplete expiration), vision is blurred with dilated pupils, and the genitals are contracted and devoid of sensation.

To maintain health the individual requires orgastic release at more or less regular intervals, depending on circumstances governing other mechanisms of energy discharge and on the amount of energy available. The orgasm is the only mechanism, except for childbirth, capable of discharging all excess energy and maintaining an economic energy level.

Human Psycho-sexual Development

There are three peaks of sexual activity in the first twenty years of life: infancy, first puberty at five years, and puberty. In the infant, contact with the environment is effected principally through the mouth, which at this time is a very highly charged, almost autonomous organ. The mouth effects its own discharge of energy at its maximum point of intensity by means of a convulsive reaction which can appropriately be called an oral orgasm. Many pediatricians, unaware of this, have made a diagnosis of infantile epilepsy when they observed this orgasm.

The oral orgasm occurs only in healthy infants who have good contact with a mother whose nipples are sensitive, warm, and alive. This contact is of vital importance to the infant and also to the mother. Most obstetricians are aware that nursing aids in the normal involution of the uterus. Frequently strong genital sensations are felt by the mother. These feelings may arouse guilt,[9] or she may be unable to tolerate them at all. They may even cause a severe anxiety known as genital anxiety.

If allowed, the infant soon discovers its genital and engages in genital play. Somewhere between three and five years of age genitality (genital primacy) is established, and from then on release is through the genital.

From the time of puberty, when there is marked increase in

[9] The guilt comes from being sexually excited by her child and believing she must have incestuous desires.

genital functioning, the structure of the organism requires orgastic release through the sexual embrace. No one yet knows exactly what the healthy sexual behavior of the individual would be in the interim between infancy and puberty; perhaps it would be both masturbation and heterosexual play.[10] However, for the most nearly complete release two organisms are necessary mutually to excite each other.[11] The infant, we remember, has another organism with which it interacts, the mother. And even the lowest forms of life reproduce at intervals by a sexual stage in addition to their usual simple division. Everyone has experienced the disappearance of exhaustion during exciting events. Excited energy gives much more power and revives the organism.[12]

In childhood, rapid growth and physical activity probably use up much of the energy built up in the organism, so that sexual discharge may not be as urgent as it is following puberty, when maturing of the endocrine system produces intense excitation of the organismic energy and a greater need for regular discharge. However, childhood is certainly not to be considered an asexual period, as Freud conceived it when he called it the "latency" period. Latency is a product of repression in our culture. In therapy, those who have had no latency period have the best prognosis. We view as pathological the child who has no sexual outlet, and milder interferences with sexual functioning are likely to be critical. The circumstances, environmental and emotional, of the first masturbatory experience, for example, are often important in setting the subsequent pattern, whether masochistic, urethral erotic, or clitoral erotic.

Unfortunately, our society is not only sex negating; it is life negating, so that few persons reach maturity with complete or-

[10] In the Trobriand Islands, sex is expressed solely by heterosexual genital play and/or intercourse from the age of four or five. Cf. Malinowski, *The Sexual Life of Savages* (London, McLeod, 1929), ch. 3 pp. 46–48.

[11] Superimposition is a basic functioning Reich saw in all nature. It is a mutual excitation, attraction, and fusion into one energy system. This process creates matter in the cosmos and new life in living things.

[12] Also in therapy, the patient needs to be stirred up by the therapist through the use of procedures or emotional display to promote release of energy.

gastic potency. Parents and teachers cannot tolerate the natural movements and functioning of childhood and adolescence. Natural ways of behaving cause them anxiety and reawaken their own sexual guilt. They therefore institute methods for stopping this natural functioning.

Neurotic Development

The groundwork of inhibiting natural functioning may be laid even before birth in a spastic uterus which inhibits movement. The birth process itself may be long and difficult with anesthesia, drugs,[13] and forceps; and birth may even be mechanically held back to await the doctor's arrival. At birth, the environment which greets the newborn is mostly unfriendly. To begin with, it is cold compared to the warm uterus. Then the baby is slapped to make it breathe, hung by the feet, and a stinging medication placed in its eyes.

But this is only the beginning. The newborn baby is separated from the mother after nine months of warmth and intimate contact and placed alone in a crib with a hard mattress, frequently with bright overhead lights shining down relentlessly twenty-four hours a day. This is followed by regimented feedings* usually from the cold, insensitive nipples of the neurotic mother or from an inanimate bottle. The environment is noisy and chaotic; the nurses frequently rough and careless. Mittens are placed over the babies' hands, so they cannot scratch themselves, but neither can they suck their thumbs, which might be necessary for satisfaction. It is pitiful to watch them try. Also they are frequently wrapped so tightly that it amounts to bundling and all their movements are restricted. The infant is blocked in all directions

13 Cf. Gerald Stechler, "Newborn Attention as Affected by Medication during Labor," Vol. 144, ff. 315–317, *Science*, April 17, 1964. Stechler found that newborn visual attention was decreased according to the amount of drugs the mother had received during labor.

* Bruno Bettelheim at the Orthogenic School of the University of Chicago states: "Time clock feedings are potentially so destructive because they rob the infant of the conviction that it is his own wail that resulted in filling his stomach." How his activity succeeds and the response it receives will strongly color all his later attempts at self-motivated action.

from reaching out into his environment. As a result, we gain a false impression of the helplessness of babies.

Classical medicine teaches us that infants do not focus their eyes for six weeks and that their breathing is irregular and jerky because the *medulla is not developed*. But healthy babies do focus their eyes as soon as they are born[14] and can follow one around the room with their eyes, and their respiratory impulse goes clear through to the pelvis, producing an orgasm reflex. Babies born in a hospital under the usual conditions will never be able to turn over in a few hours. Healthy babies who have had a natural delivery can. They are soon quite self-sufficient in movement and entertainment. But with the customary adverse environment all this development does not take place. Instead the baby contracts, the chest stops its free movement, the diaphragm blocks, the eyes do not focus, and the skin becomes cold and blue. At first they react with anger (angry crying), later with crying and whining to show their misery. Now add circumcision and the penis too contracts and remains cold and blue. I have seen it remain this way for two years.

With this effective start, life is further blocked by early toilet training, which ultimately renders the child more compliant in curbing his masturbatory impulses and sexual strivings. Sphincter control is not attained until eighteen months of age so that earlier toilet training (some mothers start at four months) requires contraction of the body musculature, especially the muscles of the thighs, buttocks, pelvic floor, as well as retraction of the pelvis and further respiratory inhibition. This is a familiar example of the armoring process. It effectively diminishes natural

14 Cf. Robert L. Fantz, "Pattern Vision in Newborn Infants," *Science*, April 19, 1963, pp. 296–297. Dr. Fantz, testing infants ten hours to five days old, found they showed an innate ability to perceive form. Also Peter Wolff and Burton L. White, "Visual Pursuit and Attention in Young Infants," *Journal of the American Academy of Child Psychiatry*, Vol. iv, No. 3, July, 1965. They state, "This study concerns the relation between organismic state and visual pursuit in the newborn infant. It is based on the observation that infants will pursue a moving object at birth . . . but that in order to pursue they must be in a condition of quiet alertness analogous to the adult attentive state. . . . A moving object can be followed by the eyes alone . . . or by a coordinated head-eye rotation."

emotional expression, and especially the pleasurable sensations from the pelvis.

Armoring is produced through the fear of punishment and the sense of guilt (mustn't touch that dirty thing) instilled in the child. This is routine and accepted training and does not include the various forms of sadism practiced by nursemaids and even mothers. One of my patients was forced to eat from his dirty diaper because he had soiled it, while another had had his nose rubbed in his diaper. And then there are the dire threats of the results of masturbation. Thus, in general, release is prevented so energy increases and tension mounts. Sexual impulses and other aggressive drives, at first tender and soft, become harsh and brutal.[15] This is the origin of the sexual sadism which society so rightly tries to abolish, but wrongly does so by further repression.

We must remember that the child originally is not harsh, he is made so. Because of the frustrations, rage develops, and it in turn must be repressed. With little release of biological energy, the individual must of necessity continue to increase his armor, which may eventually include the whole musculature. He feels a constant inner tension and anxiety. Finally effective armoring fails, the repressed sexual drives break through and are immediately warded off through symptom formation. At last spontaneity is lost, the child becomes restricted, mechanical, and confined to definite routines of living. In brief, the first cause of a neurosis is moral inhibition, its driving force the unsatisfied sexual energy.

The Therapeutic Aim

To relieve the situation it is necessary to reverse the armoring process by a dissolution of the armor, releasing and draining off the repressed emotions layer by layer, from latest to earliest blocking, until unitary function is restored and natural sexuality is reached. At this point, one sees a spontaneous tilting forward of the pelvis at the end of complete expiration. This is the or-

---

15 Reich distinguished the natural primary drives from the harsh secondary drives which have to come through armor.

gasm reflex.[16] Reich has pointed out that the severity of any kind of psychic disturbance is in direct relation to the severity of the disturbance of genitality and the prognosis depends directly on the possibility of establishing the capacity for full genital satisfaction.

[16] In some cases, particularly schizophrenics, a pelvic reflex may occur early, even in the first few sessions. This involves only part of the organism and comes through a "hole" in the armor. It must not lead one to feel that problems have been solved. The orgasm reflex implies a response in which the whole organism takes part as a unit.

2 · Emotional Development: Erogenous Zones and Libidinal Stages

THERE ARE FOUR MAJOR EROGENOUS ZONES, each important as a stage in emotional development; the eyes, mouth, anus, and genital. These major zones are paired at both ends of the organism where contact with the environment is most important and where the parasympathetic ganglia are located. The second of each pair (i.e. mouth or genital) makes direct contact and fusion (superimposition) with another organism and is capable of initiating the orgastic convulsion—the mouth in infancy, the genital later. Their development occurs in the order of position from above down through the four zones. Thus, development occurs latest in the genital; the periods of development of the other three zones are therefore known as *pre*genital stages.

During the first four years or so of life the child develops through four[1] pregenital stages to genitality or genital primacy.

[1] The oral is the only natural pregenital libidinal stage. The others are artifacts of our culture. The genital, we remember, is phylogenetically developed from the distal end of the alimentary tract—the cloaca. A major erogenous zone is one which in development may in part or wholly replace the genital in erotic excitation. The oral zone normally does this in infancy. The others do only in the presence of blocking.

The fourth of these, the phallic stage, is actually an early phase of genitality. If genitality is fully established without hooks or blocks carried along from the earlier stages, a genital or healthy character structure results. If genitality is not reached the individual remains in a stage that can only be designated as infantile. To form a neurotic character structure, an individual must of necessity have reached at least the phallic stage, even though with pregenital hooks, although this last stage may later be given up to a greater or lesser extent. Neuroses develop out of the Oedipus conflict, which arises when the genital stage is reached. The Oedipus situation is created by the adult sexual repression in our culture and is not a natural conflict necessary to human maturing.

The stages of development are the ocular, oral, anal, phallic, and genital. (There are other erotic areas as forehead, breasts, and general skin surface, which are not specifically involved in any one stage.) In normal development each stage fulfills its passing function, remains untraumatized, and in future life serves its specific role in a pleasure-giving capacity. Blocking (armoring) at any level holds energy at that level, preventing it from reaching the genital where discharge can be attained. When genitality is interfered with, the concentration of energy at the pregenital erogenous zone produces symptoms from that zone.

Emotional trauma may produce one of two results at any stage: 1) repression or 2) lasting unsatisfaction. In the former the individual never develops pleasurable functioning at that stage, largely through deprivation; and in the latter he constantly tries to obtain a once-known satisfaction. In either repression or unsatisfaction cases, armoring occurs and we say the individual has a hook or block. The circumstances surrounding the development at each stage determine the character formation. Each stage overlaps the subsequent one and there is frequently no sharp borderline between them. In fact, for example, the anal zone may be emphasized during the oral stage and produce anal characteristics. All zones are, of course, present and potentially erotic from the beginning.

The Ocular Stage

Except for general body feeling, the ocular zone is the infant's first specific contact with the environment. As a matter of fact, it remains the means of reaching out the farthest. The eyes are also the first areas to be traumatized, either by having medication applied at birth, or by meeting with cold, frightening, or hateful expressions. The latter may be even more damaging than medication. Hostile expressions imply the negation of any opportunity for warm and understanding contact. Full contact is vital to development in general. It promotes a feeling of acceptance and well-being and encourages expansion and reaching out into the environment. It is especially important for proper development of the sensory organs, all of which are derived from the skin or ectoderm. Temporary lack of contact in the baby's environment, such as from a hostile nurse, causes contraction of the body and withdrawal in the eyes but may be overcome if this situation is only fleeting. What is permanently damaging is continued lack of contact from a hostile, cold, or contactless mother. Even a mother who is not hostile but is unusually anxious, indifferent, or emotionally dead can cause irreparable damage. Development of the eyes and binocular vision is inhibited or prevented without loving contact.[2] The ultimate in lack of contact produces an autistic child, one of psychiatry's most serious problems. The infant enters the oral stage almost immediately, but the eye stage continues to develop. Normally where there is

[2] Three-dimensional, or depth vision. It is improbable that one could tolerate full binocular vision at all times any more than one could stand constant sexual excitation. The contact is too intense. That contact with the mother is necessary for development of adequate functioning of the eyes has been demonstrated by experiments on animals; cf. *Science,* Vol. 145, July 17, 1964, p. 292. *Maternal Deprivation: Its Influence on Visual Exploration in Infant Monkeys* by Philip C. Green and Michael Gordon of Chicago. They show that monkeys deprived of contact with their mother do not show the normal curiosity of looking that monkeys do who develop with a mother.

Also, *Science,* Vol. 145, August 21, 1964. p. 835. *Depth Perception in Sheep: Effects of Interrupting the Mother Neonate Bond* by William B. Lennon and George H. Patterson in Oklahoma City. They show that mothered lambs avoided running off a drop before unmothered lambs, demonstrating that the former develop binocular vision earlier.

good contact with the mother, the eyes remain open, frank, and inquiring, with a serious but trusting quality. Healthy eyes develop binocular[2] vision, which is necessary to maintain good contact with the environment and to permit adequate integration of the individual. In other words, he can place himself properly in his environment, experience pleasure from it, and respond to acceptance he finds there. Excitation from the eyes is felt directly in the genital as a pleasurable thrill. Binocular vision provides three-dimensional perspective which places everything exactly as it is and allows an objective emotional attitude. Through the eyes, the environment actually becomes an extension of the individual so that awareness of it is the same as awareness of his own body; yet at the same time he clearly distinguishes between the two, learning to pinpoint pleasurable and painful areas with unfailing accuracy. Hearing and smell fall into this stage of ocular development too, but full value of these senses has largely been lost in our civilization.[3]

If, however, the eyes are traumatized through medication or disease, or withdrawn through fear, vision is interfered with, and the eyes become dull and lifeless. Binocular vision fails to develop adequately if at all. This common traumatization is largely responsible for the general acceptance of the belief that babies cannot focus until they are six weeks old. I have seen infants focus immediately after birth and clearly follow me with their eyes as I walked about.[4] Without binocular vision the individual has to adjust to a world without perspective. It is prob-

[3] I do not wish to imply that these organs do not serve erotic functions. The erotically provocative voice of the torch singer or certain music and the interest in perfumes show they are still important. Smell is of major importance in the lower mammals.

[4] Cf. Dayton et al, "Developmental Study of Coordinated Eye Movements in the Human Infant."

(i) Visual Acuity in the Newborn Human—A Study Based on Induced Optokinetic Nystagmus Recorded by Electro-Oculography. They demonstrated instrumentally a well-developed visual fixation in the newborn and quantified newborn visual acuity at up to 20/150.

(ii) "An Electro-oculographic Study of the Fixation Reflex in the Newborn," states, "The tracings document a fixation reflex which is innately better developed than heretofore reported, with the ocular movement purposeful and well coordinated instead of aimless and unconjugated." Archives of Opthalmology, Vol. 71, No. 6, June, 1964.

able that few people have full binocular vision: most see essentially the same with one eye as they do with both. This means that they do not see with true three-dimensional vision, since it is not possible to have binocular vision with one eye. In fact people are generally divided into those who see vertically and those who see horizontally.[5] Most of us accommodate ourselves to the deficiency by gauging distances through other objects of known distance. With lack of binocular vision there is a disparity between perception and sensation, which accounts for much of the misinterpretation and delusion of schizophrenia.

I believe this lack in vision also accounts for people's general lack of understanding, and results in confusion and withdrawal from the world. It may also explain why no two people can give the same account of a jointly witnessed scene. We have to conclude that the majority of people do not really see what is before their eyes. Try looking about a room and then going out of it and describing it.

The *unsatisfied* ocular stage is produced by an initial freedom in looking which is later stopped, particularly through the means of shame. It may subsequently produce voyeurism. The *repressed* ocular stage produces inadequate perception in looking, with the resulting confusion described above.

The Oral Stage

The oral and the genital stages seem to be of particular importance because only the mouth and the genital are capable of initiating the orgastic convulsion, possibly because only these two major erogenous organs provide actual contact and fusion (superimposition) with another organism. Contact is vital for development and even for life itself. It is probable that an individual deprived of contact with any other living thing would not long survive.

Contact with the mother is particularly important to the infant. For nine months it has been part of the mother and even after birth is greatly dependent on her. The two organisms mutually excite each other, providing that sparkle and intensity

---

[5] This distinction is emphasized in industrial psychiatry in evaluating hazards of machine operators. Artists also make this distinction.

of living so necessary for development and growth. This excitement reaches its peak during nursing, if the mother's nipple is warm, erectile, and alive and frequently produces an oral orgastic convulsion in the infant. Food from a bottle can be made as nourishing from a nutritional standpoint, but it does not provide contact and excitation. Gradually obstetricians are learning and mothers are demanding that the mother and newborn baby should not be separated. However, still too few hospitals provide for this obvious need.

The newborn baby is capable of regulating itself according to its own needs and must only be taught not to endanger its life and to distinguish and respect the rights of others as well as his own. But with all the restrictions placed upon it, it soon loses this ability and its whole life depends upon outside training. Even the mother loses her natural ability to care for the newborn infant and follows instructions, however invalid. Our whole social structure seems to be built around concepts that interfere with natural life rather than assist it.

The oral zone provides means for the intake of food, fluid, and air, vocal communication, emotional expression, and erotic contact. If functioning is inhibited by repression, satisfaction is lost in all these important functions; and the joy of living is replaced by the misery of trying to survive, with eventual depression occurring.

Repression at the oral level is produced largely by deprivation, through anxiety in the mother, a cold nipple, insufficient milk, and contactlessness in nursing. The full joy of functioning is never allowed to develop. *Unsatisfaction* is produced usually by an initial fulfillment up to a certain point of development and then a sudden deprivation, such as a mother suddenly deciding to discontinue nursing regardless of the needs of the child. For the rest of his life, the child will try to make up this need through overeating, drinking, talking, and emotional vacillation.

The Anal Stage

This stage occurs between two and three years of age, after the anal sphincter has become a functioning organ. Toilet training is spontaneously accomplished during this period if the parents, especially the mother, look upon bowel functioning naturally and do not interfere with the child's progress either by early or severe toilet training or by undue interest or concern. Early and severe toilet training, particularly if started before sphincter control is attained, prevents the development of satisfaction in elimination and natural control. The development of this satisfaction is much more important to the basic character of the child than is generally realized. At this age the child is learning many skills and each brings its own reward. The sense of satisfaction and pride the child experiences when he produces a bowel movement is extremely important to him. He is at this time learning to separate himself from his mother and gaining an independent identity.

If this natural function and its accompanying emotion (i.e. pride, sense of accomplishment) are interfered with, a vital part of the child's personality is distorted. To obtain control before he is developmentally ready, the child has to tighten the musculature, particularly of the thighs, buttocks, and pelvic floor. He must pull his pelvis backward and hold his breath. This markedly diminishes sensations from the pelvis and interferes with later genital development. Such regimentation also decreases spontaneity and renders the child more compliant and even dependent on outside instruction. At the same time it creates a deep stubbornness (holding back) and inability to give freely. It is as though the child, having been made to hold back a natural function before he was ready and having been made to forego the pleasure of accomplishing something in his own right, now finds himself unable to let go even when it is desirable to do so. This results in the traits of stinginess and emotional lameness.

People who develop in this fashion can only take in, not give out. They tend to have extensive collections of things. They, as it were, have to bring the world to them as they cannot go out to the world. They develop a compulsive need for order. This tendency can be seen in small children who must line their shoes up in precise lines before going to bed or who must have everything exactly in place at all times.

Naturally, constipation is a physical concomitant. In this

country we take constipation even among children so much for granted it seems we must have forgotten that constipation is a decidedly unnatural state of affairs. Classical medicine blames constipation on diet, that is, lack of fruit or roughage or sufficient water, or on lack of exercise, seemingly forgetting that other children on the same diet and suffering the same lack of exercise are not constipated. With such restrictions on outlet, energy builds, becomes forceful, harsh, and brutal—the anal sadistic stage. But even this anal sadism is not permitted release, so to hold it back armor may increase to an unbelievable degree, producing a human machine. This is the *anal inhibited* or *repressed* stage.

The *anal unsatisfied* stage is produced by overinterest on the part of the mother in bowel functioning which fixes the child's interest and does not allow him to develop his independence. The mother worries over elimination and may praise the child for his movement, especially if done at the mother's convenience. Soon the child's being accepted centers around this ability, and he overtly tries to please for his own security. He becomes compliant and passive on the surface, but underneath he develops a stubborn tenacity and a great resentment of the need to control his impulses. Spontaneity is lost.

The Phallic Stage

This stage usually occurs at about four years of age, but may occur earlier or later depending on the development of the child. Although a stage of genital development, it is still undifferentiated. Normally it is a fleeting pride in discovery of the genital which progresses to a full appreciation of this organ's male or female functions.[6]

[6] As a matter of fact, although all previous stages are undifferentiated between male and female, the little boy and girl would be different from the beginning if allowed to develop naturally. From birth the baby girl has feminine qualities and very early seems to flirt and show her feminine wiles, while the boy seems to be more forward and aggressive. Popular tradition even tells us the two sexes behave differently during development in the uterus. We are handicapped in not yet having the opportunity to study strictly healthy development. We do know that the baby is naturally soft,

Fixation at the phallic stage occurs when the frustrating parent, in this case the parent of the opposite sex, cannot stand the proud genital exhibitionism and clamps down sharply. The anal sadistic stage has just been left, while the genital object libidinal position has not yet been established. There occurs in the male a proud self-confident concentration on his own genital; in women a fantasied penis. If development stops at this stage, the genital functions in the service of aggression, not love, since development was not allowed to proceed to full genitality, but was stopped by the nonaccepting parent of the opposite sex. What would have developed to heterosexual love turns to revenge. If one wishes to split hairs one can identify the *repressed* stage as the ascetic person, usually religious and morally righteous, and the *unsatisfied* stage in the Don Juan type of person.

The Genital Stage

If development through this stage is successfully accomplished a healthy character results in which the genital is used in its natural function of adult love. It is a differentiated stage and identification with the same sex occurs. Male and female serve strictly male and female sexual functions with natural, gentle characteristics and natural aggression. The female is concerned only with being feminine and not with competing with the male. The male is masculine only, without particularly feminine characteristics.

Even this stage can be repressed, as occurs in the hysteric, by a moralistic attitude on the part of the parent of the same sex who provides knowledge of disillusioning experiences with the opposite sex. This prevents solution of the Oedipus complex. Sex remains as a desire for incest which is forbidden.

Reaction formations[7] occur only with pregenital fixations, so

---

responsive, and gentle. Harsh and cruel qualities are instilled; they are not natural or innate. The baby is not the savage little beast that has to be civilized, as some experts teach.

[7] Change of direction of the impulse against itself through repression and counter cathexis against the goal of the drive. This results in defensive be-

that those individuals who fully develop to the stage of genitality (phallic and genital) with no pregenital blocks must solve their tensions (stasis) by aggression (phallic), or by flight or contactlessness (hysteric). They cannot solve their tensions by the usual neurotic symptom formation on a reaction basis (change of direction of the impulse). They are, as it were, stuck at the genital stage and cannot retreat to pregenital levels to solve their problems. This is due probably, as Reich states, to the amount of energy centered at the genital level which necessitates expression at this higher stage of development. In *repression* the hysteric runs from sexuality. In the *unsatisfied* stage she runs toward it (nymphomania).

---

havior toward the impulse; e.g. desire to murder changed to exaggerated sympathy, or sexual drives changed to ascetic traits.

3 · Psychic Structure

THE INDIVIDUAL'S PSYCHIC STRUCTURE was worked out by Freud, and consists of the ego, ego ideal, superego, and the id. It develops concurrently with emotional development.

The Ego

The ego is that psychic process which is concerned with reality and whose function it is to fulfill the needs of the organism in whatever manner seems best in the particular environment. It functions also in perceiving and estimating the self. It is restricted both by the environment and by the conditioning of training. Restriction may be advantageous and necessary to survival, or it may be incapacitating when it is linked with neurotic fears. We accept the fact that different individuals have different potentials; one may have a strong and effective ego in spite of severe restrictive training and an adverse environment, while another may have a poorly integrated ego although circumstances of upbringing and environment may appear favorable. However, functioning of the ego largely depends on the ability of the organism to function as a whole; that is, it depends on the degree and kind of armoring.

The ego is an important consideration in therapy. One may

wish to build it up in persons suffering from acute anxiety or depression, or may find it necessary to tear it down in overly aggressive persons.

The Ego Ideal

The ego ideal is the goal set up by the ego itself either through identification, teaching, or natural drives. It is to a great extent responsible for the relentless drive to which some persons subject themselves to attain certain goals in life regardless of their basic energy charge.

The Superego

The superego is the structured prohibitions of the environment. These prohibitions are incorporated in the individual and function on an automatic and unconscious level, blocking off certain urges and feelings from awareness, and preventing their fulfillment. *The superego is functionally identical with armoring.* If the urges are too strong to repress, their direction is changed to more acceptable, although less fulfilling, aims. The conscience fulfills a similar function in consciousness.

The Id

The id is the driving force of the needs of the body and is composed of the original instinctive drives together with secondary drives and those which have suffered change of direction by the superego. A secondary drive results when primary expressions are blocked, and is therefore made harsh by the increased pressure. Rape, sexual sadism, and perversions are types of secondary expression.

Reich has pointed out that, as a whole, the psychic structure is a resultant of conflict between instinctual demands and the demands of the outer world. The specific character has indeed developed *because of* and through conflict. Neurosis occurs when the ego's demand for pleasure is punished from the outside world whenever it is manifested. The superego, that internalization of the world's demands, maintains the conflict with the ego (even when the world is not punishing the ego directly) because it has learned to act as if all sexual pleasure were always punishable. The childhood formation of the superego is, of course, reinforced by experiences in the actual society.

4 · Armoring

ARMORING MAY BE DIVIDED into natural or temporary muscular contraction and permanent or chronic contraction. The former occurs in any living animal when it is threatened, but is given up when the threat is no longer present. The latter originates in the same manner, but because of continued threats is maintained and becomes chronic, reacting eventually to permanent inner rather than environmental dangers. In this discussion armoring refers to the latter type.

So far as we know, the origin of chronic armoring is lost in antiquity. Legendary artifacts of human behavior indicate that man was armoring before recorded history began, and no one can tell what initiated such a necessity. Certainly something of tremendous importance started armoring since it is almost universal and has persisted through all the ages. It is even questionable whether man could exist without it.

Though individuals can, masses cannot give up armoring without drastic changes in our culture and way of thinking. Probably people in general could not dispense with armor at all as long as we emphasize material ownership. Knowing how armor began is important because it can help us gauge if civilization can possibly exist without it.

Reich postulated that man armored when he became introspective; that is, when he perceived that he perceived himself, and that he perceived at all. This awareness of self-perception as an object of attention produced a split. Man became frightened and began to armor against the inner fright and amazement in an effort to control his own sensations. This sequence seems highly probable for we know clinically that people clamp down especially against the sensation of surrender in the orgasm.

Reich deduced the origin of armoring from his knowledge of schizophrenia and his observation of what he called the "universal terror of living."[1] To face the unknown is always frightening; to stand and examine it, terrifying. Pascal in his *Pensées* conveys this very well. To understand it, then, became a compulsion and thus perhaps the urge for knowledge was born. This urge, however, man seemed to divert to everything except studying his own body bioenergetically. He avoided that for millennia and even yet cannot accept contemplating his natural emotions or allowing them expression.

In the sequence of events leading to armor formation, the crucial point in holding back seems to be the terror of surrendering in orgastic convulsion where man completely merges with nature. The first orgasm is always frightening because of its accompanying loss of control. When man began paying attention to his sensations this letting go was more than he could bear and he began to try to control it. To get an idea of the process, the reader has only to pay attention to and examine his own sensations at any given moment and he will find himself holding his breath—the best way to control feeling.

Such then, we may speculate, was the starting point of man's urgency for knowledge, the craving to know, which ever since has been more important to him than his natural functioning. The latter itself, he subjected—always distorted—to formalized knowledge, control, repression, and at times an almost complete ban. This has resulted in artificial laws of behavior and mores. Man no longer dares give in to his natural organismic functioning; he holds back as if his very life depended on it.

Several legends have sprung up which seem to bear out Reich's

[1] Wilhelm Reich, *Cosmic Superimposition* (New York, Orgone Institute Press, 1951), p. 117.

hypothesis. These may well epitomize the growth of knowledge at the expense of natural love by way of armoring, as well as the origin of patriarchy.

For example, there is the bitter struggle of Aphrodite to destroy Psyche, who has ensnared the love of her son, Eros. Psyche successfully performs all the tasks set by Aphrodite and wins over the gods, immortality, and Eros. Aphrodite has to acknowledge defeat; natural love capitulates to intellect.

A further apotheosis of knowledge is seen in the legend of Pallas Athene, goddess of ancient Athens. She springs full blown from the head (brain) of Zeus. Thus she comes directly from man, not from a mother. At the trial of Orestes she casts the deciding vote and declares she always votes in favor of the man. The male assumes the favored or important position—a close linkage of knowledge and patriarchy.

The clearest account comes from the Bible in the expulsion of Adam and Eve from the Garden of Eden.[2] This narrative seems more an account of civilization's origin rather than man's origin—particularly with regard to the concomitant development of knowledge and armoring and the origin of patriarchy.

Genesis 2:16.[3] And the Lord God commanded the man, saying, of every tree of the garden thou mayest freely eat:
17. But of the tree of the knowledge of good and evil, thou shalt not eat of it: for in the day that thou eatest thereof thou shalt surely die.
21. And the Lord God caused a deep sleep to fall upon Adam, and he slept: and he took one of his ribs, and closed up the flesh instead thereof;
22. And the rib, which the Lord God had taken from man, made he a woman, and brought her unto the man.
25. And they were both naked, the man and his wife, and were not ashamed.
Genesis 3:1. Now the serpent was more subtil than any beast of the field which the Lord God had made.
4. And the serpent said unto the woman, ye shall not surely die.
5. For God doth know that in the day ye eat thereof, then your eyes shall be opened, and ye shall be as gods, knowing good and evil.
7. And the eyes of them both were opened, and they knew that they

2 Cf. Wilhelm Reich, *The Murder of Christ* (New York, Orgone Institute Press, 1953), p. 11.
3 The Holy Bible, King James Version.

were naked; and they sewed fig leaves together, and made themselves aprons.

14. And the Lord God said unto the serpent . . .

15. And I will put enmity between thee and the woman and between thy seed and her seed . . .

16. Unto the woman he said, I will greatly multiply thy sorrow and thy conception; in sorrow shalt thou bring forth children; and thy desire shall be to thy husband, and *he shall rule over thee.*

23. Therefore the Lord God sent him forth from the Garden of Eden, to *till the ground* from whence he was taken. (Author's italics.)

The "subtil serpent" or, we may say, the perceptive penis, where sensation is most acute, tempted man to eat of the tree of knowledge of good and evil. Gerhard von Rad feels that the expression, "of good and evil," is a subsequent addition and refers simply to knowledge of everything or all things.[4] But even taken at face value as a knowledge of good and evil it would imply the development of a conscience or superego, which means repression, civilization, and the birth of religion.

Thus eating of the fruit of knowledge brought armoring—fig leaves, clothes on skin, sexual shame—and drove man from his natural paradise. He lost his contact with nature and natural feelings and killed his emotional life (". . . thou shalt surely die."). This brought all the problems armoring produces (thorns and thistles) including difficult labor and a deep fear of the genital (enmity between woman and serpent).

Like Athene, Eve comes directly from man. After the Fall, God tells her ". . . thy desire shall be to thy husband, and he shall rule over thee," thus signaling the advent of patriarchy. One may postulate, then, that at an earlier time there was no patriarchal state and that man lived naturally or in a matriarchy. Von Rad cites the following passage, which he thinks may be a holdover from an earlier matriarchal culture: "Therefore shall a man leave his father and his mother and shall cleave unto his wife; and they shall be one flesh." Certainly, as he points out, it is not characteristic of patriarchy.

Still another passage from the Bible shows the ascendant role given to knowledge: "In the beginning was the Word, and the

---

[4] Gerhard von Rad, *Genesis, A Commentary*, translated by John H. Marks, (Philadelphia, The Westminster Press, 1961), pp. 77, 79, 87.

Word was with God, and the Word was God." (St. John 1:1)
This is known as the Divine Concept of Logos (Word, Idea);
that is, the idea, word, or knowledge is supreme.

A further possibility is that armoring occurred when man took
up agriculture and/or the raising of herds. This is compatible
with the first hypothesis and may have grown out of it or parallel
to it as man acquired knowledge and faced the need to obtain
more food for mere survival or a growing population. Man was
insecure and knowledge was power. He settled down, tilled
the soil, and took his mate with him—"And thou shalt eat the
herb of the field." Also from Genesis 4:16–17: "And Cain went
out from the presence of the Lord and dwelt in the land of Nod,
on the east of Eden. / And Cain knew his wife; and bare Enoch;
and he builded a city . . ."

The beginnings of agriculture[5] can be discerned in the well-
watered uplands bordering the Arabian, Syrian, and Iranian
deserts somewhere between 8000 and 7000 B.C. when men left
their caves and gathered together in more or less fixed com-
munities. Within three or four thousand years the condition
of life changed more radically than it had over the preceding
quarter of a million years. The period between 4000 and 3000
B.C. has been deemed more fruitful in inventions and discoveries
than any period in human history prior to the sixteenth century
A.D.—weaving, metallurgy, the plow, the wheel for transportation
and turning pottery, molding of bricks, harnessing of draft
animals, invention of sails, use of seals to distinguish and protect
private property. Economic organization, political controls, and
social attitudes developed, along with a more elaborate formula-
tion of religious belief. Cities grew.

Thus man settled down with his mate, tilled the soil, started the
family as a social unit, and instituted patriarchy.[6] The male was
responsible for feeding the household and did not want the
burden of any other offspring but his own. He began to place

5 Marshall B. Davidson, ed., *Lost Worlds* (New York, American Publishing
Co., Inc., 1962), p. 8.
6 Whether patriarchy may be a result or the cause of armoring, we do find
that whenever there is patriarchy there are neuroses and crime. This is true
even in tribes where only the chief's family follows patriarchial principles and
restricts sex. Only his family has neuroses and not the rest of the tribe.

restrictions on the sexuality of his wife and daughters and even set up household gods to watch his women.[7] This very likely was the origin of the double standard.

We know that armoring is more extensive in patriarchal societies, where the general attitude is sex negative, than in matriarchal societies where there is a sex-affirmative attitude. Also, in all but the most primitive patrilineal (not true patriarchy) knowledge is much more emphasized. Primarily, armoring reduces genital sensations, especially affecting the orgastic surrender in which the individual seems to merge with the cosmos.[8] Life without armoring does not seem possible in a patriarchal society, but might be possible in a matriarchal system.

There is considerable confusion as to just what constitutes a matriarchal society.[9] I have heard it stated that America is fast becoming one because of the growing influence of women; but this is a superficial view. Where women assume the same position men hold in a patriarchal system, an Amazon society is produced which is little different in effect from patriarchy. A true matriarchy is a tribal system in which the tribe and not the family is the unit. When a woman marries she remains in her tribe regardless of the origin of the husband.[10] He thus becomes an unofficial member of her tribe and assumes an unimportant role in family upbringing.

The children remain with their parents, but they receive their training from the mother's male relatives, usually her brothers.

[7] It has been suggested that this may have been done because wives and daughters were valuable property in bartering. Probably, however, it was more to ensure that only his offspring inherited his property. By this means he would attain a measure of immortality for himself. "Thou shalt surely die" was a deep and persistent fear.

[8] "Merging with the cosmos" implies complete surrender to one's bodily sensations, as though nature were simply flowing through unimpeded.

[9] Anthropologists prefer to use the terms "patrilineal" and "matrilineal" since there are so many variations of both. Some of the former are quite sex affirmative and, thus, unlike the typical patriarchal system. They seem to be very primitive patrilineal societies.

[10] In the Trobriand Islands, the wife goes to the husband's tribe, but the other factors remain constant, and the sons at puberty return to the mother's tribe. The father assumes care of the children only while they are very young. He is recognized only as the mother's husband, not as a father.

This system allows a more objective and freer attitude toward natural needs and prevents the sexual restrictions found in patriarchal systems. The competition between the parents for the children's love is minimized, and so is the competitive pressure that follows when both father and children seek a woman's attention. In such matriarchal societies neuroses and crime are unknown; frequently there are not even words for them. Strangely enough, although adolescent boys and girls are provided with facilities for being together privately and engage freely in sexual expression, the girl very rarely conceives prior to marriage. This is so striking that in a few tribes[11] the relation between sex and conception was not understood.[12]

Regardless of how it originated, armoring prevents complete orgastic release so the organism never experiences full satisfaction and constantly strives to find it. With loss of orgastic release *oneness with the cosmos* is lost; we no longer feel contact with nature, and *cosmic longing* supervenes. I believe that this longing is behind much of the thirst for knowledge and progress. According to our usual concepts, all matriarchal systems are very primitive. Their natural way of living provides adequate satisfaction and therefore members have no urge for scientific progress.[13] Where armoring exists the energy blocked from pelvic release is drawn up to the brain[14] (the organism's other end) and seeks outlet, hoping each new discovery will provide the answers to regaining cosmic contact. Particularly do we look up to the heavens and study them and contemplate them and prepare to travel there. Somewhere up there we place our God,[15]

[11] The Australian Bushmen and Trobriand Islanders are examples.

[12] One wonders how much the origin of sexual repression (and thus of armoring) may have been related to men's awareness that they are responsible for the children.

[13] Again, one can argue in favor of the reverse; i.e. the primitives have not yet become introspective and so have not developed a thirst for knowledge. The epistemological curiosity as to how we perceive that we perceive may be the basis both for armoring and for the thirst for knowledge.

[14] Reich has suggested the human brain may have become so large and complex that it is more or less autonomous and acts as a parasite draining energy from the body.

[15] It may be noted that the devil, who denotes desires of the flesh, is down in the nether regions—past the pelvis.

who will provide satisfaction, but only after death when our spirits are free of their armored bodies.

Along with armoring there is always contempt. Contempt results from pulling energy up from the pelvis to the face so that we feel superior. Contempt is basically a rejection of the genital and is expressed toward some object considered more sexual than ourselves, or toward those who differ from us sexually. This is true whatever may appear superficially to be the reason for the contempt.

Armoring is self-perpetuating, because armored parents raise armored children. The present cause of armoring is the necessity on the part of the child to accept unnatural attitudes and training conditions set up by the parents and others. It is accomplished largely by contraction, mostly of the muscles, but also to some extent by the contraction of the body tissues. It allows the child to hold back its desires and conform. In each case the specific type of armor required determines the future specific character of the individual, and one may speak of it as *character armor*. It is a result of the infantile sexual conflict and its purpose is to solve that conflict. It attempts to do so by changing the habitual attitude of the ego, especially in becoming sex negative. The end product is a reduction of the motility of the organism (much like the pricked amoeba's loss of motility), which protects the ego against internal and external dangers.

In a limited way, armor varies in response to pleasure and pain stimuli. That is, in pleasurable situations it is relaxed somewhat and in painful circumstances it is increased. But the more rigid the armor, the less flexible the behavior in the face of new situations. Even the healthy organism armors in dangerous situations but dispenses with it completely in pleasurable circumstances. Where armor is severe and chronic, the organism is tolerant only of contraction, and experiences terror when great expansion and movement occurs. It has a sensation of bursting and loss of control. This, Reich called the terror of living.[16]

If armoring prevents a child from reaching the genital level,

----

[16] The terror of living is particularly met when all armor is removed and the organism is faced with complete surrender in the orgasm reflex.

he remains at an infantile character stage. In Western patriarchal societies adult character formation begins with a particular solution to the Oedipus complex[17] which is easily identified. The solution occurs in three stages:

1. An identification is made with the frustrating reality, the frustrating parent.[18]

2. The aggression mobilized against this parent causes anxiety and is turned against the self. This creates the inhibiting aspect of the character.

3. The ego forms reactive attitudes toward the sexual impulses and utilizes the reactive energies to ward off sexual impulses, either by repression or by a change of direction.[19]

Armoring develops as the somatic aspect of repression and always involves groups of muscles that form a functional unit. Thus, a child turning his rage at unkind toilet training into an anxious effort to please his demanding parent will contract the muscles of the buttocks and the pelvic floor. The armor, resulting from a fear of punishment, is assumed at the expense of id (instinctual) impulses, and contains the very rules and demands[20] that led to it. The ego seems to be strengthened, because some of the instinctual energy pressures are held down by the armor. But actually, the armor prevents stimuli from the outside world from reaching the organism in their natural profusion, and therefore makes it more difficult to continue training in other areas. In the long run, repression (armor) is not a true solution but only an expedient that serves later as the basis for neurotic conflicts and symptom formation. That is, it does not allow a sex-economic regulation of energy, and tension continues to increase.

According to Reich,[21] character formation depends upon:

17 Malinowski found the Trobriand Islanders did not develop an Oedipus complex.

18 Identification occurs where the frustrating parent was also loved. This leads to taking over certain character traits of this parent, specifically those which are directed against the impulse in question.

19 E.g., fear of sex changed to fear of disease.

20 We swallow prohibitions as some primitives eat the animals they fear—to eat before they are eaten.

21 *Character Analysis, op. cit.,* p. 150.

1. The time at which an impulse is frustrated, i.e. early or late in its development. The earlier the frustration the more complete is the repression. Early frustration (of aggression and pleasure in motor activity) leads to marked impairment of the total activity, and later to reduction of working ability.

2. The extent and intensity of the frustration—whether it is repressed or unsatisfied and the severity of either.

3. Against which impulses the central frustration is directed, i.e. the stage of libidinal development reached at the point when inhibition (armor) is exacted.

4. The ratio between frustration and permission.

5. The sex of the main frustrating person.

6. The contradictions in the frustrations themselves (e.g. in masochism, exhibition is encouraged at the anal level but punished at the phallic level).

All of these prerequisites for illness are set within the individual's society as well as within the individual himself. It is, of course, the design of his environment that dictates how much education, what sort of morality, and what degree of gratification an individual may realize within the limits of his natural potentialities. In order to prevent neuroses in the future, individuals must be allowed to develop character structures with enough flexibility to give them the sexual and social mobility needed for keeping an economic energy level in the organism.

An impulse that has fully developed can never be completely repressed. Thus, if the child is allowed to reach genital primacy he will survive fairly well regardless of future environmental restrictions. A development just short of genital primacy produces an impulsive character, where the individual's impulses have met with a sudden, unaccustomed frustration.

Armoring develops in an orderly fashion, depending on the need to conform, and is segmental in arrangement. It contains the history and meaning of its origin. If it is due to traumatic events, it contains the memory of the events.

For example,[22] during therapy a forty-year-old woman repeatedly saw a mental image of a woman and man. She hated the woman but did not know why. She saw herself with them at

[22] Compare this case history with Wilhelm Reich, "A Cast History," in *The Function of the Orgasm* (New York, Orgone Institute Press, 1942), pp. 276–292.

three years of age. She got in bed with the man but was convinced they were not her parents. At times, she would see the man and woman on a porch at a party and thought they might be neighbors she had been left with. Gradually the woman became clearer and she experienced great hatred for her, wanting to kill her. At this point she became very excited, lying on her back and kicking, pounding, and screaming in a typical childish temper tantrum.

She had an urgency to know more, to solve the situation. The temper tantrum was repeated two or three times and she felt somewhat relieved. Following this she went home with some continued anxiety and fear of death, which gradually developed into a fear of being choked to death. She did not want to remain alone and was anxious throughout the night. In the morning while making the beds, she visualized two eagle claws clutching at her throat and became frightened when the claws turned into hands choking her. When she tried to get up after lying down on the bed to compose herself, she could not walk because her legs were too weak. She called for an appointment and I saw her soon after.

When she came in she looked very bad. Her color was gray, and her expression could be described only by saying that she gave me an uneasy feeling of death. Soon after she lay on the couch I became aware of the smell of death. She described what had happened at home, and I saw that her chest was moving very little. I mobilized it somewhat and then grabbed her throat. The picture of the hands came into her mind and she panicked and began to choke (I had touched her throat only momentarily). She could not get her breath and was becoming cyanotic, so I pried her jaw open and gently massaged her neck. She soon began to breathe, although she was rather exhausted and greatly frightened.

This event, she said, went back much earlier in her life. She was in her crib and a woman was choking her until her tongue was hanging out. Her mother kept coming into her mind, although not in the visualized scene. Shortly, she screamed, "The hands again," and choked once more. After this was relieved she choked again with her tongue out. She became cyanotic and it was with difficulty that I got her to breathe; her eyes were sunken in her head and she looked as though she were dying.

All this was repeated again and she grew very panicky. She was not able to talk and tried to write a message in the air. When I gave her a pencil and paper she wrote that she couldn't talk; I told her she wasn't expected to, she was too young. This seemed to relieve the intense fear and she came out of it again. The choking episodes were repeated, probably a dozen times. Then, she began to call for her husband and said she wanted some one to hold her and love her. I called him and in the meantime sat holding her arm and reassuring her. Finally I felt she had had enough—it seemed to go on indefinitely. I got her to dress and sit up, and she had another attack. Then her husband came and held her and reassured her. She had one further attack and he suggested taking her out to dinner to get her mind on other things. I concurred.

Although anxious and uneasy she had no more attacks, and as the day wore on she felt much better and sobbed with relief. She was afraid to go home and insisted that her husband lie down with her when she did get home. The next morning she called to say that more had come up. She was sure she had been thrown to the floor and made unconscious when she was choked. During the night she had felt she had been losing consciousness.

The following day I saw her again. She said she had had the impression of a child being thrown to the floor against the wall, and added that she had always had a tender spot in the right parietal region of her head. One winter it had bothered her so much that she had consulted a physician, telling him it was driving her insane.

She had mild choking spells this time, but they were easily stopped and she was able to keep her mouth open and so prevent cyanosis. A picture of a man over her crib came up. It was a man, a dark man, who choked her and not the woman, although a woman was there. It seemed to have happened in the daytime. "I hate the man," she said, "I could kill him." For several sessions after this time the picture of her mother hitting her with a frying pan came up and mild choking attacks continued.

Convinced of the reality of these incidents, she asked her mother about them. Her mother told her that she was illegitimate and that during the pregnancy she had tried unsuccessfully to induce an abortion. After birth, she had induced her lover to get rid of the baby, and he had choked her and left her for dead. On another occasion the mother had hit her with a frying pan and knocked her unconscious.

It is in this way that single traumatic events are contained in memory in the body's armor and reappear as the organism is mobilized. But no memory is present if the armor is the result of *attitudes* in the parents. The most malignant to overcome are the implied, unspoken prohibitions imposed gradually at each stage of development.

The specific purpose of the chronic muscular armor is to hold back and assist one to conform and thus reduce anxiety—to hold back unitary movements (emotion) and in the deepest sense to prevent the orgasm reflex, which allows complete giving or surrender to biological emotions. The armor says "no" to this surrender. Emotion must be taken literally as "moving out," and a natural emotion includes the moving-out of the whole organism as a unit. That is, the whole organism normally takes part in all emotional activity whether pleasure, rage, or anxiety. The two basic movements are *outward* to the skin and environment (aggression), which is expansion or pleasure, and movement *inward* to the center (withdrawal), which is contraction, pain, and anxiety.[23] Movement into the musculature allows the organism to fight with rage or flee with fear.

Armoring first occurs in the diaphragm in an inspiratory contraction[24] where holding is most effective, but the basic conflict involves the pelvis (Oedipus conflict). Therefore the pelvis is always last to be dealt with in therapeutic removal. If the pelvis were to be freed first the individual could not handle the sexual

[23] This is incomplete. Actually anxiety is produced only where there is contraction against expansion.
[24] The diaphragm area is where the sympathetic ganglia are located, and as previously explained, breathing in is a contraction from the standpoint of the total organism although it actually expands that area.

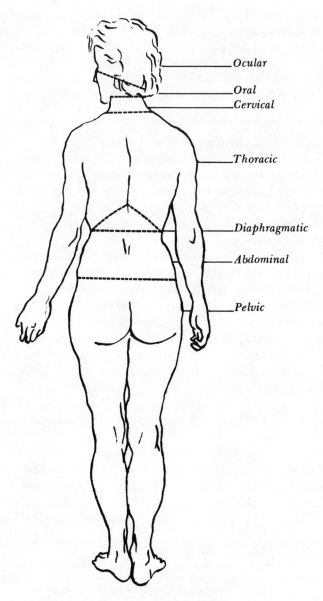

Ocular

Oral
Cervical

Thoracic

Diaphragmatic

Abdominal

Pelvic

The Seven Segments of the Body

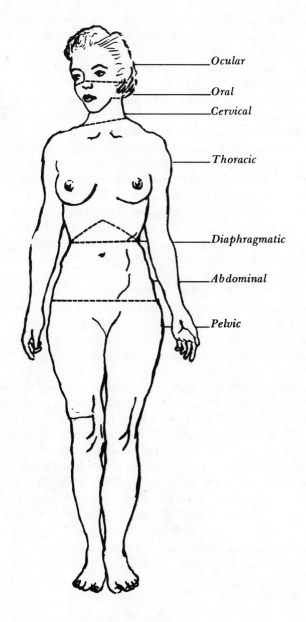

Ocular

Oral

Cervical

Thoracic

Diaphragmatic

Abdominal

Pelvic

The Seven Segments of the Body

impulse and either confusion and disintegration would follow, or else earlier problems would be carried into the sexual life (especially sadistic impulses). One exception is in depressives, where the low energy and great inhibition make early freeing of the pelvis safe.

Armor may be identified by an increased sensitivity to touch (ticklish instead of pleasant) except in heavily armored individuals where only touch is felt. Seven segments can be differentiated in the armor. Each segment includes the whole cross section at that level of the body, so that there are several rings at right angles to the spine. In addition to the rings of armor, one will usually find that one side of the body, left or right, is more heavily armored than the other. The underlying cause here is not yet understood, but it has nothing to do with right- or left-handedness. Adler speaks of the male side and the female side; and Deutsch points out the good right side and the bad (sinister) left side.

The seven segments of armor[25] are the ocular, oral, cervical, thoracic, diaphragmatic, abdominal, and pelvic. They are usually freed in that order except that the chest is most often mobilized first so that it can be utilized to build up energy in the organism and provide additional inner push to help in both revealing and removing other blocks.

Each segment responds as a whole and is more or less independent of other segments. But this independence should not be taken too rigidly, since we are dealing with a total organism which functions with an interdependence of all segments. Any one segment may fail to respond completely until further segments are freed. For example, deep holding may not appear in the throat until the pelvis is reached. With each release of a segment, armoring in earlier segments will recur and require further attention because the organism is not used to movement and tries to return to its former immobility. It must be gradually accustomed to free mobility.

In schizophrenia and epilepsy one may find little muscular

[25] Reich discusses these extensively in *Character Analysis* and *The Function of the Orgasm.*

armor, the armoring being largely in the eye segment. When this segment is freed the organism, unable to stand the increased free energy, contracts lower down and builds up a muscular armor. This in turn must be broken down. In certain cases, usually where more highly charged emotions are concerned, the organism, apparently unable to find a suitable equilibrium by armoring, withdraws energy from the part involved or even from the whole musculature. Such a withdrawal of energy is known as *anorgonia*.

It is important to determine the main character trait or attitude of the individual (the red thread[26]) because he will react to all progress through this trait and it soon becomes the main character defense. The trait may be socially acceptable (modesty, shyness, reserve, aggressiveness) or socially unacceptable (dishonesty, cheating, etc.). For example, a modest person will react to every advance modestly and never enthusiastically, while a cheat will try in every way to cheat you of success.

The principle of therapy is quite simple: merely to remove the chronic contraction which interferes with the free flow of energy throughout the organism and thus restore natural functioning. In practice it may be extremely difficult and complex. There are essentially three avenues of approach, the importance of each depending on the individual case although all three are a necessary tool in every therapy. They are (1) increasing the inner push on the organism by building up its energy by breathing, (2) directly attacking the spastic muscles to free the contraction and (3) maintaining the cooperation of the patient by bringing into the open and overcoming his resistances to the therapy and the therapist. This last is extremely important because the patient will in every way try to maintain his immobility and try desperately not to reveal himself. It may seem incredible that the patient who wants to get well fights so fiercely against therapy but behind this is intense fear of expansion and movement. He may do this so skillfully that it takes time and much ingenuity to unmask his methods. He may overtly cooperate beautifully, even

26 See "The Layering of the Armor," p. 61.

bringing out emotions that please everyone but the whole thing may be meaningless from a therapeutic standpoint. One can never work mechanically but must watch the needs of the patient by observing his bodily expression and by sufficient contact to allow yourself to feel what he is trying to express or even hide. When the patient begins to feel his own restrictions and gains sufficient contact with his organism so that he knows what he is holding back he can be very helpful in his therapy. His lack of contact is one of the most difficult problems to overcome. This is dealt with under problems of contact.

Breathing may in itself overcome minor holdings and does help to reveal and overcome more severe blocking. The patient is asked to breathe fully without forcing and to allow himself to develop a rhythm which soon becomes easier and freer. In most patients this will soon produce tingling in the fingers and lips. If this breathing continues, the sensation increases to strong and sometimes painful currents resembling sensations from an electric current. The fingers stiffen and begin to flex and become immobile. This may continue until the whole arm is involved and eventually the chest and face. At this point the patient can stop his breathing only with difficulty and the situation becomes dangerous to life. The contraction must be overcome. This is done by stopping breathing and manually mobilizing the fingers and arms.

Classical medicine calls this stiffening of the fingers and arms tetany and explains it as over-oxygenation with lowering of the alveolar carbon dioxide resulting in alkalosis and diminution of ionized calcium. We look upon it as contraction against the movement of energy which is beyond the individual's tolerance. That this seems reasonable is found in the fact that later in therapy patients may breathe as much as they like with no contractions. These may reappear after each breakthrough to a new level.

Following release of the fifth or diaphragmatic segment, soft breeze-like sensations will be felt moving down the body. These are pleasant and give a three-dimensional perception of the body. They are called streamings.

The chronic contraction of the skeletal muscles can be worked on directly, the organs and tissues only indirectly. To mobilize a chronically contracted muscle one must first increase the contraction to a point which cannot be maintained. The muscle thus overstrained must relax. This is done by direct pressure on the muscle with the thumb, by irritating or stimulating it, such as by tickling or pinching. Direct pressure is the usual and most effective means. One will find near the insertion of the muscle a very sensitive spot where contraction is greatest and it is here that the muscle responds best to the stimulus. Pressure here will relax the whole muscle. These points have been called trigger points in classical medicine, where sometimes they have been injected with novocain to produce relaxation. Of course the muscle will only contract down again unless the emotion (and ideas) that is being held back is released. For this reason groups of muscles that form a functional unit in holding back emotions are worked on together. Occasionally one muscle in this group may act as a trigger, causing the whole group to respond.

Anxiety is the basis for repression and is behind all contraction. If it were not for the anxiety the emotion would not be held back in the first place. The organism is always trying to control anxiety and cure is effected by forcing the patient to tolerate his anxiety and express his forbidden feelings. The most important emotion to elicit is rage (hate) and until this is released he cannot allow the softer feelings of longing and love to emerge. This is done in all seven segments.

Where muscles cannot be reached by the hands, other methods must be used, such as gagging, which increases the holding of the muscles involved until the gag reflex takes over and relaxation occurs. To release contraction of the brain the eyes and whole eye segment must be mobilized. Then the patient will frequently feel movement of the brain much to his surprise.

Sometimes emotions can be released and the holding will yield by describing to the patient what he is expressing or wants to do, or by holding a mirror to him, or by understanding words rather than direct work on the muscles. I have often felt that if one knew enough and were sufficiently perceptive therapy could be conducted entirely this way.

The Ocular Segment

General Description

This is the first segment and is concerned with all contact at a distance (except field reactions[27]). It includes sight, hearing, and smell. Armoring consists of a contraction and immobilization of the greater part or all of the muscles around the eye, eyelids, forehead, and tear glands, as well as the deep muscles at the base of the occiput—involving even the brain itself. I believe that the brain shows contraction to a greater or lesser extent in all the neuroses and if adequately mobilized enables the rest of the organism to tolerate expansion and movement. Contraction seems to be largely in the vegetative centers. This contraction causes and maintains the muscular contraction. It results from the original inhibition—specific "verbotens" producing specific contractions controlling various muscle groups which prevent the inhibition from expression. This is especially true in schizophrenia. Armoring in the ocular segment is expressed in an immobilized forehead (it appears flat) and eyelids. The flesh at the side of the nose is smooth and waxy. The patient is unable to open his eyes wide. Indeed, he will seem to be peering from the eyeholes of a false face. In schizophrenia the expression is empty, or as if the individual were staring into space. The more emotion brought up in looking, the less able is the individual to see clearly. The schizophrenic may see clearly but does so from the safety of his withdrawn shell. It is as if the neurotic looks but does not see, the schizophrenic sees but does not look, and the voyeur looks unseen.

One sees patients who, from an early age, have been unable to cry. Frequently one finds myopia and other visual disturbances that are not organic. The pupils may be dilated, particularly in schizophrenia, indicating deep anxiety. Anxiety or suspicion may be overtly apparent (suspicion is seen best by having the patient

[27] A field reaction is exemplified by that sensation we feel of someone's presence though we cannot see him, or by the awareness we have when we are near a wall or other obstacle in the dark. The blind become particularly alive to field reactions.

look out of the corners of his eyes). The eyes may show hate or pleading like a cowed or cornered animal's. The majority of patients have an inhibition against healthy flirting, which leads to a holding across the brows. This is often replaced by a neurotic unconscious flirting, especially in hysterics. The eyes generally hold anxiety and when open are a mirror of the emotional state of the organism.

Signs and Symptoms

Frontal headaches are the most common symptom, and are caused by chronic raising of the eyebrows to express anxiety or surprise. The patient may complain of a band around the head. Occipital headaches are due to a spasm of the occipital muscles produced by a chronic "ducking" attitude caused by a fear of a blow from behind. Fear of being hit on the head results in a flat or expressionless attitude. Haughtiness may be a defense against a frightened or attentive attitude, and the appearance of one engaged in deep reflection often is a defense against anxiety about masturbation. Symptoms of dizziness are caused by insufficient armoring, which allows movement of more energy than can be tolerated.

Therapeutic Principles[28]

Dissolution of the armor is accomplished by having the patient open his eyes wide during inspiration of breath, as in fright; and by mobilizing the forehead and eyelids through forcing an emotional expression. Mechanical exercises are of little value. The therapist should have the patient look suspiciously from side to side, roll the eyes while focusing and expressing anger, sadness, etc. Grimacing and direct work on the occipital muscles are helpful. It is sometimes necessary to move the forehead manually or open the eyelids to start the process or have the eyes focus on your moving finger. He should encourage the patient to open his eyes wide while breathing out, and to reach out with the eyes by flirting, smiling, longing, and other alive expressions. One can sometimes bring out emotion in the eyes by having the patient

[28] Here as in all cases one must never overlook the possibility of organic disease.

repeatedly look at you and away. The movement prevents holding and allows the expression to show itself.

Recently, Dr. Barbara Goldenberg developed a further technique in mobilizing the eyes by the use of a moving light upon which the eyes focus. This seems to be an important breakthrough in therapeutic technique. Here she offers the following comments on the use of the light:

I believe the light affords a unique opportunity for getting at the deep armoring in the brain parenchyma, hitherto untouched except indirectly through mobilizing the eyes. One may postulate two factors at work: (1) the direct photic stimulation of the brain substance itself, and (2) the pushing of the patient beyond the visual stimulus threshold so that he is forced to give up holding in the eyes.

During an infant research field trip I had occasion to observe the visual stimulus threshold demonstrated[29] and decided to see if it existed in other age groups as well. I noted that if one has a child or adult patient follow a target (such as a pencil) moved randomly ten inches in front of the eyes, there is frequently a strong emotional reaction after about fifteen minutes. The time factor appears critical and a shorter time span may elicit nothing. This does not seem explainable by fatigue alone. Following this maneuver one can often elicit strong affective reactions in patients—reactions which used to take months of painstaking work to uncover. If a two-battery pen light is substituted as the target, in a darkened room, the added factor of direct photic stimulation on the brain markedly intensifies the patient's reaction.

After fifteen minutes of such photic stimulation I have sometimes obtained spontaneous abreactions. There is almost always a sharp increase in affective responses and the release of unconscious material. One has the impression that the organism feels more integrated and therefore "safer" in letting go of the holding. The up-coming material is usually that which is closest to the ego and ready to surface—not chaotic bursts from deeper layers.

In lightly armored or unarmored patients, use of the light may elicit a partial or complete orgasm reflex. The effects on the eye segment and on contact are quite striking at times. For example, there was a marked difference in scholastic performance in two students (one a college physics major, the other in high school), both of whom went from failing to honor grades in the space of three months. One, an ambulatory schizophrenic, reported "a clearing in my head for the first time in my life," and a new found ability to grasp and assimilate what was taught in class. Two child patients, age 1½ and 6, respectively, who manifested severe eye block by crying without tears developed a flow

29 By Dr. Gerald Stechler of Boston University Medical School, who postulates its existence.

of tears after one session with the light. A borderline schizophrenic reported clearing of the chronic haze and yellowish cast before his eyes. Two migraine patients were entirely free of headaches after a few sessions.

There is some evidence the light may be useful in reaching hitherto untreatable patients—for example, those with hooks, or those incorrectly treated by premature loosening of the pelvic segment while the eyes were still heavily armored. Two of my patients showed mild symptoms referrable to the pelvic segment following use of the light (pruritus ani and bleeding hemorrhoids), while the eye segment was opening up. One 63-year-old passive feminine developed streamings and hard erections after twelve years of impotence but it is still too early to assess if adequate functioning is present.

Both eye functioning and eye motility have received some attention in psychiatric circles. For example, Goldfarb of Ittleson found that schizophrenic children show a preferential neglect of distance receptors (eyes and ears) which may be reversible in part by treatment.[30] He also noted their inability to have dissociated head-eye movements (i.e. if they follow a target with the eyes, the head also moves involuntarily). In my experience, some adult schizophrenics show this too. Goldfarb also observed that OKN (optokinetic nystagmus) is absent in schizophrenic children. Getman of Luverne, Minnesota, pointed out the absence of eye motility in non-readers or slow readers and advocated exercises to mobilize the eyes.[31] Doman and Delacato of Pennsylvania stressed the importance of creeping in infants and the concomitant side-to-side head movements in developing good eye motility and thus good reading ability.[32]

The experiments in expanding consciousness and "op" art may also be related to eye segment armoring phenomena. It is possible that LSD may dissolve the deep armoring in the brain precipitously and with chemical insult to the tissue. This may be followed by a more severe re-armoring when the drug has worn off. A patient of mine who took one dose of *peyote* against my advice showed evidence of this. Oster produced LSD-like effects by having a subject look through a square pane of glass ruled with concentric circles.[33] Some experimenters use flashing lights, and the alpha brain wave synchronizer of the hypnotists is fairly well known.

[30] William Goldfarb, *Childhood Schizophrenia* (Boston, Harvard University Press, 1961).

[31] G. N. Getmen, *How to Develop Your Child's Intelligence* (Luverne, Minnesota, 1962).

[32] Robert J. Doman et al, the Doman–Delacato Institute for the Achievement of Human Potential, Philadelphia.

[33] Gerald Oster, *"Moiré Patterns and Visual Hallucinations,"* from mss. of lecture given at Research Center for Mental Health, New York University (Washington Square College), Dec. 18, 1964.

"A word of caution regarding use of the light. There is no substitute for empathic contact with the patient. If the light is used as a mechanical "gimmick" instead of in a contactful way, it will accomplish nothing or may do harm. Overuse is dangerous though most patients eventually build up a threshold of tolerance and may require longer time exposure (20–25 minutes). Some patients learn to defend very successfully against the light or may even flee therapy. Most of them respond very positively and will comment on the difference it makes. A feeling of integration and well-being is commonly reported. However, sometimes a patient cannot tolerate the light organismically and this must be respected and not necessarily dismissed as resistance. Often one combines the light with other maneuvers, such as having the patient scream, hit or cry out words. The patient should be kept in contact and not allowed to drift off hypnotically. If used contactfully, the light is an extremely useful catalyst and means of reaching the deep cerebral armoring. Without contact it degenerates into a "gimmick." It can shorten and catalyze treatment but does not eliminate the need for the usual careful character analysis and segmental removal of armor from the head down.[34]

Sound is also important but we have not yet developed any special means of applying it.[35] Of course we use it routinely in the tone of our voice which is frequently very effective in producing responses from the patient.

Throughout therapy, one never ceases to be aware of the eyes, but watches them constantly. They may have a different expression from the oral segment. For example, when the face is looked at as a whole the total expression may be one of anger; but when the eyes are looked at alone they may only appear sad, and the anger is found in the mouth.

One cannot overemphasize the importance of mobilizing the eyes and should never proceed further until the eyes can tolerate further release of energy. They are actually an extension of the brain and our only means of mobilizing the brain. I have seen too many cases in consultation where the eyes were neglected and armoring removed from the remainder of the body. The patient gives a picture of panic, expressed in the eyes, a mask-like face and acute distress. This is not an easy situation to overcome.

[34] Personal communication to the author.
[35] Recently a technique for utilizing sound in therapy has been developed by Dr. Goldenberg. It seems to be of importance in some cases.

The Oral Segment

General Description

The second segment includes the muscles controlling the chin and throat, the annular muscle at the mouth, and the muscles of the occiput. Together, they make a functional unit, so that dissolution of one part of the armor affects all the rest. For example, dissolution of the armoring of the masseters will lead to clonisms of the lips and jaw and the release of emotions natural to the area—crying and a wish to suck. The whole oral segment may in some cases be mobilized by eliciting the gag reflex. This is done by having the patient put his finger down his throat without stopping breathing. Full expression of the oral segment depends on the free mobility of the ocular or first segment and, sometimes, on loosening of lower segments. For example, crying may not be complete until the two subsequent segments are free. The jaw may be tight with clenched teeth or unnaturally loose; the lips may be thin and determined or thick and sensuous.

Signs and Symptoms

One may observe a silly grin, a sarcastic smile, or a contemptuous sneer. A timidly friendly smile may be present or the mouth may be sad or even hard and cruel. The chin may sag, or be flat, pale, and lifeless. It may be pushed forward, giving a pugnacious appearance and causing a tightening of the floor of the mouth which holds back crying. A tight jaw leads to a monotonous, restrained voice. A tight throat leads to a whining, high, weak voice and harsh breathing. The mouth may be dry (from anxiety) or there may be excessive salivation (from unsatisfied oral needs).

The patient may speak little or talk constantly under pressure, or even stutter. The facial expressions as a whole should be observed carefully; the depressed face, the artificially beaming one, the one with stiff and sagging cheeks heavy with tears, or the one with masklike stiffness from suppressed crying. A wooden expression may be the result of an early attempt to avoid "making faces." Children are taught not to make faces, or "they will freeze that way." Also, the "face at the window," seen or imagined in early childhood, may be found frozen in a patient's expression. Children learn very early that faces must be rigidly controlled.

The oral segment generally holds back angry biting, crying, yelling, sucking, and grimacing. During expiration in some patients one will notice a progressive closing of the throat. This is the same mechanism that is active during the initial stage of swallowing. They must swallow back each impulse. Severe holding in the jaw may cause temporal headaches.

Therapeutic Principles

The therapist should stop the patient's talking, if excessive, and keep him from making extraneous or aggressive movements. Have him accentuate the expression he is showing. If this accomplishes nothing, stop it. Exciting the patient causes a push of energy and eliminates *voluntary* defenses, allowing *involuntary* expressions to come out. Encourage these expressions. Direct work on the masseters and chin may be indicated, or having the patient make sounds that tend to mobilize the lips and throat may help. If crying is being held back the patient will try in vain to talk with a loud and resonant voice. Suppression of crying is frequently associated with nausea due to tension in the muscles of the floor of the mouth. Working on the submental muscles or on gagging may bring out the crying. Sometimes having the patient imitate crying causes release. The need to bite is almost always present and the patient may be allowed to bite a suitable object such as a towel. Sometimes in depression the expression remains depressed even after armor is dissolved. This is from habit and can be overcome by having the patient smile.

In stutterers the jaw, lips, tongue, and soft palate may each have to be dealt with separately, making the sounds *puh* for the lips, *wah* for the lips and jaw, *lah* for the tongue, and *kuh* for the soft palate.

The Cervical Segment

General Description

The third segment comprises the deep muscles of the neck, the platysma, and the sternocleido mastoids. It also includes the tongue, which is inserted mainly on the cervical bone system. The emotional function of armoring in the neck is to hold back anger or crying. The result is a stiff neck, a stubbornness, "I *won't* cry." Anger or crying is literally swallowed without the patient's even being aware of it. A fear of being choked leads to a lump in the throat and covers a desire to choke someone else. It is seen frequently in hysterics in connection with a fantasy of the father's penis in the throat, and of being choked by it. Their desire to choke leads to guilt and to a fear of being choked, a displacement of energy from lower segments upward (from hands and arms to throat). Some patients have a very sensitive larynx from a fear of having their throat cut.

Signs and Symptoms

Frequent swallowing, voice changes, harsh breathing, coughing, the sensation of a lump in the throat, and choking sensations (fellatio fantasies) are the major indications of armor in this segment.

Therapeutic Principles

Elicit the gag reflex and reduce spasms of the sterno mastoids and deep muscles of the neck. Also elicit screaming and yelling. *Remember the neck is very vulnerable,* and one must proceed with great caution as there are many important nerves, vessels, and the larynx—all of which can be easily injured. I had one patient who suffered a severe bradycardia from pressure on the vagus due to armoring.

The Thoracic Segment

General Description

Although the chest segment can be divided into upper and lower parts, it can best be considered as a whole. It consists of the intercostal muscles, pectorals, deltoids, muscles of the scapula, spinal muscles, the chest cage and its contents, and the hands and arms. It is the most important segment because it contains the most vital structures, the heart and the lungs. It is the first segment to be blocked, by holding in inspiration to reduce anxiety. Thus expiration is never complete. Blocking places pressure on the solar plexus and reduces sympathetic excitation. In schizophrenia, the eyes have been damaged as well as the chest in the first ten days of life.

A chronic attitude of inspiration is the most important means of suppressing any emotion. In the majority of cases, this armoring should be reduced first in order to build up energy in breathing, and to put more inner pressure on blocks. If the chest moves freely one has increased functioning even though further progress is impossible. In depressives the chest must be mobilized quickly to build up energy and reverse the dying process. In patients with a high charge,[36] however, mobilization of the chest may be dangerous so that an outlet for energy must be provided first (such as the lower limbs).

Asthma is a special condition occuring in chest armoring in which there is a parasympathetic over-excitation to overcome sympathetic contraction. The patient assumes a calm and brave façade to cover up his deep anxiety. In other words, he refuses to be anxious. Deep rage is behind this façade, a rage caused by an inability to show anxiety; behind the rage is a deeper layer of anxiety. Thus, we have a calm façade, superficial anxiety, rage, deep anxiety. To overcome the condition one must make the patient anxious or make him imitate anxiety; in a sense, one must cause him to back away from the block. If the attack is slight, it can be relieved by having the patient vocalize— ahhhhhhhhhhhh. (According to Reich every asthmatic has a fantasied penis in his throat.)

In coronary or other heart conditions one must proceed with great caution or *heart failure may occur*. In coronary cases, the chest is very rigid and great caution is necessary in mobilization. If pain or pallor occurs one must stop, and one should always have cardiac stimulants handy. Once the chest is mobilized, however, a great strain is removed from the heart.

[36] Energy charge can usually be estimated by the appearance of the individual, color of the skin, and ability for sustained effort. However, accurate estimation is made by examination of the red blood cells. The higher the charge, the fuller are the cells, the redder their color, and more extensive their energy fields.

In the average patient the chest is usually rigid and does not move in respiration. It is held high in the inspiratory position and eventually gives rise to emphysema. If the chest does move, it may be high or low, rigid or soft, but with small excursion. In schizophrenia the chest is soft but movement barely perceptible.

The shoulders are held either back or forward but do not respond to breathing, and the head, instead of falling gently backward in expiration, usually comes forward or is jerked back forcibly. The spinal muscles may be acutely contracted. These are important regions of holding back and may prevent the chest from moving. They contain spite, a frozen anger. The intercostals are sensitive and painful and the patient may be very ticklish.

The emotions held in the chest are heartbreak, bitter sobbing, rage (stronger than that found in the oral segment), reaching, and longing. These are deep emotions which when expressed afford much relief. ("A weight has been lifted from my chest.") The hands may be cold, clammy, and weak from withdrawal of energy. Armoring does not interfere much with manual dexterity, but withdrawal of energy does. The latter is an indication of more emotionally charged material and of more explosive emotions.

Laughing seems to come from the chest and is the least understood of the emotional expressions. Animals do not laugh.[37] Primarily laughter is probably an expression of joy, but it seems to be a response to any excitation above the tolerance level. Laughing and crying may be interchangeable for any other emotion or for each other in addition to their basic functions. Natural crying is a result of need; as a secondary reaction it is a socially more acceptable vehicle for emotions such as rage.

Signs and Symptoms

An armored chest basically expresses restraint and self-control and will give a feeling of being unmoved or unaffected by events. Where there is no armor, the expressive motions of chest and

[37] The higher apes as experimental animals apparently do laugh and play tricks. These, however, are not living in the natural state and are subjected to human conditioning.

arms give a free buoyant feeling. Typical armor is a chronic inspiratory expansion, as if one had taken a very deep breath and not let it out, and it can be accompanied by high blood pressure, palpitation, and anxiety. Continued for a long time, a disposition to tuberculosis or pneumonia may develop, or the heart may become enlarged.

For the patient with an armored chest, rage is cold, crying is unmanly, and longing is too soft. Reaching out or embracing are not felt vegetatively. The hands lose their orgonotic charge and are cold, clammy, and painful (leading to Raynaud's disease). Behind the clamminess of the hands, there may be an impulse to choke which is armored off in the shoulder blades and hands.

Women who are armored in this segment have insensitive breasts and are disgusted at nursing. A knot may be felt in the chest from a spasm of the esophagus, behind which is a holding back of angry yelling. The related anxiety can be elicited by pushing on the chest and having the patient yell. The chest holding is mainly "I won't," and the ability to give and surrender depends on mobility of this segment. Early memories of disappointment and mistreatment may come out with release of the emotions of the chest, which is usually blocked very early. Memories seem bound in plasmatic immobility and are reactivated when excitation occurs.

Therapeutic Principles

Increase breathing with instructions to follow through in expiration, exert pressure on the chest during expiration or press gently on the epigastrium, and work directly on the intercostal muscles, deltoids, and spinal muscles. Elicit hitting, choking, tearing, scratching, yelling, rage, and sobbing, and finally, reaching with longing. Opening and closing the hands softly may bring out otherwise unnoticed anxiety. I saw one case of severe chronic headache produced through holding back impulses in the hands and arms. Where there is doubt between two emotions, use the more aggressive expression. For example, if a patient wants to cry he will do so after rage; but if he wants to get angry crying will inhibit his expression. The patient may continue one emotion to avoid another. When he appears to be enjoying it, it is time to stop it.

The Diaphragmatic Segment

General Description

The diaphragm separates the body into upper and lower parts and may be compared to a height of land. Above the diaphragm, expression is upward to the eyes, mouth, and arms. Below, the expression is through the pelvis. The stomach contents may be expelled in either direction.

The fifth segment includes the diaphragm and organs under it and does not depend on the mobility of the chest for functioning. The diaphragm may remain immobile even though the chest moves, and vice versa. It comprises a contraction ring over the epigastrium, and lower end of the sternum, and goes along the lower ribs to the tenth, eleventh, and twelfth thoracic vertebrae. It contains the diaphragm, stomach, solar plexus, pancreas, liver, gall bladder, duodenum, kidneys, and two muscle bundles along the lower thoracic vertebrae. Armoring is expressed by lordosis of the spine (hollow under the patient's back). Breathing out is with effort and the abdomen balloons. The first four segments must be free before it can be loosened. For this, repeatedly eliciting the gag reflex without interrupting expiration is effective. When this is free, wavelike movements occur in the upper part of the body with a feeling of giving; that is, the torso tends to fold up with each expiration. This segment holds severe murderous rage.

Signs and Symptoms

Symptoms are nervous stomach disorders, more or less constant nausea with an inability to vomit, peptic ulcer, gall bladder disease, liver conditions, and diabetes. The major abdominal organs are at the diaphragm, and blocking causes many psychosomatic diseases.

Therapeutic Principles

Relieve the block by gagging and respiration. When the segment is opening, vomiting occurs.

The Abdominal Segment

This is the sixth armor ring. It includes the large abdominal muscles, the rectus, transversis abdominus, and muscles of the back (latissimus dorsi and sacro spinalis). The muscles at the flanks are especially important because in them one first finds tension from stasis[38] in an unarmored person. Armored flanks produce ticklishness and hold spite. Stasis can be relieved by freeing tension in these muscles. Fear of attack is found in tension in the lumbar muscles, and is similar to tension in the neck from a desire to duck. Therapy is simple if the higher segments are open. Masses in the abdomen may appear and disappear during treatment of this segment.

The Pelvic Segment

General Description

The seventh and last segment contains all the muscles of the pelvis and lower limbs. The pelvis is usually pulled back. The muscles above the symphysis are tense and painful and so are the superficial and deep adductors of the thighs. The anal sphincter is contracted and pulled up, as is the whole pelvic floor. The gluteal muscles are contracted and sensitive. The pelvis usually is rigid, immobile, and asexual. Sensations and excitations are absent.

Signs and Symptoms

Symptoms from pelvic armoring are constipation, lumbago, growth in the rectum, ovarian cysts, polyps of the uterus, benign and malignant tumors, vaginal conditions, irritability of the bladder, irritation of the urethra, and vaginal and penis anesthesia. In the male, low energy in the pelvis (anorgonia) leads to erective impotence or premature ejaculation, and in the female to anesthesia or vaginismus. The feet and legs may be cold and swollen, with numbness, tingling sensations, and varicosities.

[38] See "Stasis," p. 104.

This segment contains anxiety and rage. The latter is of two types: anal or crushing, and phallic or piercing. (Examples: anal—kicking; phallic—striking with the pelvis.) Pleasure in the pelvic area is impossible until the anger is released. Also present may be contempt of the sex act and of all the pelvic structures.

Therapeutic Principles

The various spasms must be freed by mobilizing the pelvis and eliciting anxiety and rage. This may be followed by having the patient repeatedly contract and relax the pelvic floor. When this is accomplished the pelvis moves forward spontaneously at the end of each complete expiration, giving the orgasm reflex. It is then capable of reaching out and taking over during the orgasm with the complete surrender of the organism as a whole. This capacity gradually develops into reality during the year or two following therapy. The patient's health must be structuralized.

The Layering of the Armor

There are three basic layers in every armored individual:

1. The superficial veneer or social façade.
2. The secondary or great middle layer where the sum of all the repressions has built up, resulting in destructive forces such as rage, spite, hate, contempt, etc. There are usually many subsidiary layers here.
3. The healthy core, the rational self-regulating protoplasmic movement and excitation, which expresses itself when all blocking has been removed. Here lies the simple, decent individual below all irrational training and environmental influences.

Presumably the infant is born with a healthy emotional structure and without chronic armor. It has a basic energy charge and a natural aggressiveness depending on its freedom of growth in the uterus. The more spastic its developmental environment, the more its aggression is restricted. The higher the energy charge, the more the effect of the spastic environment is counteracted. Right after birth occurs, however, the organism is subjected to repeated restrictions of its natural and even secondary functioning. Each prohibition or inhibition becomes part of the character, through contraction due to anxiety (fear of punishment or rejection). Contraction causes an increase in inner tension and the outward push of all repressed material under more pressure increases. This ever-increasing pressure produces harshness which expresses itself as hate. Hate must again be repressed, so only modified expressions such as contempt or disgust are allowed to come out.

Each emotion or urge is originally repressed by prohibition (fear) from the environment, which eventually is incorporated in the organism as the superego. The energy behind the repressed feeling is utilized in the repressing by maintaining contraction of the muscles. The feeling is, as it were, split in two; part of the energy is used to hold back the other part, and thus immobility is established.

If the repressing force is not equal to the push outward, then an alteration of the drive to a more acceptable, but less fulfilling, one is attempted. This is called reaction formation. Since the original feeling remains unexpressed and is still there, a constant pressure must be maintained to keep up the altered outward expression of the drive. The original drive itself absorbs energy (libido) and becomes stronger, so that the reaction formation gradually must spread to substitute for more feeling.

To relieve the situation this equilibrium must be disturbed, either by reducing the holding of energy (breaking the muscle spasm) or by increasing the inner push (breathing) or both.

The second or great middle layer is usually very complex; many sublayers pile one on another until a social adjustment has been reached which is presented as the social façade or personality. The personality is, then, the end result of all the social and educational restrictions placed upon the original healthy core. This may be a comparatively stable or unstable façade, depending on the effectiveness of the defenses in the middle layer and the degree of satisfaction the organism can still attain.

The social façade contains one (sometimes more) basic character trait as its means of meeting the environment. This trait carries throughout therapy and causes the patient to react consistently in the same way to each problem he meets. It becomes the main character defense. Reich calls this trait the *red thread* and it must be recognized to understand and evaluate the individual. The basic character trait is never dissolved but remains always an integral part of the personality, although it may be modified. It may be socially acceptable—kindness, modesty, reserve, shyness, correctness, righteousness; or socially unacceptable—dishonesty, cunning, or cheating.

Therapeutic Principles

The three layers are dealt with in each segment as it is mobilized and its armor dissolved until the final core of unitary vegetative functioning is reached. The most important thing is to mobilize and allow expression of hate. Each segment of the armor may contain a great number of subsidiary layers within the secondary layer. When a subsidiary layer yields, it is called a breakthrough. This may or may not be a dramatic event, but it is felt as a temporary relief. Sometimes a layer involving one segment cannot be removed or even discovered until other segments are freed. For example, some crying may come out with loosening of the first two segments, but deep sobbing comes only after freeing of the first four segments. In unlayering, one works from the outside in and from the head down to the pelvis. Even this cannot be held to rigidly. One must watch the needs of the organism.

The depth of the layer on which one is working is recognized by the extent to which the organism is involved in the response (emotion) and the ability of the patient to function. If the first four segments are free one is always working at a deep layer. Every warded-off impulse also serves the function of warding off a more deeply repressed impulse. Blocking of the outward flow of energy by contraction from the surface (armoring) leads to frustration. This results in a forceful push of energy from within because of increased pressure and autonomic excitation, thus producing rage. Rage is a forceful push of energy occurring when the natural soft flow is blocked. If energy instead of pushing out is withdrawn, weakness of the part results. An organism may, after a long time, cease building up energy when outlet is blocked and then it rapidly becomes weakened. This occurs particularly in severe depressions and is known as shrinking.

Where anxiety is felt, it means that there is an inefficient contraction (armoring) against the outward push of energy and it signifies an unstable equilibrium. This state is deliberately produced during therapy in breaking down armoring. A patient gets well by standing or facing his anxiety. Anxiety occurs only where there is movement; that is, during the process of expansion or contraction. When contraction is complete and effective, anxiety ceases. An affect block[39] represents a successful armoring or contraction.

Adiposity. Excessive fat can be looked upon as a form of armoring. The fat soaks up energy (1 gm. fat equals 9 calories as compared to 1 gm. protein equals 4 calories) and also acts as a protection against stimuli. It interferes greatly with therapy. Behind it is a great deal of anxiety.

Guilt. Guilt is frequently a serious problem to overcome and has not been easy to understand from a bioenergetic viewpoint. We know of course that behind it is rage. Konia, in a personal discussion, has offered a possible explanation in that the energy carrying out the impulse remains stuck in the muscles short of completion. Excitation of this energy revives the feeling of guilt. For example, suppose a child is caught masturbating and commanded to stop immediately because it is felt he is doing something bad. The energy behind this pleasurable experience is frozen in the muscles participating. Anything reviving a repetition of the act will reawaken the "verboten" and the guilt. Pressure is built up producing rage at the frustration. To overcome the guilt the muscles involved must be mobilized, expressing the rage, and the situation discussed, allowing a new guilt-free evaluation of the act.

Anorgonia

Anorgonia appears to be a condition alternate to that of armoring, and is a reaction by the organism to very emotionally charged situations. Perhaps it would be better to say that armoring produces an immobilization by muscular contraction, while in anorgonia it occurs through immobilization of the plasma

---

[39] See "Anal Character Types," especially the compulsive character, p. 124.

system. Whether energy is actually withdrawn from the area, or merely lacks excitation, or receives too strong an excitation from the vegetative system is not clear. I believe that, in most cases at least, the last is the case and that it may result in paralysis of the vegetative system, as well as of the tissue plasma generally.

When very vigorous excitations which travel fully to the genital (natural pleasure impulses) meet and conflict with disruptions of the orgasm reflex that are equally strong, anorgonia follows. The organism responds to the conflict with a block in plasma motility to control the strong, unfamiliar plasma excitation.[40] The block is shown in weakness, falling anxiety, failing equilibrium, or collapsing. It is as if the expansion were to start and be unable to follow its natural course—as if the impulse itself were suddenly extinguished, and with that came loss of contact with the affected part.

Anorgonia may be a chronic condition from a gradual plasmatic shrinking. That is what occurs in cancer[41] where there is resignation, and also in depression; the result is a gradual lowering of the organismic energy level. It may also be an acute condition; an example is the falling anxiety which is a frequent component of orgasm anxiety.

In any case, an anorgonia condition in an adult can be traced to a childhood need to repress pleasure, that is, to stop expansion. Possibly the infantile prerequisites for the condition were met when a strong desire for physical contact was left ungratified. In most cases, anorgonia is not severe and can be overcome without too much difficulty. At other times, especially in cancer, it may be an extremely grave symptom.

Although in many cases of anorgonia there is undoubtedly a withdrawal of energy from the part affected, the basic mechanism seems to be that too strong an excitation produces paralysis of the plasma system.

Much still needs to be learned about anorgonia, but I have

40 Plasma excitation comes from the vegetative system as a nerve impulse. The nerve impulse produces a movement of the plasma which is seen as a wavelike motion, but if the excitation is too strong paralysis may occur instead. Movement of the plasma is perceived as sensation or emotion.

41 Cf. Wilhelm Reich, *The Cancer Biopathy* (New York, Orgone Institute Press, 1948).

the impression that it is primarily a muscular problem. People suffering from this condition have struck me as consisting largely of internal organs and skin. That is, the muscles seem to be passive or unable to participate in an emotional flow of energy to the genital. Whether the organism cannot stand the flow of energy in the muscles themselves or whether this passivity allows too great a flow to the skin is not clear. In any case, the result is a severe vegetative contraction with resulting weakness, coldness, and collapse. In principle at least, the condition seems to be an inability to *tolerate* aggression; since where the organism can tolerate aggression but cannot *express* it, armoring occurs.

One severe case of anorgonia occurred after intense feelings of hate followed by genital excitation. The area affected extended from the legs to the chest. The patient responded quickly when I had her dance to a record she was fond of. My rationale was that it would be beneficial to encourage excited energy to flow into the muscular system. Almost any activity that was safe, easily available, and usually enjoyed by the individual concerned would likely have had the same effect.

5 · Problems of Contact[1]

Contact

With the Self

CONTACT REQUIRES MOVEMENT OF ENERGY above a certain minimal level plus excitation. Where the organism is free of blocks there is a free-flowing plasmatic movement which gives rise to sensations (organ sensations) and a three-dimensional perception of the body. Sense impressions and emotions flow together in a functional unity and are felt as pleasure streamings. The individual becomes fully aware of the body, its sensations, desires, and needs. We say he is "alive." He feels alive and is joyous in that life. He likes himself and his body and becomes independent. He has attained contact with his core, i.e. his primary drives. Where blocks are still present awareness of those free parts makes him acutely aware of lack of contact with the blocked parts and gives rise to frustration. He feels his armor as a restricting foreign body and wishes to be free of it. This is a very favorable sign in therapy. Self-perception in the armored is either greatly diminished or distorted. It is the most difficult and deepest problem to solve.

[1] Reich has treated this subject more extensively in *Character Analysis, op. cit.*

With the Environment

Our environment is accessible to our understanding only through sense impressions, i.e. sensations (plasmatic movements), as with self-perception. Our emotions are the answers to the impressions of the environment. If the environment is pleasant we feel pleasure—if menacing or unpleasant we respond with anxiety or unpleasure, and tend to withdraw contact even completely under certain circumstances. Armored individuals are disturbing and felt as unnatural to the unarmored. Unarmored contact is simple, straightforward, and direct. Full contact with the environment goes with streamings in the body and true binocular vision and a feeling of responsibility. Love is an expression of full contact, even thoughts of the loved one can produce streamings through the body centering in the genital. It must be remembered that most of what passes for love is really not love at all but is based on the anxiety or hate present in armored man where all natural impulses, particularly love, are inhibited. The degree of contact or lack of it may be judged in therapy by having the patient describe the therapist. Does he do it mechanically as though you were just an object or does he see you as a living, feeling person? In the latter case he is quite aware of your presence, attitudes, and feelings. In complete contact one even is aware of the exact thoughts of the other person. This occurs infrequently.

With the Cosmos

This is the ultimate contact of the organism in reaching back to his origin and feeling a part of it; that is, contact with nature, with the universe. This is attained in the full genital orgasm and undoubtedly in babies during the oral orgasm. But beyond this one becomes intimately concerned with nature, its beauty, its marvels, and its wonder. One decries its destruction by irrational man and wishes fervently to preserve what is left of its beauty, its forests and wild life. One reaches out to the heavens and feels oneself a part of the throbbing, whirling universe, the cosmic ocean from which one came. One belongs.

Cosmic feeling (core contact) is the basis for all religions.[2] This perception compels one to reach out to something beyond man, an unknown from which he sprang and to which he wishes to return. Where contact is not blocked or distorted, but ignorance is present, anamism results. Distorted contact gives rise to mysticism and the various religions. Full contact with sufficient information results in functionalism (thinking as nature functions). Where cosmic contact is lacking we find a mechanistic approach to all natural functions. This has largely been the pattern until recently in modern science. Now a few functional concepts are forcing their way in. Mechanistic science has reached a dead end. Mechanism is sufficient for man-made machines but is inadequate to explain nature.

Contactlessness

General Description

Contactlessness appears when the push from within is equal to the contraction from without; that is, when the repressing and the repressed forces are equal and there is a stoppage of energy movement. There is no contact without movement; and contact is established through the free movement of energy. Biophysically, contact is an energy charge (above the minimal level) plus excitation. This gives rise to sensation, which in turn must be properly perceived. There is some degree of contactlessness in every case of armoring.

Healthy people, in fact, can withdraw contact when faced with painful or unpleasant surroundings such as a shocking disaster, or even such a minor occurrence as listening to a boring lecture or conversation. We must remember that all of the mechanisms used in neuroses are natural and exist in healthy individuals to meet specific occasions. It is merely the extent to which they are used in neuroses that makes them pathological.

In therapy, as each layer of armoring is removed, three things appear in sequence: First, anxiety occurs. Then, emotion is re-

[2] Wilhelm Reich, *Ether, God and Devil* (New York, Orgone Institute Press, 1951), pp. 62-96.

leased—rage, contempt, spite, crying, etc. After the emotion is expressed, there is a sense of relief. Third, contactlessness appears. There is no desire to move and the patient is temporarily stuck. A stage where the repressed and repressing forces are equal has been reached.

Contactlessness may also occur where excitation is avoided by withdrawal in the eyes. This occurs naturally in sleep. Also, it is a major factor in schizophrenia. But it is more important in all the neuroses and more prevalent in the general population than is realized. The eyes, ears, smell, and touch are all important factors in excitation. I believe the eyes are by far the most important, and contactlessness can be produced by dulling the eyes regardless of whether the origin of the stimulus was sound, smell, touch, or even pain. Withdrawal of energy also results in contactlessness—as in anorgonia and shock.

Signs and Symptoms

A feeling of inner loneliness or deadness are usual symptoms. Schizophrenics will feel that they are splitting and everything will seem not only strange and alien, but also uninteresting and unrelated to themselves. Contactlessness includes genital anesthesia and orgasm anxiety. In therapy, the latter is the last form of neurotic contactlessness to show itself and the final hurdle that must be surmounted before health is established.

At bottom, it is the fear of orgastic contact that is the source of all fears of contact with the world. In therapy, a feeling of emptiness of life or experience will accompany the orgasm anxiety. Also, superficial communications and a disinclination to speak of genital desires. a sudden deepening of reserve, fears that the body will come apart, falling dreams and fantasies, flight from meaningful relations with the world (including sexual relations), and a return to infantile reactions and to earlier symptoms—all characterize the final contactlessness. Paresthesia and depersonalization are examples of contactlessness.

Therapeutic Principles

To overcome contactlessness, the individual's equilibrium must be disturbed by increasing the push outward, or reducing holding, or both. This creates anxiety. The therapist should point out the contactlessness to make the patient aware of it and prevent substitute contact. Describe his behavior and point out the difference between the ideal he sets for himself and the emptiness in which he lives. Dulling and withdrawal of the eyes must be overcome.

The following letter indicates a growing awareness in the writer of her contactlessness. I had previously pointed out her snobbery as a defense.

Dear Dr. Baker,

I am thinking a lot about my snobbery. Does it boil down to that?

I am too snobbish to be someone's wife, too important to spend my time having babies, too snobbish to be a person working from 9 to 5, too precious to become a member of a collective farm, too preoccupied with "higher" things to clean my finger nails or polish my shoes.

I have not given of my highness to anything or anyone, I have preserved it for something much more important. I don't know for what but I am waiting. Someone like me is not meant for the mundane things in life.

There never was a job that I did well; efficiency is for secretaries. I shine so, one must overlook such trivialities as an unclean apartment or messy hair.

No man has ever heard me say, "I love you". Whenever it was said to me I turned my face away.

I am too good to be an office girl or farmer, and I suppose too good to sit down and work at anything.

I love music, but not enough to practice, love to write, but not enough to exert myself to learn how; loved John, but not enough to give myself to him. I play at being a siren, yet am afraid of water, for I don't trust that I can swim in it, I can only drown in it.

I demand: respect, love, esteem.

I am headed for fame. My dramatic life cannot end without someday coming to everyone's notice. Fame is so certain I don't even have to work for it.

I was in a youth movement, yet was never part of the group; I went to school without being part of the student body. Always alone. Ever since I can remember, alone.

I am a woman who cannot love, a pianist who cannot play, a friend who cannot give, an "artist" who does not work, an idealist who does not act.

Why doesn't a roller run over me and spread me out thin and make me usable as a dish rag.

I should go to Israel and make myself useful. I don't deserve my freedom, I don't exploit my opportunities.

I dreamt that I was one of many trees. They all opened and bloomed, but my branches remained bare and dry.

How can I have any respect for myself?

Don't accuse me to trying to entice; I am above such things. I am above anger or passion or love, I suppose. I shall not be seen crying uncontrollably, helplessly, by you or anyone else. I will not accept anything or ask for anything.

If ever I ask you why I am unlovable, show me this letter.

Contactlessness becomes intolerable when the patient has begun to experience the first sensations of orgastic streamings in the body and genital. In genital anxiety an exact analysis of attitudes and sensations during masturbation and the sexual act must be brought out, and if unduly increased friction movements are present during sexual activity they must be stopped.

Substitute Contact

General Description

To distinguish substitute contact from true contact one can stop the behavior designed to make contact. When substitute contact is stopped, anxiety occurs; when true contact (legitimate response) is stopped, the patient remains at ease.

Substitute contact occurs when immediate vegetative contact is destroyed to a greater or lesser degree so that the remainder is insufficient to maintain relationships with the outer world. Substitute functions and artificial types of behavior are developed in an attempt to establish relationships. True, they are based on movement of energy, but it is below the minimal level and comes out of reaction formations rather than genitality.

Signs and Symptoms

Substitute contact can be recognized in any sort of insincere or hypocritical behavior, whether assumed for the occasion or a habitual mode of expression. The salesman's brash geniality, the hostess's forced smile, the tired teacher's patience are commonly noticed forms.

Other substitutes for genuinely felt contact with another person would include casual promiscuity or coquetry, bragging of sexual prowess, or dirty wisecracking or a giggly rather than involved attitude toward sexual expression. Affectation in speech and behavior (condescending, dignified, lukewarmly friendly, childishly wooing, grandiose, markedly modest or immodest) usually signal a state of contactlessness. People who mangle the hand instead of shaking it, or always scream with delight and surprise on meeting, or talk forever about something no one else is concerned with are out of touch. Contactlessness can, in general, be seen in embarrassment and unnatural movements and gestures; that is, in attitudes that stand out and are disturbing. Genuine contact is simple and pleasing. Substitute contact is a substitute function and acts as a defense.

Therapeutic Principles

The symptoms are pointed out and the patient is requested to stop such behavior. Problems of contact are particularly met during the stages in therapy when castration and genital anxiety are dealt with directly.

Castration Anxiety

This is an anxiety produced originally through the threat of castration, either with words and implications, or by circumcision. Evidence may be found throughout therapy and may be a prominent factor behind attitudes and symptoms, but it usually becomes clearly defined toward the end of therapy when one reaches the pelvic segment. It is characterized by a feeling of threat from the outside, an attack usually related to employers or to other people in authority and eventually to the therapist; finally it is felt as a direct attack on the genital. Patients will protect their genitals, cover them with their hands, etc. Fear may be intense, and some patients will relive the terror of their circumcision.

I have also had women who put their hands over the genital, and when at last they felt compelled to look at it, they screamed with horror, saying, "It's gone. Nothing sticks out. Please help me." Some have said, "My penis is gone." They later confide that they had the feeling that their genitals were bleeding wounds (men frequently think of the female genital in this manner). Such an episode represents the final relinquishment of a fantasied penis.

Genital Anxiety

Preorgastic Anxiety

Preorgastic anxiety arises when genitality is being reestablished and orgonotic sensations reach the genital. The individual cannot tolerate the expansive process. Contraction occurs, causing earlier symptoms to reappear and patients avoid discussion of sexual desires, become superficial in their communications, and present ideas of falling and sensations of disintegration. They complain they feel as badly as ever, therapy has accomplished nothing, and all is hopeless. Genital contact may be avoided or, when contact is made, sensations may disappear after an initial excitement. Anxiety is felt in the genital at sexual approach.

One young man brought the following dream: A beautiful, young woman entered his room and immediately removed all of her clothing and made advances to him. He became very excited sexually and was about to proceed to intercourse when he became frightened and had the feeling that something in the vagina would injure his penis, so he thought he would investigate first with his fingers. Then he looked at his hand to contemplate which finger he could best afford to lose. At this he awoke with anxiety.

Genital anxiety may occur spontaneously, following childbirth, since pregnancy produces an increase in energy, a softening of the muscles, and delivery opens the pelvis. If this is not understood, serious diagnostic errors and incorrect treatment may result. Frequently this sort of spontaneous genital anxiety is diagnosed as schizophrenia, depression, or post-puerperal psychosis.

Orgasm Anxiety

Orgasm anxiety is a fairly well-circumscribed anxiety produced by final and complete surrender of the organism. The sexual act is successful and pleasurable to the point of orgasm, when in males pain may occur in the tip of the penis—in women, spasms of the vagina or anesthesia. Feelings of impending death, insanity, or disintegration may occur, sometimes falling anxiety as well. Encourage the patient to proceed with the sexual act to completion in spite of pain or reluctance to continue. Get out exact details and stop any rigid or harsh movements.

6 · Genitality

GENITALITY IS REACHED in the final stage of development following the establishment of genital primacy. This occurs usually at about four or five years of age, but one must remember that long before this the genital is an erogenous zone with pleasure-giving capacity. Even the young baby plays with its genital and certainly receives pleasure from the contact and excitation. This is, presumably, only a local phenomenon, since the infant is still in a pregenital stage and more complete satisfaction is available through the oral zone. However, following development into the genital stage, pleasure is directly concerned in the response of this organ and release of tension is obtained through its conscious excitation and manipulation.

We have still too little experience with healthy children to make any dogmatic statements about the nature of childhood sexuality or about what it should be like before puberty. However, those individuals who have practiced self-gratification for long periods in childhood have the best outlook in therapy and the least difficulty in establishing satisfactory genital functioning. It seems reasonable to assume that, in our culture at least, masturbation is a necessary prerequisite for later genital primacy and a satisfactory sexual life, and thus for emotional health generally. I believe, however, that heterosexual play and actual intercourse between children is a more natural expression and would be general in a sex-affirmative society, as it is in the Trobriand Islands.

Reich distinguished three groupings of individuals, with regard to self-gratification in childhood:

1. Psychoneurotics who fully reached the stage of phallic development with genital masturbation, but later either repressed genital eroticism and became sick hysterically or withdrew libido from its genital position, regressing to earlier levels, and developed a pregenital type of neurosis. These are the average neurotics.

2. Psychoneurotics who reached the genital level only incompletely or not at all because of powerful pregenital blocks or because of severe castration trauma which blocked development into the genital stage. In these the genital becomes emotionally charged with pregenital wishes and fantasies, acquiring the significance of some other erotic zone such as the anus, breast, or mouth, losing thereby its own importance. The result is the severest form of impotence and any history of childhood masturbation is lacking. These are most difficult cases therapeutically.

3. Individuals who were symptom-free, and gave a history of long periods of undisturbed masturbation in childhood. These are the so-called normal in our society.

The kind of orgasm that takes place in children is important. Reich has described the orgasm in a child as having no sharp peak. This seems to be generally true, but in the infant the oral orgasm does appear to have a sharp peak; the oral orgasm appears to be similar to the genital orgasm following puberty. In between these periods, the orgasm one observes usually involves a smoothly rising and declining curve of excitation which has no acme, although a few of my patients have insisted they experienced a sharp peak in this age period. In these cases, the penis was lubricated with saliva, which gives a much more intense excitation. Since the oral contact of the infant with the breast is moist, as is contact in intercourse, and since few children discover this method of excitation, the common lack of moisture may explain the smooth excitation curve found in most childhood masturbation.

Masturbation should occur with regular, gentle friction movements of the genital. In girls up to the age of puberty, the clitoris is stimulated; following puberty excitation should shift to the vagina. Equally important are the accompanying fantasies of wishing to penetrate with the penis in the case of boys, or in girls of wishing to surrender to some male (the father). The pregenital masturbation (where full genital primacy has not developed) is accomplished by squeezing or rolling the penis between the hands; definite friction movements are lacking. Cases presenting this pattern are difficult therapeutically.

Adult sexual makeup may depend on the child's first masturbatory sensation. Masochism may be the final result if an initiatory excitation appears when a child is spanked. Or, urethral pleasure and enuresis may predominate in the adult if a child who was bladder trained strictly meets his first excitation when he urinates. Or, there may always be an anxious expectation whenever genital excitation occurs in a person who met excitation when he overheard his parents in intercourse or when he was in some other anxiety-producing circumstances.

The sexual problems inflicted on children come from the forbiddings and dire threats of consequences which cause guilt and make complete satisfaction impossible, or even cause them to retreat from sexual expression altogether. It seems generally known in this era that masturbation is never harmful, even the so-called "excessive masturbation" (which is merely a persistent effort to obtain some relief and satisfaction in the presence of severe genital blocking). However, too often our attitude is that children should try to keep interested in subjects other than sex. From puberty on, certainly it is more natural to prefer intercourse to masturbation since the former offers a more complete release.

Masturbation is pathological where an adult prefers it to the sexual embrace and demonstrates a deficient ability to make full contact. Two important preconditionings for this pattern are an emphasis on the dangers of disease in intercourse or an emphasis on the sexual act as a sadistic one.

Adult genital love is an expression of a mutual attraction between two individuals of the opposite sex, with energic lumination, and with the goal of sexual union. Love is felt primarily in the genital. This is true even of healthy love between those of the same sex, except that in this instance genital union (even the thought of which would be distasteful) is not a goal. The difference is not well understood biologically, although it seems apparent practically. One may even speculate as to why there are two sexes. The lower forms of life do not have them. It is probable that sex differentiation is due to nature's tendency to specialize in complex forms of life. However that may be, it is normal in the human for sexual attraction to be limited to those of the opposite sex. It seems likely that there is a deep biological basis for this, centered in the behavior of the energy in the organism.

We are so accustomed to taking natural events for granted that we forget to ask why. It seems so obvious that males should be attracted to females that we do not bother to wonder what really causes the attraction and mutual excitation. Furthermore, the healthier the individual the more specific becomes the attraction. Why a specific mate? Certainly training and conditioning have much to do with the selection, but this is largely on an armored basis. Yet some animals are just as selective. We also find individuals who are mutually attracted to each other sexually but who are highly unsuited in all other respects.

I believe Reich found a possible explanation when he discovered that individuals had different rates of orgonotic pulsation. This has apparently no relationship to the rate of pulse or respiration. It varies slightly from day to day (apparently from atmospheric and emotional changes), but each individual seems to have a specific range. The significance of different rates is not yet known, but they are easily determined on an oscillograph. Male and female with harmonious rates may be attracted to each other whereas discordant rates repel.[1] (We can understand a correlation or harmonic relation among sound vibrations.) Most of us have been disturbed by some person without being able to determine why and have been able to relieve the situation only by leaving his presence. This may well be a field reaction where pulsation rates are disharmonious and therefore disturbing.

I had a young husband and wife in therapy. The wife came

[1] I believe that a similar mechanism may appear in conception. The ovum accepts or rejects the sperm either with or without the x chromosome. The woman may thus be responsible for the sex of the child after all.

to me first with rather severe hysterical symptoms and complaints about her marriage: it was very unsatisfying and largely on an infantile level, including even talking baby talk to each other. Later the husband entered therapy also with some serious symptoms. As the wife improved she found it less and less possible to remain with her husband although she insisted she cared for him. She simply became upset whenever he was near her.

They remained separated for a couple of months, during which time the wife showed marked improvement. Then a well-meaning but blundering friend persuaded her to go on a trip with her husband against my advice. She came back very upset, contracted, and with a return of her symptoms. The vacation, she reported, was a horrible failure. Slowly she again improved and started making dates with her husband, but each time the date ended drastically. She would become irritable and depressed, freeze on sexual contact with a feeling that she could not stand her husband even to touch her. An occasional date where they went out only to dine could be pleasant for her.

This went on for two years and I was greatly puzzled by what appeared to be such neurotic behavior toward her husband while she seemed so well when away from him and did not react this way with other men. She continued to feel love for her husband although it became more and more evident that something was seriously wrong with the marriage and the question of divorce was raised. Eventually after some time away from her husband she seriously considered divorce and marriage to another man. Though interested in this man she could not feel for him the love she felt for her husband but rather a "quieter but pleasant feeling." Clinically she was very well. When she visited her husband to discuss divorce the old feelings of love for him returned and she decided once more to try and make a go of the marriage. On the first date, as her husband approached her sexually, with her encouragement, she again became very upset, irritable, and felt she literally wanted to kill him when he insisted on his attentions. She decided she could never see him again. As she was describing this episode in session, it suddenly dawned on me that the difficulty had nothing to do with neurosis but was energetic. Their fields were disharmonious. It explained what had puzzled me for so long—how clinically well she seemed to me but how seemingly neurotic her behavior whenever she was close to her husband. She loved him but biophysically they were incompatible. Both had to accept the fact. She felt relieved to find that it was not her neurotic behavior that caused the distress to both. She could then accept the divorce as necessary and with concern only for the hurt her husband must feel. Her attitude and behavior has been markedly mature and healthy—in retrospect, it had been for some time. The husband, too, who had grown quite mature, accepted the dissolution rationally but with real sadness.

Courting exists in all higher animals and seems to be for the purpose of getting acquainted or "smelling each other out." Fear is deeply rooted and is necessary for survival; until it is eliminated the organism cannot expand fully nor surrender completely to another organism voluntarily and spontaneously. Courting establishes trust. It may be long or short, depending on circumstances and the individuals involved, but the healthy individual does not consider sexual union without some degree of courtship.

Once sexual union becomes an urgent goal, the activity may be divided into three stages: foreplay, genital union, and the orgastic convulsion. There are no rigid natural laws for the first two. Foreplay allows whatever may be mutually acceptable and pleasurable, with the exception of sadistic acts. Nothing can be considered perverse so long as the goal remains genital union. Foreplay may be long or short; usually the male rushes to genital union while the female prefers more foreplay. Both should be sexually excited (streamings in the genital) before even foreplay is considered. In a healthy relationship it consists largely of body contact and gentle caresses of the loved one's body. Frantic manual excitation of the genital plays no part.

The sexual act can hardly be completely satisfying if one or the other must be excited by artificial means. Such an individual is not biologically ready for the sexual act. Either his free energy has not reached the point of lumination, or it is bound by anxiety. Or, it may be simply that the partner is not desired.

Foreplay contrives to increase the excitation to the point of urgent union (desire for penetration), a desire which should be present in both partners. Erection in the male is an obvious and accepted requirement.

Erection in the female is not so obvious nor so well considered a requirement. Yet in adequate sexual readiness the labia become erect, also the nipples where the breasts are responsive. Further, there are two types of vaginal secretion, watery and mucous. The latter offers a higher degree of contact and excitation, and unless it is present a woman is short of full sexual readiness. Too long foreplay with clitoral stimulation will tend to produce a clitoral orgasm and interfere with full vaginal response.

Many marriage counselors, psychiatrists, and psychologists have gone into detail concerning the proper way to excite the clitoris and have detailed sexual positions in which the clitoris is stimulated, reminding readers that the clitoris is the counterpart of the penis and needs to be stimulated just as the penis does.

This advice is based on a mistaken premise. It is true that the clitoris is a vestigial penis, but being so it has lost its function. It is replaced by a much more satisfying organ, the vagina. The clitoris is important only in those cases where the female is arrested at the phallic stage and the clitoris has assumed the importance of a fantasied penis.[2] Interest and excitation at this level detracts from and may completely prevent a vaginal response. In healthy development, the clitoris assumes little or at least only fleeting importance, just as does the phallic stage in the male, and in maturity it is of minimum significance for sexual pleasure. Instructions for properly exciting the woman by clitoral stimulation, and the caution that lubricants should be used if the clitoris is dry, miss the basic point that in such cases the woman is not ready for sexual union in the first place, either because of emotional problems or present environmental or physical conditions. Correction should be aimed at these more basic issues.

One further point against such interest in clitoral stimulation is that during sexual union for the clitoris to come in contact

[2] This group unfortunately comprises a large portion of the adult female population, so that one can understand why the importance of clitoral stimulation is taken so much for granted.

with the penis requires that the pelvis be retracted; and that in itself inhibits pelvic and more particularly genital sensations.

It is still debatable whether the female feels pleasure in the vagina itself[3] or whether this is an illusion from the pleasure felt in the labia and introitus. The posterior wall of the vagina seems to be the most responsive. There is, however, a definite urge toward penetration and the vaginal orgasm as opposed to the clitoral orgasm. The latter produces only a local response, while a vaginal orgasm results in a total response of the whole organism with more complete satisfaction. Also, where there is genital potency, the vagina becomes an active organ, sucking the penis much as a mouth sucks a nipple.

Actual genital union where contact (streaming) is present carries an urgent need for friction movements, soft but aggressive and in response to breathing. Rapid harsh movements are due to contactlessness and cover up any natural sensations of surrender. Timid movements or lack of movement may be due to anxiety or to cut down sensation.

The actual sexual act lasts from three to twenty minutes, with a continued feeling of natural gentleness. The position requires only that freedom of movement be not interfered with. One may or may not proceed directly to orgasm. One may pause, alter position, etc., but at a certain point the act becomes automatic and initiates the orgastic convulsion. At this point stopping or otherwise interfering with smooth progress, such as one partner interrupting rhythm, becomes very painful and disturbing. This may occur when one or the other cannot tolerate the full swing of the orgastic convulsion and interferes by rapid, jerky movements or even withdrawal, or becomes frozen and immobile or even loses sensation entirely. The sexual act should be devoid of fantasies, which are in themselves a running away. Fantasies must be prohibited even at the risk of loss of desire. In the end phase of therapy, all of these problems must be gone into in detail and corrected.

[3] Cf. Arnold H. Kegel, "Sexual Functions of the Pubococcygeus Muscle," *The Western Journal of Surgery, Obstetrics, and Gynecology,* Vol. 60, pp. 521–524, October 1952. Kegel believes that deep vaginal sensations come from the insertions of the pubococcygeus muscle in the vagina.

One of the greatest difficulties to overcome is to remove the compulsion from sex and to accept it as a pleasure only when really desired. Women are taught to believe that men want sex all the time and must be satisfied, so they feel obliged to feel ready to submit at all times. Men must demonstrate their manhood and satisfy women. If they could be honest with each other most would find that neither desired sex nearly as frequently, except in new relationships. Normal sexual activity varies from three times a week to once every two weeks depending on health, work, and other environmental conditions and one may abstain for as long as a year with no serious stasis disturbance.

The full orgasm depends on complete absence of holding in the organism. At a certain point, excitation grasps the whole personality and its increase is not subject to voluntary control. Having spread to the entire organism, it then concentrates in the genital area and a warm, melting sensation follows. Involuntary contractions of the muscles in the genital and the pelvic floor occur in waves; the crest of each wave of contraction coincides with deep penetration during expiration. The spasms that produce ejaculation follow. In women, there are contractions and elongation in the vagina which are accompanied by a desire to receive completely. Because of the invagination, this is comparable to the expansive urge of the penis to penetrate fully. Next, there is a clouding of the consciousness and an increase in contractions which involve the whole body.

After the convulsion the two organisms remain united for a time while energy, which has been concentrated at the genital, flows back through the organism, which is experienced as gratification. Separation then occurs with relaxation and sleep and a tender, grateful attitude toward the partner.

Excitation dulls with constant contact; therefore husbands and wives should not always be together. They should sleep in separate beds or they lose the ability to excite each other and become emotionally sticky. In this state they feel anxious when separated, but are lacking in excitement when together.

The genital union fulfills two of the basic functions in all nature. One is universal, both in the non-living and the living.

The other is essential for functioning in the living. These two are: *superimposition,* where two energy systems mutually excite and attract each other and fuse into one energy system—in the living organism this revives and provides the sparkle of life—and the *orgastic convulsion,* which discharges excess energy to maintain a normal energy level. This process occurs in all energy systems confined within a membrane, i.e., all the living.

There has been considerable confusion about the emotions accompanying charge and discharge in the sexual act. The orgasm formula can be expressed:

$$\text{TENSION} \longrightarrow \text{CHARGE} \longrightarrow \text{DISCHARGE} \longrightarrow \text{RELAXATION}$$

When energy moves outward to the skin (expansion), pleasure is felt. When contraction against this outward flow occurs, anxiety is produced. In both cases, a state of tension exists. TENSION → CHARGE is an expanding movement. If it is uninterrupted as in genital potency, pleasure is experienced. When this expansion is not tolerated, contraction against it occurs and anxiety is produced as in genital anxiety. When now discharge occurs, tension is removed and relief (from tension) is experienced.

SUPERIMPOSITION   ORGASM

$$\text{TENSION} \longrightarrow \text{CHARGE} \longrightarrow \text{DISCHARGE} \longrightarrow \text{RELAXATION}$$
(pleasure)   (relief)

In certain conditions, relaxation is not tolerated following discharge and contraction takes place instead. If discharge has been minimal (orgastic impotence), there is still considerable tension and anxiety is produced. Where discharge has been appreciable, tension is removed and contraction without obstruction occurs, giving rise to unpleasure (sadness). This is a frequent finding and has led to the axiom that "every animal is sad after the sexual act."

Here, the formula would be:

$$\text{TENSION} \longrightarrow \text{CHARGE} \longrightarrow \text{DISCHARGE} \longrightarrow \text{CONTRACTION}$$
(pleasure)   (unpleasure)

I am not considering here the further complications possible where rage, sadism, or other neurotic mechanisms are active.

Genital Disturbances

Genital energy is the regulator, the safety valve which is closed to most people. Genital disturbances fall into two groups: the social (or non-biopathic), and the biopathic (those due to chronic armor). Desire may be greater than in the healthy because of lack of adequate satisfaction.

Social Disturbances

Non-biopathic disturbances and people who have them react to education with relief. Biopathic disturbances, on the other hand, are not affected by education. Biopathically disturbed people ward off any such influence, and even tend to build up rationalizations to strengthen resistance.

Social disturbances are usually due to ignorance, sometimes supplemented by economic problems. One of the most frequent problems is living conditions that do not allow privacy either in masturbation or in lovemaking. This situation creates anxiety and tension and interferes with satisfaction. In handling these disturbances, a detailed description of the circumstances surrounding sexual expression is necessary.

For example, where does masturbation occur? Is guilt present? Is masturbation satisfying? Do others occupy the same room? Even after marriage, is there privacy? Must the sexual act be hurried because of the danger of interruption by others? In such cases, intercourse is frequently attempted in clothes and even while standing up. Such practices interfere with contact and freedom of movement and should be eliminated.

Commonly, there is a fear of pregnancy which causes holding back. Here, one discusses the attitude toward contraception. Some are opposed on religious grounds, while others do not trust contraceptives. Those who can accept advice readily have a better prognosis. Coitus interruptus and coitus condomatus both interfere greatly with satisfaction and should be given up.

The same can be said for petting without the final act; tension builds up with no relief.

Satisfaction is also interfered with when people with dissimilar energy levels attempt to relate to each other. Individuals are born with high or low energy charges and too great a disparity between partners leads to sexual incompatibility. An individual with a comparatively low charge may be healthy in every sense of the word, but will have a lesser sexual need than a partner with a higher charge.

One cannot expect that the genital embrace will be completely satisfying to both partners in the first few experiences. Frequently considerable time and patience are necessary for partners to adjust to each other. The healthy male may be premature and the female fail to be adequately excited because of the anxiety from the new experience, particularly if the environment is not favorable.

Biopathic Disturbances

Difficulties here are due to chronic armor which inhibits the full convulsion. Particularly inhibitory are spasms of the throat and anus, which are the primitive openings of the alimentary canal. Difficulties fall into two groups:

1) Functioning has been satisfactory but has ceased to be so.

2) There never has been satisfactory genital functioning. Those in the former group have the better prognosis. We usually expect at least to return a person to the level of his best former functioning. It is very important to elicit details of functioning though the patient tries to evade them. The following information is essential:

First, has there ever been any genital functioning, and to what extent? Has masturbation ever been pleasurable, and through what means and what fantasies? Especially heed fantasies that are sadistic, homosexual, or otherwise perverse. In the female, look for fantasies of rape.

Has there been reluctance to touch the genital? If manipulation has occurred, has it been with more or less rhythmic movements, or with pressing and squeezing which are pregenital forms of masturbation? What have been the type and regularity of genital manipulation in childhood? Puberty? Marriage?

In intercourse, is there desire before the act, or is it a duty and is artificial stimulation necessary? Is it done compulsively, such as every Friday night?

Usually the woman requires considerable foreplay while the man rushes to the sexual act, and this disparity may make it necessary to have the husband or wife come for further questioning. Or, the man may not develop an erection unless stimulated. That may be non-neurotic because he does not desire the woman or because his energy is below the lumination point, or it may be neurotic.

What restrictions are placed on the partner? For example, the man may resent the woman moving during the act or he may prefer entry from behind. These are usually due to a running away from full contact except during the later months of pregnancy when this position is preferable. Does either have to fight to have intercourse?

Hardness in the embrace may be present, especially squeezing, which the healthy individual will not tolerate.

The therapist must examine methods of avoiding strong excitation:

1. holding the breath,
2. controlling sounds,
3. controlling movements or engaging in rapid jerky movements,
4. arching the chest,
5. straightening and stiffening the legs,
6. holding the anal sphincter.

There are two types of sexual embrace: 1) with orgastic streaming in the genital, or 2) without it. Streaming is felt as a sweet, melting sensation and a drawing out. If streaming is present there is a very good prognosis. If not present, one is faced with orgastic impotence. Inquire as to sensation in the tip of the penis, whether it is dull, anesthetic, or painful. Sometimes it is dull because of the woman.

In orgastic impotence, the orgonotic charge in the genital is lost and contactlessness supervenes. To compensate for this, movements may be rapid and harsh, or there may be no impulse for friction movement at all and ejaculation will be produced mainly through pressure. In some cases even an urge for penetration is lacking. Only touch is felt. Pleasure in the genital is absent. The individual may be erectively potent but cannot surrender either to his partner or to his own organism.

Premature ejaculation occurs because of anxiety. One sneaks in and out quickly as though getting away with something. Here, the contraction due to anxiety, combined with the sexual excitation, increases pressure and squeezes out the seminal discharge without allowing a true orgastic convulsion. In the deepest sense a fear of the father's penis in the vagina.

Reich states that premature ejaculation also occurs where the energy is low. Apparently the excessive excitation necessary for the act in the presence of low energy produces anxiety and so increases pressure and squeezes out the semen.

Homosexuality results from identification with the parent of the opposite sex. The identification is based on fear, and the basic cause of homosexuality is fear of heterosexuality. Extensive therapy is usually required to cure this condition. The first overt homosexual experience usually occurs at sixteen years; this is the age at which reactions against the initial push of puberty have consolidated and final sexual patterns begin to emerge. Before the age of sixteen, homosexual play may have been experienced— as it often is in young mammals—but such early play has little significance for adult patterns. In homosexual cases, I have usually found that there was a desperate attempt toward heterosexual adjustment before the final surrender to homosexuality at sixteen.

These are the common biopathic disturbances. Occasionally one meets with rarer forms of perversion; all of them are subjects for extensive therapy.

7 · The Adolescent Problem

THIS IS ONE OF, if not the most, important problem in the world today. It is talked about constantly, solutions are offered, even gestures are made for adolescents here and there, but no one dares really touch it. One would be looked upon with horror if one seriously advised or put into practice what everyone really knows is the solution, since few can admit it even to themselves.

Society persists in a more irrational attitude toward adolescent sexuality than toward any other period in the sexual life of man.[1] Except for Reich[2] and possibly a few others[3] no one has even bothered to listen to the misery of those who, for the five to ten years between puberty and marriage, are allowed no acceptable genital expression. The natural genital embrace is considered evidence of delinquency and self-gratification is universally frowned upon; yet, during this period, genital urgency is the greatest of any period in life. We spend so much time correcting sexual problems of adults while completely neglecting the period in which these neuroses are fixed.

[1] Sweden is a notable exception. There, great strides apparently have been made toward accepting adolescent sexuality.

[2] Cf. Wilhelm Reich, *The Sexual Revolution* (New York, Orgone Institute Press, 1945).

[3] Alfred C. Kinsey, in a lecture in New York City, clearly expounded the adolescent sexual problem.

The child matures sexually during adolescence, experiences a strong surge of sexual feeling destined to be the most intense he will ever experience, and society and the law say "don't touch it." According to society, the church, and the law, the adolescent is not supposed to have any sexual outlet. I have seen those who fulfilled this obligation and they were very crushed and sick. Surely we cannot believe that this is the solution; but it is one means of handling the problem. There are two other possibilities: masturbation and the genital embrace. With the former, I would include mutual masturbation and petting. Everyone knows that the vast majority of adolescents engage in one or the other or both of these outlets. However, we still pretend that we do not see it and that the adolescent is asexual. If he is careless enough to be caught expressing his sexuality he is severely punished, and any adult who condones his expression is contributing to the delinquency of minors.

With such conditioning the adolescent must, of necessity, feel guilt over his sexual urges and expressions. Conventional psychiatry has concluded that it is the guilt and not the masturbation that is harmful, but still takes the attitude that the adolescent should be encouraged to get his mind off sex. On the other hand, for those few adolescents who can marry, sex becomes permissible and not harmful.

The simplest solution would be to permit adolescents to live as their sexual needs would have them, but that course would often lead to disaster. In our society the great majority are not prepared for sexual expression, although many seek it just the same. In Reich's work with adolescents, he estimated that over two-thirds were unprepared to assume such responsibility even if society would permit it. Half of these could assume the responsibility if given sufficient knowledge and counseling. The other half would require extensive therapy. However, nature intended genital union at this stage. The fault is in our culture.

Genitality is everyone's right, but each must pass through babyhood and early childhood without trauma or major blockage if he is to achieve it and handle it responsibly. For only the emotionally healthy or those who could feel what emotional health should be can experience the genital embrace as love rather than as pornography or guilt. There is no easy solution and there will not be until we learn to bring up healthy children and to change our own attitudes and the attitude of the law. Adults are afraid of the intensity of genital feelings in adolescents, and so kill the feelings or suppress them.

Has anyone investigated what harm derives from sexual expression in adolescents? I do not mean in cases of rape, but where there is mutual desire and consent. One obvious objection is the possibility of pregnancy. Many girls do become pregnant. Seventeen did in a single class in one school. Was that better than to have taught them contraception and thereby contributed to their delinquency? I am sure that most readers will not like either alternative and will be appalled at both. Everyone prefers abstinence in adolescents. There again, nature takes over and brings in a safety valve in the form of night emissions and erotic dreams. But at best these afford only temporary relief.

Can we learn nothing from the Trobriand Islanders, whose attitude is sex-positive and who make arrangements for adolescents to be together?[4] They have no crime, no neuroses, and no insanity or obesity among their tribes. This prenuptial liberty is not an end in itself. Actually it is a preparation for marriage allowing a natural choice based on personality and compatibility rather than merely on sexual appeal. I understand that following such marriages both partners are remarkably faithful. My experiences have been in keeping with this in my practice. Those patients who are well integrated and have had considerable premarital sexual experience have been consistently more faithful in marriage than those who have married with little or no previous experience.

The demand made on youth for sexual abstinence in our culture is responsible for their sexual misery, the conflicts that occur in adolescence, and the sexual problems of the adult. The adolescent reaches sexual maturity, experiencing the necessity for sexual outlet and having the capacity for reproduction, while he is still structurally and economically incapable of creating the framework demanded by society for genital union—marriage.

[4] Other tribes who follow this policy are the Igorot of Luzon, Akamba of East Africa, and the Munski of northern Nigeria.

In matrilineal societies in primitive situations, the sexual misery that plagues our adolescents is never seen. Puberty rites introduce the adolescent to a full sex life and there is much emphasis on sexual happiness. Authoritarian societies, on the other hand, emphasize abstinence. Let us consider in more detail the three possibilities[5] for the adolescent in our culture.

Abstinence

With the development of the genital organs and the increase in activity in the endocrine glands, it is evident that sexuality enters a very active phase at puberty, with a normal urge toward sexual expression, specifically toward the genital embrace. But sexual ideas, particularly those involving intercourse, must be repressed or distorted if total abstinence is to be possible. More often than not, adolescents do not repress the idea of intercourse but think of it without feeling or attach so many fears and disgusts to the idea that it loses all real significance. However, to ensure abstinence, there must also be repression of sexual excitation. If that is achieved, the adolescent avoids the painful conflict about masturbation and the dangerous struggle with his environment.

In general, adolescents' attitudes toward sexuality change after the first steps into puberty. After sixteen or seventeen they are more negative toward it; they have replaced a striving for pleasure by a fear of pleasure. This anchors an increasingly defensive attitude toward sexuality. The inhibited pleasure turns into unpleasurable or even painful genital excitation. This forces the adolescent to suppress his sexuality. Suppression always leads to psychic and somatic disturbances, but it helps him avoid the conflict with society and with his own developed morals.

If the sexual energy that is being suppressed does not manifest itself in illness, it will be channeled into daydreams and moodiness—any of which interfere with normal activities. If the neurosis does not develop immediately it surely will when he is later confronted with the demands of "legal" sexual activity in marriage. Therapeutically, those patients who never dared to masturbate have the worst prognosis.

5 For a more complete discussion read *The Sexual Revolution, op. cit.*

Popular custom suggests athletics to divert the sexual energy and release it in activity. However, not all the energy can ever be released, and repression is necessary anyway. Abstinence surely results in sexual atrophy, the flow of energy back into infantile and perverse activities, and in nervous disorders. Actually, abstinence is in itself already a pathological symptom indicating severe repression. It always damages the future love life and reduces achievement in work.

Masturbation

Masturbation is a substitute, lacking sexual intercourse. However, it has only a limited value. It may be useful if it helps a youngster through the early upsets of puberty. But only a few adolescents reach puberty with a relatively unimpaired functioning; most of them are so damaged by education and upbringing that they cannot masturbate without guilt. Usually they fight the impulse. If unsuccessful, they masturbate with severe inhibitions and harmful practices, such as trying to hold back the ejaculation.

Eventually, even successful masturbation becomes disturbing because the lack of a love object is painful. Further repression becomes necessary because fantasy is forced into infantile and neurotic reactions long since given up. At this point, the infantile repressions and those acquired at puberty meet and reinforce each other. The more severe the infantile damage to sexuality, the less chance has the adolescent to take up a normal sex life. Guilt feelings with masturbation are more intense than they are with sexual intercourse because it is heavily burdened with incest fantasies, while a gratifying sexual act makes these fantasies superfluous. Also, contact with a second energy system causes more excitation and therefore greater release.

There are many transitions between the extreme of the one type, who is incapable of taking the step from his infantile parental fixation to a rational sex life, and the opposite type, who seems to do so easily. The first represents the "good" youngster who gives in to all the demands made on him. He becomes the resigned marital partner and provides the main quota of neurotics. The other is rebellious, ambitious, adverse to parental restriction, and of above average intelligence. These, society may force into psychopathic behavior if their needs are not understood and properly handled.

Adolescents who achieve the development from masturbation to sexual intercourse are always the ones who are vigorous, bright, and competent. However, most adolescents are shy and awkward.

Sexual Intercourse

To begin with, the adolescent has to overcome his own inner inhibitions, the result of his sex-negative upbringing, so that usually he is not equal to the task of establishing a heterosexual relationship. His fixation in infantile attitudes toward his parents creates a discrepancy between psychic immaturity and comparative physical maturity. Not only is there a strict social taboo against adolescent sexuality, but, even more, every kind of active measure is taken to prevent him from sexual intercourse. For example, factual education is rarely given. He is given physiology and told how the sperm and ovum unite to form a new being, but not that he is biologically ready for intercourse.

On top of this he is never allowed opportunity for privacy, and his knowledge of contraception is likely to be incomplete or inaccurate. The adolescent who dares has to do so in cars, in corridors, in the bushes, always with the possibility of detection or resulting pregnancy, to say nothing of the law.

Obviously, in a society that does not recognize sexual expression outside of marriage, and without a rational sexual education of children, and without privacy and knowledge of contraception, it would be both foolhardy and unhelpful to advise adolescents to ignore rules not consonant with health. Such advising would be no less harmful than preaching abstinence.

However, we can at least affirm the sexuality of adolescents in principle, help them where we can, and work for an eventual sex-affirmative solution. Now, we can only present their problem fully and honestly to them and let each find his own solution.

Even knowing the facts, and that their feelings and urges are natural, will give them some help in their effort to survive.

The average adolescent today has too much life and health in him to repress but has not learned responsibility, nor has he the knowledge of how to handle his problems. He knows only rebellion; so we have juvenile delinquency. The youth no longer will be denied their rights. Society must recognize this and help them to assume the responsibility of these rights.

PART II

.

CHARACTER TYPES:

The Effects of Armoring

8 · Genital Character Types

INDIVIDUAL CHARACTER DEVELOPMENT depends on the degree of fixation or armoring at the various erogenous levels where the major part of the energy is concentrated. Symptoms characteristic of these levels are present whenever there is an increase in energy concentration or block at that level. The great majority of persons fall into one of the specific character types although most of them have elements of other character types. There are a few who are difficult to place in any category. They either have no major block or their structure is difficult to understand. Some can be diagnosed only after months of therapy, others not at all with our present knowledge. No two people are the same. They vary in energy, in training, in background, and in inherent basic characteristics. Both the infantile sexual demand and the defenses mobilized against it are embedded in the neurotic character. The defense or armor may belong to the same stage of development as the instinctual demand or to a different one.

Blocks (or hooks[1]) may occur at any of the erogenous zones

[1] In the strict sense of the terms hooks and blocks are not synonymous. Actually, a hook is a block that, for some reason either in its development or in a particular significance to the individual, is peculiarly difficult if not impossible to overcome. It is sometimes produced accidentally in therapy when the pelvis is opened too early, especially in persons with a high energy level, rendering the organism incapable of yielding pregenital holding.

and are of two types, repressed or unsatisfied. The term *block* refers to the fact that the individual has been able to develop beyond a given level but has been unable to give up that zone or level completely. Symptoms from it affect the personality and interfere with genital functioning. Only the genital release can give complete satisfaction.

When energy is blocked from the genital it can never be completely discharged. It is either felt constantly as a need (manifested in overeating or drinking as the result of a block at the oral unsatisfied stage, for example), or the organism has to defend itself against any expression at all from the blocked zone (laconic speech or lack of interest in food in the oral repressed stage, for example).

A block is functionally identical with muscular armoring in the zone in which the block is present; i.e. with an oral block we will find a spasm in the masseters, orbicularis oris, and muscles of the floor of the mouth. The particular blocks of the major erogenous zones determine the character type. Blocks in the non-erogenous segments produce variations of rigidity of that character type. Except for those persons who remain infantile, all have at least reached the phallic stage, though they may afterward have given it up and returned to earlier fixations. Where there are no major blocks and genitality is established, a genital character results. The characters that function at the phallic and genital stages are the least complex and do not show reaction formations (change of direction of drive). Reaction formations occur only at the more infantile or pregenital levels (e.g. anal, oral, and ocular).

Armoring is more complete in the repressed than in the unsatisfied stage. In unsatisfied blocking, strivings are felt and impulses get through but the zone cannot yield sufficiently to fulfill needs. (Therefore, we have overeating, overdrinking, overtalking, none of them with any satisfaction.) There is a constant demand for expression. When these impulses are consciously restrained, anxiety results. The more the individual withdraws to a pregenital level, the more his appearance and functioning assume characteristics of that level. (For example, depression and retardation when withdrawal to the oral repressed stage occurs.) The following illustrates very roughly the major characteristic that results from blocking at each erogenous zone. (This of course is only a schematic outline and cannot be taken as absolute.)

	Stage	*Repressed*	*Unsatisfied*
1)	Ocular	confusion	voyeurism
2)	Oral	depression	overindulgence
3)	Anal	restraint	submission
4)	Phallic	righteous	Don Juan behavior
5)	Genital	flight	nymphomania
		(or freezing)	(or frantic behavior)

Genital Characters

The Genital Character (Orgastic Potency)

The genital character is that individual who fulfills the criteria of health. That is, he is well enough integrated and free enough emotionally so that he can sufficiently express and satisfy himself in life. Because satisfaction is available to him, he does not build up tension and develop chronic armor. Ideal health is, of course, merely a concept and is not found in nature; but functional health is fluid and allows a wide range of expressions.

If the greater part of an individual's energy is centered at the genital level, he functions as a genital character. This means that he has reached the post-ambivalent genital stage with no blocks at earlier levels that are capable of interfering with functioning. The wish for a parent's death (father or mother) and incestual desires have been given up; genital interests center on a heterosexual love object free of incestual identification—therefore, the Oedipus complex has been solved and not simply repressed. Any residual pregenital impulses find suitable expression in sexual foreplay or in cultural pursuits. (Significantly, modern society provides more or less constructive and harmless means for gratifying any conceivable pregenital impulse—stamp collecting, amateur theater, civic reform, window box gardening, and so on indefinitely.) However, in the genital character, most of the energy finds expression in the genital orgasm, since it is the most complete, gratifying, and bioeconomic release. Aggression[2] is at the service of the ego for rational goals but is not an end in itself.

Ego and superego are in harmony. The superego sanctions a sex-affirmative way of life; it is not harsh and punitive as it is to the neurotic. Since orgastic potency reduces the instinctual demands on the ego and gives it greater autonomy to feel and act in the outside world, there is no need for a genital character to prove himself a man through socially noticeable exploits. Unconscious guilt and inferiority feelings are absent, so he does not have to bind them up in symptom formation and irrational strivings. The armor is pliable and at the service of the ego, which can call it forth or dispense with it as objective situations require.

The affect is characteristically natural. A resilient organism, the genital character can run the gamut of feeling from intense joy to deep grief, from love to hate, from pleasure to unpleasure. He reacts with deep sorrow to an object loss but does not let it overwhelm him. He is not ashamed or self-conscious in expressing feelings and can surrender to them fully. He loves and hates rationally, and can withdraw from the world completely when he so chooses or can involve himself wholeheartedly in affairs.

An ordered sexual economy is the basis for his fundamental character traits. Having reached the genital stage of development means that there is more energy available to the ego because there has been no need to use it up in repression (body armoring, symptom formation, neurotic character traits, etc.). Rather, the genital character may direct his energy toward rational aims, deep affective expression, and regular orgastic convulsion and discharge. Orgastic potency gives him self-confidence and determines his sexual behavior and attitude; since he is quite sure that he is a man, he needs no tricks or bragging to impress himself on others in any situation.

---

[2] "Aggression" in the popular sense refers to behavior that is pushy, offensive, assaulting, and even hostile. That is neurotic aggression. Here, "aggression" refers to natural aggression, which is active, spirited, and animated, but never offensive.

The genital character is basically moral in sex but not moralistic. He accepts full responsibility for his acts and knows the difference between freedom and license. Promiscuity and asceticism both seem emotional ills to him. He enters the genital embrace because he loves his partner and surrenders himself fully and earnestly without fear or restraint. He is never jocular or pornographic in the sex act. His monogamy is spontaneous; he makes love to one partner because that course fits his feelings, not because social rules or customs coerce him. If need be, he can change his sexual object—or even, under special conditions, accept polygamy (or polyandry). His self-regulation leads him to withdraw energy from a desire that cannot be satisfied by shifting his attention to other goals or other partners.

Because his primary drives are fulfilled, he has a natural decency. He is unafraid of life, and therefore does not have to compromise with his convictions if his own are opposed. He knows what others want and can accept their needs. Never dogmatic, he thinks functionally and objectively; his motives are rational, undisguised, and directed toward self-improvement and social improvement. He gives himself freely and with pleasure to work he can believe in, but he cannot work mechanically. He accepts responsibility for work, but never dictates. Willing to live and let live, he is genuinely pleased by the happiness others obtain. He affirms the natural sexuality of children and adolescents, and is easily on good terms with them. He is indifferent to perversions and repelled by pornography.

The body of the genital character is strong. His skin is warm and radiating, the eyes sparkling, the lips full and sensuous, and the limbs and torso well formed. He is relaxed and his behavior is calm. He can express emotions of any kind freely, which is a major indication of free-flowing bioenergy. He can cut ugly faces, sneer, growl, scream, and show anxiety in his eyes (many neurotics cannot do this). He can open his eyelids fully, wrinkle his forehead, bite, and hit strongly with his fists at an imaginary hated object. The gag reflex is fully developed. The eyes are deep, serious, and penetrating with full contact; the pelvis is free and well developed. The genitals and breasts are well developed, but not overdeveloped. There is no extraneous fat.

Stasis

Stasis occurs when for some reason genital release is not possible over a period of time. Tension builds up and is held by tightening the muscles of the lateral abdominal walls, holding in the spinal muscles, and holding the pelvis rigid. The individual becomes irritable and cross, with increasing irrational tendencies. Stasis can easily be overcome therapeutically, and is sometimes overcome spontaneously through renewed sexual activity. Where stasis is present, there is a tendency toward a quick climax in the sex act. Stasis may build up when the partner inhibits complete release by holding or by disharmonious movements.

If stasis is not corrected it may continue to increase, causing withdrawal to pregenital levels, and develop into a neurosis. The dammed-up energy floods the organism, reactivating pregenital erogenous zones seeking means of discharge. This produces infantile fantasies and revives the Oedipus problem, which only reinforces defense mechanisms. Thus caught in a vicious circle, the organism has no outlet until the energy overflows in symptom formation.

The Hysterical Character (Genitality with Anxiety)

Hysteria has been known since ancient times and was the first emotional disorder to be recognized as having a sexual connotation. It has been pandemic at certain periods in history, especially during the Middle Ages. It was extremely common at the turn of the last century. It is still common but the marked manifestations earlier writers described, such as fugues, fits, and paralyses, are comparatively rare today. A few decades ago only the severe cases sought therapy. Today we see earlier cases and also milder cases because of the widespread acceptance of therapy. However, except that symptoms are less marked, hysteria possesses the same characteristics it has always had, and Reich's description is as accurate today as it was thirty years ago.

Characteristics and Symptoms

The hysterical character, usually female, has reached the genital level but with anxiety. Thus there is genitality, but genitality which cannot be accepted. There is a constant push toward genital contact with a simultaneous flight from it, so that one finds a constant approaching and running, even during the sexual act. Complete sexual satisfaction is not possible, so there is never a complete discharge of energy. This leads to stasis, which only increases the turmoil and results in an organism which is alive, but restless and flighty.

Sexual energy floods the whole organism. The body movements are not compulsively hard nor phallically self-confident, but soft, provocative, rolling, accompanied by a specific sort of agility of a definitely sexual flavor. The total impression given by walk and attitude and body shape is very sexual. Flirtatiousness is notable in female hysterics, either plain or covert, in the way of glancing, speaking, moving. Male hysterics will add a feminine facial habit to feminine behavior, seeming too polite and too soft in a masculine context. Both male and female are apprehensive, most particularly when their provocativeness produces the normally expected response. When the sexual goal seems close to attainment, they turn passive or withdraw. In actual intercourse, they will frequently increase activity to overcome anxiety, but feeling will not increase with the increased activity.

They have a tendency to be strongly suggestible and to alter their behavior in unplanned and unexpected ways, together with strong disappointment reactions. They swing from compliance to quick deprecation and groundless disparagement. Suggestibility predisposes to flights of imagination as well as hypnosis and pathological lying.

Pregenital zones in which there are fixations, such as the mouth and anus, are genitalized. A fearful need to protect the self against the desire to commit genital incest creates the armor; the sexual behavior increases as the hysteric becomes more fearful and apprehensive. The sexual attitude is an illusion, however, because the female hysteric is cut off from sex and cannot accept it. The sexual provocation is actually a testing out of danger, and at the first sign of sexual aggression toward her she runs. It is true that she desires sex, but simultaneously she has an anti-sexual attitude.

Armor is present but is always soft and light and shifting. The body has a good general tone. Symptoms occur when there is an overflow of energy which can neither be bound by the armor nor expressed. The hysteric has little capacity to bind energy by armor and is therefore prone to the development of symptoms. Symptoms other than genital mechanisms are due to pregenital fixations, such as depression from an oral block. There is little direction toward accomplishment in intellectual or cultural areas or toward sublimation. Reaction formations do not appear as often as they do in other character types. In the hysteric, sex energies are neither discharged sexually to relieve stasis nor are they anchored in character armoring. Instead these energies are largely discharged in apprehensiveness and somatic innervations.

Fully developed genital excitations lend themselves only to direct gratification. Where there are no pregenital blocks the hysteric has available as defense only contactlessness and flight. This may manifest itself in two ways: (1) *Frantic behavior,* in the unsatisfied blocking, such as hysterical fits, laughing, crying, running about, and delirium (from going away in the eyes); or frantic sexual behavior, including nymphomania; or tics (partial frantic behavior); or plain flight to or away from the threat. (2) *Calm behavior,* in the repressed block, such as paralysis and withdrawal. This may be partial as in hysterical paralysis and anesthesia, or total as in amnesia and fugue states or in passivity (freezing). Any ocular, oral, and anal blocks give symptoms of these stages.

Overt homosexual activity may be found in some hysterics. This is not true homosexuality, which involves identification with the opposite sex, but is due to a deep fear of the opposite sex and to suggestibility, which allows the hysteric to comply with homosexual advances. Also the Oedipus situation is avoided. Genital sensations reactivate the Oedipus complex and the threat of the competing mother. The hysteric thus must run from the man and, as if to prove further her lack of interest in the father, may take a woman. The hysteric can accept a man either if she has no feeling or is forced. The latter relieves the sense of guilt. Also what is frequently overlooked—it reaffirms her need to fear men as dangerous and not to be trusted.

Genesis

The hysteric has grown up essentially healthy and looks healthy until the sexual push at puberty. The father and mother are accepting in early childhood and the child identifies with the parent of the same sex. She could not reach genitality unless the parents were reasonably accepting of the pregenital phases. The hysteric, usually a girl, finds her mother (the boy, his father) moralistic and represses her sexual drive through identification. The problem is a prime Oedipus situation and the child's rejection of sex revolves around the incest barrier, and every man becomes a symbol of her father. Any genital excitation leads to a reaction of "no" in the organism because it awakens the incest prohibition. The Oedipus complex occurs when the natural attraction of the child to the parent of the opposite sex is stopped by the moralistic attitude of the parent of the same sex.

Therapy

The hysteric does not know that she uses her genital strivings to feel out danger, nor does she know she is sexually provocative. She must be unmasked and the infantile anxiety dissolved for effective therapeutic results. The hysteric must be cornered and prevented from running. Some milder cases of hysteria may recover spontaneously through marriage with an understanding partner.

Common Types of Hysteria

1) The *pure hysteric*. She has no pregenital blocks. This is the typical, curvaceous, sexually attractive, doll-like creature with normally developed breasts and pelvis prominently displayed.

2) The *hysteric with an ocular block*. She is usually tall and slender but with proportionately well-developed thighs and breasts. Where there is severe ocular blocking, the ego is weak and she has poor integration. These are difficult cases and there

is frequently much actual running from therapy. They may be difficult to differentiate from schizophrenics.

3) The *hysteric with an oral repressed block*. The pelvis and thighs are well developed but the upper part of the body is slender with small breasts. This type is more serious in attitude and shows varying degrees of depression.

4) The *hysteric with an oral unsatisfied block*. She is usually short and heavily built with broad shoulders, well-developed breasts, heavy shoulder muscles, and an overeating problem from a need to fill the feeling of emptiness in her stomach, behind which is a fellatio fantasy. Fat is built up to absorb the excess energy. Dieting produces acute anxiety. One such patient who had a very persistent overeating problem and could not tolerate the anxiety produced by dieting brought the following dream: She was in a session with a former therapist. She remarked that she was hungry. The therapist left the room and brought her some food.

She reported that she woke from the dream feeling anxious. At this point she told me that she presently had a peculiar feeling in her stomach. It was not hunger but she had an overpowering urge to eat. I told her the feeling was a displacement from some other part of her body and asked what sensations she had in her mouth. She replied that she had an urge to suck. I encouraged her to give in to the sensations; she was very embarrassed at first but soon gave in to sucking movements. Shortly this urge ceased and she reported that she had developed genital sensations. The peculiar feeling in her stomach with the urge to eat had disappeared.

5) The *hysteric with an anal block*. Compulsive symptoms, and sexual fantasies of an anal type are present.

All of these types seem attractive to men. Their pelvis and thighs are sexually provocative, the mons pubis is prominent, and the genitalia are well developed.

The Intellectual ("Big Brain") Hysteric

I describe this type separately since it is neither common (I have treated only seven cases), nor does it follow the pattern of indifference to intellectual achievement seen in the usual hysteric. Here the intellectual achievement is the major characteristic. This is a type identified by Reich as one who uses her intellect as a tall phallus to defend herself against all men. Apparently this condition is confined to females.

These individuals are highly intelligent with exceedingly high IQ's and every one of my cases had either a Ph.D. in psychology or was an M.D. specializing in psychiatry. Two of them had both degrees. I do not presume that this is necessarily invariably the case, but it is probably usual. The special interest is under-standable. Although these patients are truly hysterics, and the more emotional do show typical hysterical qualities, they tend to be more serious, aggressive, and efficient than the usual types, and all possess a rather old-maidish quality. They are usually heavy about the hips and thighs with a tendency to underdevel-oped breasts.

Scholastically, their record is rather below what one might expect from their intelligence, but they are quite efficient in their subsequent work. Their driving interest is to find a man who loves them and to whom they can respond. In this they have little success. They marry quiet, ineffective, passive men who tolerate all of their idiosyncracies with indifference, and whom they in turn despise. Otherwise, rather than being pur-sued, they do the pursuing and usually select an aggressive, phallic type of male who rapidly loses interest although they go all out with their feminine charms.

As patients they are determined, persistent, and flattering as long as therapy does not touch them deeply. Then they deprecate the therapist and the therapy in ways that grow less subtle as therapy becomes more effective. A favorite trick is to consult other psychiatrists impulsively and then inform you later, con-tritely promising never to do so again but doing so at the first impulse. The combination of their intelligence and tendency to deprecate can be quite devastating.

One such patient reached the point of feeling she used her head as a phallic weapon, smashing everyone about her. She then developed the orgasm reflex and was able to surrender to her spontaneous functioning on several occasions, once holding this level for seven days. Then she suddenly turned on me with all her fury and intelligence, left her boy friend, returned to her despised husband, and decided on the more intellectual approach of psychoanalysis. However, for the short period of apparent health (she later said bitterly that even that was not real), the potential she showed made any effort worthwhile and created a tremendous challenge to cure her.

Such patients display many paradoxes; for example, one finds an efficient specialist pleading for assurance about her ability to perform simple tasks. They constitute one of the most difficult problems in therapy and are not cases for the beginner or for therapists lacking strong egos. Dr. Reich has said that one has two choices—tell them that they are too smart for you and send them away, or smash their intellectual defense. One patient whose intellectual defense had largely been broken clearly used her breasts as a second line of defense, using them as a phallic symbol.

In the seven cases of intellectual hysteria that I have treated, each of the five common types of hysteria has been represented, although three were pure hysterics. A common event in their histories has been a seeming desertion by the father when the child was four years of age. For example, in one case the father migrated to a new country ahead of the rest of the family in order to prepare for their eventual reunion. In another case the father was a salesman absent six months at a time. I do not know how important this may be in producing this condition or whether what is involved is largely a matter of native intelligence. I am inclined to believe that this is an important event leading to incorporation of the father which serves the basis for the mechanism of the large phallus. It is extremely difficult to get these patients to give up the father.

9 · Phallic Character Types

The Phallic Narcissistic Character (Genital Revenge)

AT THE GENITAL LEVEL there is a differentiation between the sexes: the genital is used for sexual love, the female as female and the male as male. There is no competition. At the phallic level, undifferentiation still exists. Where fixation at this level occurs, both sexes use the genital as a weapon against the other sex. The female has a fantasied phallus or fantasies of taking the penis from the male. Sex is used as a means of revenge.

Characteristics and Symptoms

The phallic character will be athletic in build, with a hard, sharp masculine face—although he will quite frequently have a girlish face in spite of his build. Aggression often shows not so much in what he says or does as in how he says or does it. He is bristly and anticipates an expected attack by attacking first. This aggression is a defense against surrender and against finding himself weak. The erect phallus is his bulwark of confidence, and erective impotence causes him to fall to pieces—he becomes anxiety-laden, cringing, and helpless. In behavior toward a love object, he has always some sadistic traits, more or less disguised, and the narcissistic element in his loving is more important to him than his actual partner is. The more neurotic he is, the more obtrusive his behavior becomes. His impressive self-confidence, vigor, and flexibility move toward arrogance, hauteur, cold reserve, and deriding aggressiveness.

He resents subordination unless he in turn can dominate others. He has an exaggerated self-confidence, with a grand manner and a sense of his own superiority, through which his narcissism is expressed. Rarely infantile in his display, narcissism represents pride in his erect phallus and he survives through life on this confidence. He often forms personal attachments, but from irrational motives. He displays an aggressive courage to ward off opposite strivings. He often manages great achievement, but shows less attention to details than the compulsive.

His energy level is above average. Such men are highly potent erectively but impotent orgastically and possess contempt for the female. They use the sex act to degrade women by piercing and destroying them—and by that prove their own potency. The more potency is disturbed, the more labile the mood and the more work is disturbed. There is a homosexual potential because of identification with the parent of the opposite sex. The male varies from nearly healthy, including the hero, the successful businessman, and athlete, to the very sick—the active homosexual, the psychopath, the drug addict, the depressive, and paranoid, depending on the number and the intensity of infantile blocks.

In women, the less neurotic individuals have great self-confidence, physical vigor, and beauty. With deepening neuroses, clitoris sexuality and active lesbianism appear. The female has a fantasied penis or fantasies taking the penis from the male. For her, the sexual act is equivalent to depriving the male of his penis and incorporating it into herself. She takes vengeance on the man, castrating him, or making him impotent or apparently impotent. She competes strongly with him and constantly tries to cut him down to size with very effective remarks or actions. A favorite habit is to taunt the male into sexual union and then ridicule him for being unable to satisfy her. She is adept at finding fault with everything and puts herself across so well that she is difficult to refute.

Both men and women of this type have a strong ego defense as long as there is effective libido gratification. Anal passive tendencies will appear, either in symptoms or directly, if absence of gratification allows the ego defense to break down over a period of time. The most successful defenses are found in active homosexuality and in phallic sadism and in the psychopath. The least successful defense is found in paranoids and erythrophobia. The shakier the defense, the stronger the rages and tantrums. Behind the aggressive façade is a weak, dependent, timid person. The unsatisfied block manifests itself in Don Juan behavior; while, in repressed blocking, the individual tends to be morally righteous, ascetic, and protective toward sexual morality.

Armoring is usually general, being particularly marked in the chest, diaphragm, and legs and heavy in the shoulders. In phallics, as in all types of character, the pattern of amoring in the non-erogenous segments is not related to the character type as such, but creates the individual variations within that type. In all cases, it is *only* the armoring in the erogenous zones that determines the character type. For instance, among phallics an eye block produces a paranoid; an oral repressed blocking leads to a chronic depressive; and an oral unsatisfied block produces a manic depressive, an alcoholic, or a drug addict. The more dominant the earlier blocks become, the less evident become the phallic features.

There is a point here which must be clarified: We can speak of a phallic with an eye block who is not a paranoid or a phallic with an oral repressed block who is not a chronic depressive. The distinction lies in the degree of importance of the pregenital blocking. Where the characteristics remain definitely phallic and the pregenital block merely modifies the picture we would call such individual a phallic with a particular block, but where the pregenital block gives the major characteristic then we speak of a paranoid or chronic depressive or manic depressive and so forth. One may blend into the other gradually and the dividing line is a matter of judgment. For example, we can speak of a phallic with an anal block. The extreme case would be the compulsive where the phallic level is largely given up.

Chest armoring on the other hand would produce only a variation in the specific type particularly in regard to rigidity.

Genesis

In healthy development, the phallic stage is the stage of getting acquainted with the genital. The phallic character is severely disappointed by the parent of the opposite sex at around four years of age. In the male, the mother cannot tolerate the exhibition of the boy's erect phallus and clamps down on his phallic expressions. This rejection of the phallus is equivalent to a castration threat. The mother's stopping of the child's expression produces rage which stimulates the urge for revenge, at the same time producing harshness of attitude and expression. The child's development on to genitality is stopped but there is sufficient push to avoid retreat back to anality, which has just been abandoned.

Behind the phallic surface, however, one finds anal surrender (in the female a pregenital vagina), and finally oral tendencies. Therefore, the phallic struggles constantly to defend himself against going back to anal surrender and to maintain the phallic position—because it is not secure.

Genitality is the only secure position as it is the only stage that allows release without stasis. The phallic position is insecure because there is only partial contact with the genital and a constant danger of total loss of this contact. The phallic identifies with the parent of the opposite sex, who is the frustrating parent in his case. He must identify with the frustrating parent for survival. "If you can't fight 'em, join 'em." In the male phallic, the mother was the dominating parent. The patient will be angry at her for rejection (rejection of phallic exhibition) and therefore will want to use his phallus against her as a weapon of revenge. This attitude is a defense against the deeply repressed original love of the mother who frustrated and disappointed him.

The closer a character is to genitality, the less complex he is. The hysteric and phallic have no reaction symptoms; that is, they have no symptoms which are not an exaggeration of normal patterns. Reaction formation is found only when there is a fixation at a pregenital level.

Therapy

The therapist breaks down the aggressive defenses back to the passive anal level where the patient becomes cringing and helpless—then the patient develops by healthy pathways to genitality. If the revengeful erective potency is not destroyed in therapy, one has made no headway. The therapist unmasks the aggression as a defense against passive feminine tendencies and eliminates the unconscious tendency to seek revenge against the opposite sex. In resisting, the patient will deny that he has any passive tendencies and will denigrate both therapy and the therapist; frequently he also will attempt to assume control of the interpretative process.

An example of the sort of cringing helplessness that may appear follows.

A forty-eight-year-old athletic man, married, a successful businessman, and a classical Don Juan type, during the course of therapy, called me one morning for an emergency appointment because of acute upper abdominal pain, nausea, and weakness. There were no psychic manifestations so he doubted that I could help him but wanted me to see him before he went to his family doctor. He remarked at the clearness of his thinking; he had no confusion like that experienced in a similar previous attack.

The skin was cold over his abdomen, the chest and legs were warm, pulse rapid and of fair volume. There was rigidity and tenderness over the upper abdomen; he had not contracted anywhere else. I gently massaged the upper abdomen and produced gradual relaxation. The abdomen became warm, the pain ceased, and he felt much better. His awareness of the true nature of the condition became clear. This state lasted for a few minutes, then suddenly abdominal cramps again overtook him. His whole body became cold, his pulse weak and rapid, and his face ashen. His eyes were sunken and his voice weak; he became pleading and anxious and complained that he was very ill. I agreed. It was pitiful to see so powerful a man suddenly become so helpless, pleading, and frightened. I again gently massaged his abdomen, and worked vigorously on his thighs, which had now become spastic, and reassured him. I had him gag two or three times and then he grew suddenly sad; tears came to his eyes and I encouraged him to turn over, sob, and give free vent to his feelings. At the same time I released the spasm in his dorsal muscles. He burst into pitiful sobbing, calling for his mother—who had died when he was ten years old.

He said he had been lonesome; she was kind and had loved him. After her death he knew only cruelty; he recalled that after every trying day he had dreamed of her, and he felt something deep had been struck. The sobbing continued for five or ten minutes until he felt better.

He was relaxed but weak and said he wanted to go home. Starting to dress, he was again overcome by abdominal cramps and I had him lie down so I could massage the abdomen again. He again began to sob and said that now he longed for his wife; he wanted her to comfort him and be near him. I called her in and, explaining the situation to her briefly, left them alone for fifteen minutes.

When I came back he had dressed with his wife's assistance and said he was very tired and sleepy. I cautioned her to drive and told her to put him to bed and give him some hot tea when they got home. She was to call me if there was any recurrence of the symptoms.

The next morning he called again for an appointment. He looked rather exhausted, but good. There was only vague pain in the abdomen, slight spasticity of the recti abdominus and thigh muscles. I massaged the abdomen a little and told him I did not think we should disturb him further just then.

From this time on, this man, who had been a classical Don Juan type, showed no further interest in pursuing other women. I might mention that when he first came to me, he told me that he had over twenty women on his active list.

Paranoia and Paranoid Conditions
(Genital Revenge Distorted by Ocular Blocking)

I describe these conditions merely for the sake of completeness, since these people do not usually come for therapy. They do not recognize their difficulties as coming from within themselves, but they rather see them as all due to environmental injustice and persecution. Paranoid symptoms or rationalizations vary in plausibility depending on the general degree of integration of the individual and the severity of the eye block which prevents rational perception of the self in its environment.

Characteristics and Symptoms

The paranoid individual has always been irritable, stubborn, sullen, suspicious, resentful of discipline, moody, and unable to engage in sustained harmonious relationships. Hypochondriacal symptoms may be present and the individual spends a lot of time observing his sensations. He is often of superior intelligence but he spends so much time striving after satisfactions he cannot achieve that his constructive achievements are minimal. He begins to seek an explanation of his failures in the jealousy or enmity of others. Experience is misinterpreted; there is a hidden meaning in what goes on around him. He imagines slights and indignities and attaches far-reaching significance to trivial details in the behavior of others. Vague feelings of fear tend to increase his suspicion.

Paranoid ideas may vary widely, from slight exaggerations of everyday life situations to easily recognizable, bizarre delusions. Persecution ideas may develop into grandiose ones in which a transformation of the personality appears. The individual may even attempt to play the role his ideas assign to him; for example, a prophet may take to wearing a beard, long hair, and peculiar dress, and to forgiving his enemies. However, his underlying hatred will be but superficially buried.

In all paranoid conditions, the individual is confident he is right and clings obstinately to that opinion. He cannot *see* things any other way.

A not uncommon form of paranoia appears in the litigious type. Because of dissatisfactions he initiates more and more ill-advised legal actions; this is always an attempt to prove that he is right and superior and to strengthen his basically insecure and weak ego. Occasionally, paranoia assumes an erotic form, and an individual may believe that a woman of wealth or prominence is in love with him. He may pester her with letters, telephone calls, and even visits right up to the point where she asks that he be legally restrained. Or, a husband may become very jealous of his wife, accusing her of unfaithfulness and believing in the truth of his accusations quite genuinely.

Genesis

The paranoid is a phallic character with a repressed ocular block. The degree of integration and thus the degree of deviation from normal displayed through symptoms probably depends on the age at which the blocking occurred.

Therapy

A discussion of therapy for such cases is more or less academic, since few seek it. The better integrated paranoids are, the more rational their symptoms will be and the more difficult they would be to handle in therapy. For example, the severest blocking and the most bizarre symptoms are found in paranoid schizophrenics —who are frequently good candidates, therapeutically speaking. In any case, the suspiciousness and the eye block must be attacked consistently.

The Chronic Depressive Character[1]
(Genital Revenge Blocked by Oral Inhibition)

The chronic depressive is a phallic with an oral repressed block. He has all the basic qualities of the phallic—colored by the degree to which the oral block is effective. When the oral block is very powerful, phallic qualities are given up entirely and depression becomes the dominant feature. His ego, which is always weak, is caught between the punitive superego and the demanding goal of the ego ideal, usually a phallic image. Chronic depressives seem to be prone to developing skin cancer.

Characteristics and Symptoms

This is one of the least understood of the character types and one of those most frequently diagnosed incorrectly. Chronic depression has been called anxiety hysteria, phobia, compulsive,

[1] For a very excellent description of this character type and the manic depressive, which follows, see *American Handbook of Psychiatry*, 1959, Vol. 1, article on manic depressive psychoses by Arieti, pp. 419–452. Arieti does not, however, distinguish the chronic depressive as separate from the manic depressive, depressed, which I feel he should; so that in reading his article, which is well worth reading, one must select the material which belongs to this type from all the information he gives on the manic depressive, depressed.

and even schizophrenia. From the symptoms one can understand this confusion.

The depressive is caught between oral repression and phallic narcissism. The drag back from the oral block may reactivate many compulsive features, as well as others which appear to be compulsive but really are not. For example, his rigid, righteous, usually moral, attitude may well make one think of the compulsive; actually, this is his method of expressing his phallic core, inhibited as he is by oral repression. His great inhibition makes overt aggression next to impossible.

He is easily distinguished from the compulsive, however, in that he is acutely sensitive, very much alive in his feelings but unable to show them. In the compulsive, heavy armor has created a dulling and anxiety is not as acute. Here, on the other hand, compulsive-like symptoms are usually in the form of phobias fraught with acute anxiety. Occasionally, typical compulsions may be present.[2] Unlike the compulsive, the chronic depressive is generous, not stingy, even though like the compulsive, he is frequently interested in collecting.

He may be mistaken for a schizophrenic because his timidity and modesty make him seem introverted, but a Rorschach will show he is extroverted. He is in a cage and cannot express himself, and is therefore considered cold and aloof. His independence is apt to accentuate such traits. His characteristics depend on the pull of the oral block; the greater the oral influence the more evident his depression becomes, while his phallic or compulsive traits become less evident. In his best moments, he approaches a restrained phallic. Overtly, the depressive may seem well adjusted but his inner life is torment.

Depression ordinarily is not obvious, but seriousness is always present. When depression is marked there is a rapid lowering of energy, loss of weight, and shrinking. There is usually a history of depressive periods, and the patient reacts to disappointments with depression and self-blame. He is inclined to blame himself for most difficulties, while the usual phallic blames others. He is tolerant toward others but intolerant toward him-

[2] Anal characteristics are activated by the drag back from the phallic to the oral level.

self. He is righteous, determined, extremely responsible, and rigidly honest, possessing a strong, relentless drive even though his energy is usually below average. His lips are thin and his jaw is tight. He has little ability to defend himself aggressively as his own sense of guilt forces him to agree with his accuser. He is meticulous, orderly, and above average intelligence. In spite of his handicaps he usually gives a good account of himself but feels inadequate since his inhibitions prevent him from functioning anywhere near his capacity. It is the disparity between his achievement and his basic capacity that produces the feeling of inadequacy over which he feels much guilt.

Most depressives possess a rather good sense of humor, although it is inclined to be cynical or self-depreciating in type; and in speech they are often brief and caustic. Life itself is a trial, but their drive and great determination keep them going. Ideas of suicide are seldom out of their minds but they do not consider it seriously, except as a last resort solution. Sometimes they show hysteria-like manifestations in their desperation. The ultimate necessity for suicide seldom comes to them. Their critical ability is usually better developed than their creative ability, and life leaves them filled with bitterness—which may lead to gall bladder disease.

The depressive is well-meaning but is frequently misunderstood because he expects others to understand with little explanation. He is usually a poor eater, fussy in what he eats, and gets little satisfaction from the oral zone.[3] He is inclined to be very temperate, but may overindulge in an attempt to break his chains (or at least appear to break them). He envies the phallic and longs for freedom from his restrictions, but cannot break through strong inner inhibitions. He has the strong sexual drive of the phallic, but is inhibited by moralism and concern for propriety, as well as by an inner feeling of inadequacy and a fear of being ridiculed by the woman. As children and adolescents, depressives are well behaved, quiet, idealistic, and sentimental. They prefer

[3] This is to be distinguished from those cases, usually hysterics, who defend themselves from oral pleasure, especially kissing, and react with disgust because of their rejection of sex. In these cases the mouth has become sexualized.

intellectual pursuits to sports or other physical activity. Lincoln, Mark Twain, and Hamlet are representative examples of the chronic depressive.

Genesis

The chronic depressive has reached the phallic stage with an oral inhibited block. The block is brought about by oral deprivation. The depressive does not give up the phallic level as the compulsive does, but tries desperately to cling to it. The phallic characteristics are more or less an ideal to be attained; this may account for the relentless drive of the depressive. Actually the depressive is forever trying to win the love and approval of the mother he always needs because of his early deprivation. Failure he always blames on himself with devastating guilt and goes to extraordinary lengths to succeed. He can accept any punishment rather than loss of love. He survives by being needed. He marries a mate who needs him. There is one point worthy of mention and that is the emotional advantage of depression. During depression anxiety usually disappears. His concern is thus directed outward rather than on himself and he thus feels more like an average person with a problem. Where the depression is not too deep potency is frequently improved because of replacement of the anxiety by the depression.

Therapy

In depression there is a rapid lowering of the energy level which is dangerous. The chest must be mobilized at once to build up energy, and the inhibited rage which has produced the depression must be released. It is difficult to mobilize aggression, and even more difficult for the depressive to maintain it. His drive, however, compensates and makes him a responsive and helpful patient. Nausea may be a prominent symptom; it is due to repressed crying, and is relieved when crying occurs.

The Manic Depressive Character
(Genital Revenge Masked by Oral Strivings)

The manic depressive is a phallic with an oral unsatisfied block. He differs from the chronic depressive in being less well integrated. He is unstable and volatile, flowing back and forth with wide mood swings from elation to a depression deeper than the chronic depressive's and with more retardation.

Characteristics and Symptoms

Characteristically, this type is rotund, with a tendency to breadth rather than height; but he is agile, impatient, and intolerant. The body gives an impression of flabbiness and poor substance; the more the depressive characteristics dominate, the less rotund it is.

Usually manic depressives are talkative and energetic, but changeable and with poor ability to persist at one task. The more manic they become the more restless, flighty, jerky, and pushy is their behavior, with increasing excitability and loud, boisterous, and boastful speech, frequently rude and vulgar. Their judgment is poor and their insight at best is only fleeting. They seem to have been wound up and let go without guidance.

This condition may suddenly change to a hopeless, reproachful depression. All activity then becomes slowed, including speech, and the face appears sad and hopeless, the body seems to shrink, and the shoulders droop. This may increase to the point of immobility and total neglect of all bodily needs. In the manic phase, eating, drinking, and talking are excessive; in the depressive they may all be stopped completely. Compulsive symptoms may be present, especially when neither phase is too marked. One sees all degrees, from slight variations from normal to the extreme where hospitalization is necessary. In some individuals the depressive side dominates, in others the manic; while in still others the two alternate quite regularly. As the years pass variations tend to become more marked and longer in duration.

Genesis

The manic depressive has reached the phallic stage with an oral unsatisfied block. The oral craving tends to make him unstable, demanding, and intolerant. A sudden yielding of the block creates a manic phase. The body is unused to handling the increase of energy and, with the armoring present, the organism responds in a jerky, disorganized way. The manic is filled with elation from the newfound freedom and goes all out to satisfy the oral craving. At other times, holding increases to the point of stupor.

Therapy

One must watch for the possibility of suicide, both when the patient is going into and when he is coming out of a depression. As in the chronic depressive, the depressed phase requires immediate mobilization of energy through releasing the chest, but unlike the chronic depressive, the manic's rage must be controlled because his poor judgment and expansive attitude may get him into a great deal of trouble.

The Alcoholic

Any character type may produce an alcoholic from oral unsatisfied blockings, but the typical alcoholic belongs to the phallic group. The drug addict also fits into this group. Whether or not the individual is an alcoholic is determined, not by the amount or frequency of his drinking, but by the reason for his drinking. Characteristically, he contains a great deal of helplessness and lack of aggression and is prone to give up easily.

According to Reich, the frustration of his phallic exhibitionism together with psychic castration by his mother led to identification with her. Therefore, relinquished anal attitudes reappear and strengthen the passive feminine behavior patterns. The passivity, in turn, is counteracted by aggressive exhibitionism. Thus he is held away from masculine genitality both by regression to anality and by identification with his mother. His penis unconsciously comes to have the meaning of a breast. From that, he quite naturally develops a maternal attitude toward younger men and leanings toward fellatio. Women alcoholics will take the same sort of interest in younger women. Oral regression masks the phallic traits as it does in the depressive.

If the patient will stop drinking and depend on treatment to handle his anxiety, therapy is greatly expedited.

10 · Anal Character Types

The Compulsive or Anal-Inhibited Character
(Phallic Sadism Held by Anal Caution)

THE COMPULSIVE is the human machine. His outstanding characteristic is caution, and the general function of the character is to defend against stimuli and to maintain psychic equilibrium. On the deepest level, it is actually a defense against soiling. The general impression is one of great control.

Characteristics and Symptoms

A pedantic concern for orderliness is prominent. The compulsive's whole life, even to minor details, is run according to plans laid carefully ahead of time. Any change is felt as a disturbance or even with anxiety. Because he is thorough, he may be efficient, but he cannot adapt to changes or new situations.

A trait never missing is circumstantial ruminative thinking. This ruminating may be an effort to take his mind off forbidden urges and to free himself of the strain of holding back, functioning as an escape or relief. He always divides his thought fairly equally among details, regardless of the comparative importance of the matters being considered. For example, as much time is devoted to unimportant details as to crucial matters. He is invariably careful of money and goods, if not absolutely stingy, and he is better at criticism and analysis than at creative activities —he makes a good scholar but a bad artist. The compulsive cannot give but must hold on to everything. There is also a tendency to collect things, to be acquisitive. He cannot reach out so he must bring things to himself. All of these traits derive from anal eroticism; they are reaction formations from anal erotic tendencies.

If reaction formation is not successful, one finds traits of an opposite nature which are breakthroughs of original tendencies (soiling)—producing sloppiness, inability to handle money, etc. Other reaction formations are sympathy and feelings of guilt; they come from anal sadistic impulses rather than from anal eroticism. Hostile and aggressive impulses are quite frequently even satisfied in the symptoms derived from anal eroticism. In very severe cases, the compulsive will have an affect block; ordinarily he is lukewarm in his affects. There is a corresponding outward restraint and control which is quite marked. Because of his fear that he will lose control and be unable to hold in (control his anal sphincter), he is always inwardly indecisive, doubting, and mistrustful.

The central fixation is on an anal sadistic level. He was toilet trained too early and had to develop stringent reaction formations. Because anal sadistic feelings must be avoided, very great self-control is a typical early reaction formation. The compulsive develops to the phallic stage, but the anal repression has led into a notable (anal) stubbornness that forces the development of anal sadism. Because of the early repression and because the parents will have been distinctly anti-sexual, genitality is barely reached before it is relinquished. The genitality will have been reached only in the form of aggression of the phallic sadistic type, however. Attached by guilt and by the early inhibition, the compulsive drops his phallic sadistic sexuality and returns to anal aggression and eroticism.

Reaction formations are intensified and form the character during the typical compulsive's well-developed latency period (between five and twelve years of age). The whole process of developing and relinquishing phallic sexuality is repeated at puberty under the pressure of organic development. Violent sadistic impulses occur, commonly directed toward raping and beating women, but are usually confined to fantasy. They are accompanied by an affective weakness and feelings of inferiority. Ethical and aesthetic reaction formations develop in response to the inferiority and are basically a narcissistic compensation. A progressive affective flattening occurs, so the compulsive looks like a model adolescent. The patient, however, feels an inner emptiness and a desire to start life anew and may attempt to do so repeatedly.

Compulsions and obsessions may be prominent and are a compromise between holding and yielding. The typical mode of repression is the dissociation of affect from ideas so that it is possible for the compulsive to think and dream of incest and rape without excitation. Affect block, the ultimate in compulsive repression, is really one great spasm of the ego. All the muscles of the body, but especially of the pelvis, pelvic floor, shoulders, and face, are spastic. This gives the typical hard expression and awkwardness. Contact is mechanical.

The first layer of armoring consists of aggressive impulses turned into holding back—the holding both is aggression and holds in aggression. In the passive feminine, also an anal character, anality works in the original libidinous direction; but in the compulsive, anality functions as a reaction formation, a holding back against anal libidinal urges. There is constant fear that self-control may be lost because of the urge to let go in the face of the necessity for self-control.

One does not usually find physical diseases in the compulsive because of the high energy level and the methodical, quiet life. Occasionally, depression is present from oral blocking; it is usually not a dominant feature.

Genesis

Compulsives are produced by severe toilet training before the child has attained adequate ability to control sphincters; that is, before one and a half to two years of age. This training demand leads to contraction of the whole body musculature in order to conform. Severe anxiety results from the requirement beyond the capacity of the child. The body becomes tight and rigid and heavy armoring results. The patients are walking machines, especially those with affect block. They literally hold back for dear life. This holding back with no release leads to tremendous pressure, which produces rage—which again must be repressed. The compulsive does finally reach the phallic stage, but with much sadistic aggression and brutality. It is given up because of the intolerance of the parents and the individual reverts to anality.

At puberty, the phallic level is revived with sadistic aggression, but because of the holding the sadism is not acted out but exists only in fantasy of rape, murder, etc. The fantasies and the phallic level are soon given up and the compulsive becomes a model adolescent, but at the expense of affect. Most compulsives are males because the repression comes usually from the mother. Identification with her occurs at the holding level, not at the erotic level as in the phallic or anal unsatisfied. The anus is not used as an erotic substitute. It is true that there is a homosexual potential through identification with the opposite sex, but this is a much more complicated and repressed factor than in the passive feminine character.

Therapy

The doubting should be attacked first. This reaches back to the love–hate ambivalence. The hate soon predominates and one concentrates on it. Rage is worked through on two levels: the more superficial (anal squashing and kicking and meanness), and the deeper phallic level (piercing and stabbing). Most patients come to therapy because of distress about their symptoms or because of lack of satisfaction in life. Their lives are empty.

The Passive Feminine or Anal-Unsatisfied Character
(Phallic Sadism Given Up for Anal Submission)

The passive feminine character is essentially a phallic who has given up the phallic level. The phallic narcissistic defends himself against his anal and passive homosexual impulses by phallic aggression, but the passive feminine wards off his genital impulses with the aid of anal and passive surrender.

Characteristics and Symptoms

This character type is exclusively male. Overtly he is passive, retiring, modest, polite, compliant, and weak. He appears soft and mild and resembles the male hysteric, but differs from him in that, underneath, he is tenacious, stubborn, spiteful, sly, vicious, and contemptuous. He has a viper in him. This is a result of the greatly repressed (squeezed) rage arising from his necessity to comply. His anal attitude is directed toward women and leads to insistence on satisfaction at the anal level by being waited on and shown attention. Although compliant, he cannot give and hates the woman. Homosexuality is usually expressed by fellatio and anal intercourse. He has identified with the female (mother) at the anal erotic level and is attracted by male sexuality. If he enters a homosexual relationship he accepts the passive role, whereas the phallic homosexual assumes the active role.

Where the father has been particularly severe, the picture is that of an overly polite, obsequious, ineffective, servile individual. Sexually, he is ineffective and feels very inferior; homosexually, he offers himself to strong men to placate the angry father from whom he fears castration.

Genesis

The passive feminine character reaches the early phallic stage with a strong drive but is slapped down severely by the mother. He retreats to the anal level, where overinterest has been shown, and identifies with the mother at the anal erotic level. He then defends himself against the phallic qualities which had caused him such disaster.

With a severe father, a father-identification in the superego develops. This leads to a very critical superego superimposed on a passive feminine structure, producing a strong sense of inferiority and an accentuation of all the passive feminine characteristics.

Therapy

The therapist mobilizes the anal sadistic rage and encourages aggression. One has to be prepared for considerable venom. A great deal of character work is necessary to bring out awareness of the hate and spite behind the overtly compliant, cooperative attitude.

One passive feminine character, a young man of twenty-two years, came to therapy because of sexual problems and his feminine physique, about which he was very sensitive. He thought it would be impossible for a girl to love him, so his only outlet was masturbation. Even that was unsatisfying. If he masturbated in the morning it tired him for the rest of the day and prevented him from sleeping in the evening. If he masturbated in the afternoon it also tired him. He had tried to sublimate in schoolwork, but couldn't concentrate. He was very self-conscious and cautious; his shoulders were narrow, his hips broad, and his thighs and buttocks fleshy. He talked in a rather high weak voice. His one sexual experience with a prostitute had disgusted him. There had been no homosexual experiences, but he had felt a feminine melting sensation in the presence of some men.

Although his initial expression was one of contempt, it soon changed to suffering and he said he liked to make himself appear helpless. I told him he was helpless like a fox. Although he would comply with requests in therapy, he complained that nothing meant anything and that nothing made him feel.[1] I pointed out what a good compliant boy he was, so I was to blame for any lack of success. He doubted whether I was competent and admitted that he did not really want me to be successful. At the end of each session he would hide a smile of triumph at my lack of success in making him let go.

At the same time he was afraid I would harm him because he laughed at me.

Sometimes vicious hate would momentarily appear, and once he remarked that therapy was like a game of chess. He could block every move I made and felt guilty about making a fool of me. I pointed out that he wanted to be understood, but feel-

---

[1] That is, he was contactless from immobilization.

ing that no one did understand he played games to avoid exposing himself.

After this he brought a dream of poisoning his mother and began to feel overt hostility for me. He would like to bash my head on the floor, he explained, and started coming late and missing sessions. He doubted my sincerity in wanting to help people, and told me I charged exorbitant fees and drove around in a Cadillac. Further, I was myself very awkward and the reason we made no progress was that I made mistakes. Moreover, I failed to recognize his cooperativeness just so I could "get" him in a vulnerable spot, and he didn't think it was fair of me to hit him in his vulnerable spots. He said he fantasied that he would go to another therapist and that I would commit suicide over it.

Then, he began bringing out fantasies of strangling women. When I asked him if that gave him any idea of why he was so passive, he admitted that he was afraid of his destructive tendencies and of cracking up. Quickly, he added, "I don't quite believe it, because I am armored against it, just as I was when I brought up the dream of poisoning my mother."

As time went on, he looked more and more hateful, threatened to beat me up if I continued, and admitted he was afraid to hate because of his murderous impulses.

The Masochistic Character
(Phallic Exhibition Given Up for Masochistic Behavior)

Erotic demands may be made from any erogenous zone at any stage of development. Frustration of these demands leads to a destructive impulse against the frustrating person mixed with the corresponding sexual demand. That is sadism. When this impulse is again blocked, it turns inward against the self and becomes masochism. This is what has happened to the masochistic character. While one may look upon the average neurotic as a cripple, he is ambulatory and can do a good deal for himself. The masochist, in contrast, can be considered a bedridden cripple because he must depend on others for any release of tension, no matter how slight.

Although the masochist strives for pleasure as everyone else does, a disturbing mechanism specific for masochism causes his striving to fail: every pleasure sensation, when it reaches a certain level of intensity, is perceived as a threat (fear of punishment). The pleasure sensation is then inhibited by this mechanism and turned into unpleasure or pain. Behind this is his intolerance of expansion and movement which renders it impossible for him to discharge tension. For this reason he suffers more than any other neurotic. Masochistic characters are not common, but masochistic symptoms in other neuroses are extremely frequent. During the end phase in therapy every patient goes through a masochistic period, depending on the therapist for relief, that is, to make him burst.

The greatest damage to children is caused by contradiction between or inconsistency from the parents. Either leads to immobilization of the child, and is a vital factor in masochism. Also prominent is guilt resulting from a conflict between love and hatred for the same object. Dynamically, it corresponds in intensity to an inhibited aggression. Through the solution of masochism, Reich proved the death instinct does not exist.[2]

Characteristics and Symptoms

There are several key traits which make up the masochistic character and single him out from other anal types. Neurotics will often show one or more of these traits, but a full-blown masochist has them all and they give his character its peculiar stamp. The clinical diagnosis of masochism is made only when all the traits listed below are present.

First, there is a constant whining and complaining which mirrors an inner sense of chronic suffering, always present and real.

There are several reasons for this trait. Foremost is the fact that the anal holding (armoring) is of an especially spastic type—really an expression of the mother's anal permissiveness and the father's prohibition; hence, a constant letting go and holding back, or push and stop, push and stop. (This spastic holding is

2 Cf. Wilhelm Reich, "The Re-Emergence of Freud's Death Instinct as DOR Energy," *Orgonomic Medicine*, II, No. 1 (April 1956). Here Reich postulates evidence of Freud's death instinct in DOR energy.

in contrast to the compulsive holding which is much tighter, a consistent "stop," as it were.) The push and stop stymies and freezes the masochistic character; he is trapped and immobilized between two counter-directives and cannot free himself. He must therefore coerce and provoke people around him to do it for him. That is why he resorts to the annoying habit of nagging and complaining to those closest to him. He torments them into striking back at him, because this behavior gives a little relief from tension and also puts the person who strikes back in a bad light. He then has justification to hate and provoke further in an endless, vicious circle.

Disguised exhibitionism also plays a role here. The masochist is caught between the mother's encouragement to show off anally and the father's opposition to it. (The mother herself clamps down on the later phallic display.) The complaining becomes an oblique way of showing off and drawing attention. Since proud display is forbidden, he turns it into the opposite, as if to say "See how miserable I am; you don't love poor little me!"

The second trait, the compulsion to torture others, is really an offshoot of the first. Provocative in the extreme, it is designed to wring from the object some violent relief of tension—like getting someone to puncture a tightly blown-up balloon. The masochist is really asking for *decompression,* not pain, but is willing to suffer the pain if only the unbearable tension can be abated. He longs to be relieved of his load, but dares not seek relief directly lest dire punishment befall him. Someone else must take the responsibility and accept the guilt.

Another typical feature of masochism is the awkward, atactic behavior. Outwardly the masochist is both physically and socially clumsy, while inwardly he feels painfully stupid and ugly. This too stems partly from repressed exhibitionism, but it also reflects a very specific tension in the psyche and the genitals. This peculiar spasticity is the essence of the masochistic character, stuck in a "bog" between counter-commands. He is the most helpless and the most immobilized of all the character types and is totally dependent on outside sources for relief from his tension. The push-and-stop nature of the armoring leads to this characterological ataxia—it pervades every level of his functioning.

The fourth characteristic is a variant of the second: it is a chronic need to damage and derogate the self. Here again, one sees the defense against exhibitionism. Like all anal types, the masochist has had to give up phallic exhibition and slip back to an earlier (anal) libidinal position. His anal structure makes him feel inferior and ashamed because his ego ideal is still phallic. The shame adds to and reinforces his suffering, for the more he wishes to exhibit, the more he must repress and the smaller he must make himself. So he proclaims his insignificance, loudly, and even behaves as if he were stupid and retiring. He does not dare to risk punishment by asking for love directly, but can only show how miserable he is and hope that the love object will respond. Behind this pattern of behavior, he always is fearing rejection and disappointment.

Because of his helplessness the masochist has an intense fear of being abandoned which he expresses in an excessive demand for love. This is the fifth of his special traits.

Somatically, he is oversensitive to cold because he is chronically contracted at the skin surface by anxiety. He is unable to expand by himself and so cannot relieve the contraction. He clings to the warmth of the bed and craves constant contact to warm and protect him. His need for love (warmth) is as boundless as it is unattainable. Oral fixations may heighten the insatiability of his demands, but play no role as such in shaping the masochistic structure. However, at an anal level, too much coddling as well as too little love may lend to this sort of excessively demanding behavior. In line with this trait, there is another feature specific for masochism; i.e. skin erogeneity. In fact or in fantasy, the skin undergoes beating, pinching, burning, piercing, shackling—the goal being warmth, not pain. (Also present is the need for decompression noted above.) The masochist feels cold because chronic tension and spasticity contract the surface blood vessels. Body contact with the love object, or any kind of skin activity, relieves anxiety by expanding the biosystem.

Finally, there is the masochist's specific sex behavior, stemming from all of the above traits and set in the framework of his anal character structure. The anal orgasm has a flat curve of excitation with no sharp rise and no acme. Owing to the push-and-stop nature of his armoring, the masochist takes hours to masturbate. He is wont to hold back ejaculation and begin anew over and over again because he cannot stand any strong excitation (expansion). Finally the ejaculum flows out instead of spurting and he is left with a joyless, miserable feeling. The activity is typically pregenital and may include rolling on his stomach, kneading and squeezing the penis between hands or thighs, and fantasies of being tortured or degraded.

Heterosexual experience is similar, with typical holding back whenever excitation mounts. An anal libidinal organization never permits full orgastic discharge and release of tension. It produces more anxiety which further hinders adequate discharge, so that tension keeps mounting in the organism. The masochist, trapped between permission and prohibition, dares not take an active role in relieving the tension—on penalty of castration. For this reason he cannot stand the pleasure feelings of mounting sexual excitation (expansion of the biosystem). Passive beating fantasies convert this pleasure to unpleasure and at the same time spare him the responsibility of the punishable active role. Decompression, not pain, is again the goal. He merely accepts the pain as a necessary precondition for relief of tension and for escaping castration.

Corollary to all this is the masochist's special way of perceiving end pleasure itself. To his intensely spastic organism it seems a kind of bursting. But since bursting equals castration to him, the longed-for orgasm itself comes to mean execution of the highest penalty. This explains, too, why any sharp rise in pleasure becomes intolerable and must be changed into pain.

Bioenergetically, pleasure is functionally identified with expansion of the organism, while anxiety is a contraction against pleasurable expansion. The cardinal trait of the masochist is that *he cannot tolerate any expansion of his biosystem* (i.e. pleasure). Expansion immediately becomes a danger signal to which he responds by clamping down in a contraction. The pattern mimics his early experience when he was caught between parental counterdirectives. He preserves the early experience energetically and characterologically in a crippling intolerance of expansion (pleasure) and a total dependence on outside sources for relief. The somatic counterpart of the psychic situation is severe spasm of the pelvic floor, anus, and genital.

To review briefly, the masochist presents:

(1) A chronic sense of inner suffering with constant outward complaining. This comes from having no satisfactory outlet and experiencing a constant state of tension from a simultaneous inhibition and encouragement of his efforts to let go. The tension of the masochist is greater, for example, than that of a compulsive, because in the former there is a push and then a stop while in the latter there is no push, just inhibition. Complaining shows the self as miserable and is a masked exhibitionism.

(2) A tendency to torture others—on a superficial level, nastiness serves to justify hatred by getting other people angry and showing them in a bad light. On a deeper level the masochist releases tension by means of anger and attack from outside himself.

(3) Awkwardness and clumsiness. These symptoms stem from the great physical tensions of the masochist.

(4) A tendency to injure and deprecate himself. He appears stupid or remains quiet and mild in a corner. This is a defense against the exhibitionism which has been forbidden.

(5) A fear of being left alone or deserted and an excessive need for love. This is due to the masochist's minimal ability to expand by himself. He requires another person to cause expansion of energy out to the skin (a field reaction). His skin is cold and he wants it to be warm; he is contracted and cannot expand and is therefore never satisfied. Clinging also comes in here and lying in bed does too.

(6) An impulse to have the skin injured (beaten, burned, etc.). This activity brings energy (warmth) to the skin.

(7) In sexual behavior, release with low excitation (squeezing and pressing without friction movements) and prolonged masturbation, avoiding the orgasm to keep down sensation. In intercourse, a masochist is seldom erectively potent, and if he is he is reluctant to move the penis in the vagina. The genitals function at an anal level and genital feelings are intolerable because they

entail marked increase in sensation. The pelvic floor is spastic, as are the anal sphincter and genital.

Genesis

The conflict between sexual desire and fear of punishment is the cause of every neurosis. The masochistic character, based on a peculiar spastic attitude in both psyche and genital, immediately inhibits any strong pleasure sensation and thus changes it into unpleasure. This constantly nourishes the masochistic suffering which is the basis of the masochistic character reactions.

The suffering sensation is created mainly by the conflicting behavior of the mother and father. The mother shows excessive interest in the child, especially in his excretory functions; she watches him, even his excretory movements, keeps him near her not only without repressive training but, in fact, with encouragement in elimination. This leads to an erotic fixation of the child's interest on excretory functions and a sticky relationship to the mother. The father's attitude is just the opposite. It includes violence and beating for soiling. Thus, there is a contradiction between the parents, with the mother praising and the father punishing excretion. The child develops an anal fear of the father together with an anal fixation on the mother. So he depends on the mother for permission and cannot obtain gratification himself without fear of punishment. This fear is identified with the release and gratification afforded by evacuation, which is punishable. So he learns, in effect, to beat himself to obtain relief.

The masochist does reach the phallic stage, but only at the level of exhibitionism. Then he is slapped down severely by the mother. This is another contradiction, within the mother this time, instead of between the parents. Exhibition which was not only permitted but encouraged at the anal level is forbidden at the phallic level. Thus the phallic level is given up and the child returns to the anal level, with the chronic tension of being dependent on outside sources for relief. He functions on the principle that "you must relieve me; I am helpless."

In masochistic perversions there is the threat of castration as the phallic level is approached with concomitant beating. Since it is only beating and not castration he suffers, the beating relieves the castration fear and allows some sexual release.

The suffering of the masochist is real, objective, and not subjectively desired. Self-degradation is a mechanism of protection against genital castration. Self-damaging acts are an acceptance of milder punishments as protection against castration. The fantasies of being beaten are the only remaining possibilities of relaxation without guilt.

Therapy

The first object of therapy must be to turn the masochism back into the sadism from which it started. When the patient attempts to force the therapist into displaying qualities that will justify his hate, he must at first be encouraged in order to develop some ability for self-expression. As the sadism returns, infantile genitality and castration fears will reappear, together with great anxiety. All increases in sensation will cause anxiety, and this must be clearly explained and sympathetically repeated. If the patient will accept the therapist as a partial safeguard against his anxiety, it is easier to get him to express the anal rage, kicking, and squashing that he is inhibiting. He will probably retreat toward masochism repeatedly, particularly when orgastic sensations or movements awaken his anxiety.

Therapy for masochists is one of the most difficult of problems for a therapist, largely because even at the most advanced stages of therapy the masochism will reassert itself. The general progress of treatment requires, first, the conversion of masochism back into sadism; second, the usual progression from pregenitality to genitality; and third, the elimination of the anal and genital spasticity which is the acute source of masochistic suffering and inability to bear pleasurable sensation. Genital anxiety must be eliminated as well as the need to put the therapist in a bad light. This must be exposed as a masked aggression.

11 · Oral Character Types

ORAL SYMPTOMS ARE PRESENT in practically all neuroses treated, especially in the pregenital characters. They are particularly prominent in the chronic depressive, manic depressive, and alcoholic; in the severe manifestations of these neuroses the individual has retreated essentially to the oral stage. There is, however, a character type which functions basically at the oral level, the oral character. He is best described as inadequate; he lacks the drive of the phallic. The world is just too much for him. He is frequently considered schizophrenic because of his lack of drive, his inability for sustained effort, and his living much below his potential station.

Characteristics and Symptoms

The oral repressed character is usually tall, thin, sallow, and lacking in energy. He is a poor eater and food is tasteless to him. He is quiet, laconic, and speaks with an unusually low voice, through which nevertheless come caustic, biting comments. He bites his lips, swallows frequently, and is prone to sulk. He carries a constant air of resentment, usually has little to say, and easily retreats into his shell of inaccessibility. He is very sensitive and is easily slighted. He needs constant praise and encouragement. He hopes for understanding and love without effort on his part, but never feels he gets either. He complains constantly about this and feels he is not sufficiently appreciated.

Secretly, and often openly, the oral character asserts he has abilities never shown, but when given opportunity to show them he fails miserably, giving some excuse or other. He is inclined to strive for goals he does not have the energy to attain or maintain. He has little ability for sustained effort; thus he feels the world treats him badly. He does not make friends, is lonely, and has little to give. He may overtly admit he wants to be taken care of, and secretly all such characters feel they should be cared for as the infant is at the oral stage. In spite of grandiose ideas (infantile narcissism) his ego is weak; he holds a poor opinion of himself—and with good reason, in view of his weak showing in the struggle for life.

Such characters mostly content themselves with a marginal existence, persisting in waiting and hoping for grand success in their chosen field, which is frequently one of the performing arts. They have a passive stubbornness, a great degree of "I won't," and immobility. These characteristics make them unpleasant to live with and extremely exasperating. You wish you could shake some gumption into them. They cling and suck and are content to run up debts they have neither the ability to pay nor the concern to worry about. Such characters frankly expect support from more ambitious members of their families. They are especially inclined to depend long on their parents; spouses usually give up and leave in disgust.

They are chronically depressed but usually not too obviously so, although they constantly talk about suicide. This seems to be more out of a desperate effort to be understood than out of any serious consideration of ending their lives.

Characteristics and Symptoms: Oral Unsatisfied

This type varies from the oral repressed type chiefly in being more changeable. He is subject to periods of elation, overeating, alcoholism, and drug addiction. The alcoholic and manic depressive are essentially phallic characters but insofar as they give up the phallic level they become oral unsatisfied characters and return to the breast.

In therapy the oral character frequently refrains from admitting any improvement, presenting the same picture week after week, although friends and relatives may note remarkable changes. Sexually, he is inadequate and timid with the opposite sex. In the oral unsatisfied character, activity consists in considerable oral manifestations both heterosexually and homosexually.

Genesis

Repressed or unsatisfied, either oral character reaches the phallic level with a strong oral fixation, resulting in his identification with the mother, the phallus becoming identified with the breast. He clings to this level through his strong tendency to suck, contrary to the phallic who develops a strong drive for revenge. The alcoholic substitutes the bottle for the breast.

Therapy

It is important for the oral character to understand that his difficulties are due to his own inadequacy. He needs considerable character analysis but also encouragement. He needs to grasp his bona fide potential and give up his grandiose aims. His energy level must be raised.

Some of these cases are extremely difficult. I have the impression that they were emotionally deprived to such an extent that they never learned to reach out because there was nothing there to reach for. They do not even experience longing and cannot tell you what they want in life. They grew up in an emotional drought.

12 · Ocular Character Types

Schizophrenia (Ocular Repression with Panic and Splitting)

SYMPTOMS FROM THE OCULAR STAGE are prevalent not only in all neuroses but in the general population as well. Few people seem to have full development and integration of the eye segment. The schizophrenic, however, has certain basic characteristics stemming from this zone which stamp him with specific differences from other characters.

The schizophrenic, except in extreme cases, does not withdraw to this segment as the oral character does to the oral segment or the compulsive to the anal segment. Complete withdrawal would produce an essentially intrauterine picture with a foetal position and a complete shutting out of the environment. This is seen in some cases in psychiatric hospitals.

The exact difference between the eye block in the schizophrenic and that in other neuroses seems to be a result of the *time* at which blocking occurred. Reich states that in schizophrenia the block occurs in the first ten days of life, before any development takes place. In other neuroses blocking occurs later, even at puberty. Whatever its cause, the difference is quite evident[1] and

[1] William Goldfarb, *Childhood Schizophrenia* (Cambridge, Mass., Harvard Univ. Press, 1961), pp. 9–10. Goldfarb states ". . . observers became impressed by the receptor behavior of schizophrenic children, who demonstrated an un-

one can clearly differentiate the schizophrenic types, which comprise the major character types affected by this specific ocular block.

The types of schizophrenia are:

> *Hebephrenic—Hysteric with a repressed ocular block*
> *Paranoid—Phallic with a repressed ocular block*
> *Catatonic—Compulsive with a repressed ocular block*
> *Simple—Oral character*[2] *with a repressed ocular block*

The severity of the eye block determines how much other characteristics of the character type are given up and to what extent withdrawal to intrauterine existence supervenes. Schizophrenia is determined in the first ten days of life but, although some children develop schizophrenia, most cases are not fixed until puberty and overt symptoms do not present themselves until this period or later in life. Symptom development at puberty or later occurs in other character types as well.[3] As

---

usual pattern of receptor preferences in which the distance receptor modalities (hearing and seeing) were not used, and the proximal receptor modalities (touch, taste, and smell) were the chief bases for orientation to the environment. This failure to utilize the distance receptors affected adversely the children's ability to conceptualize and contributed to their uncertainty about their personal identity. Experience gained in the course of therapy concerning the reversal of phenomena such as visual avoidance or auditory exclusion (pseudo deafness) enhanced understanding of phenomena such as . . . the child's intrinsic capacity for perceptual stimulation. . . . In any case, it became clear clinically that unusual receptor preference could be reduced and that the child could be helped to use all sensory modalities for self-orientation. An example is the following excerpt from one child's psychiatric record: 'When approached during his first week at the Center, Philip would stare blankly and unseeingly. His pupils would remain dilated even as one moved to within a few inches of his face and peered closely into his eyes. He also seemed not to hear. At times he would actively cover his ears if merely approached visually. After a year of treatment he would dash into my office to greet me. He would look directly into my eyes and show a quick responsiveness to all of my spoken words.' "

2 This last classification is presumption based on previous knowledge of simple schizophrenia. I have had no experience in treating this condition in the light of the energy concept.

3 This statement is not to be taken as implying that children do not show neurotic symptoms. Most children do have symptoms (I have treated dozens, from infants to adolescents). The symptoms, however, do not appear in the developed form they take in typical neuroses; therefore, in psychiatric nomenclature, "behavior disorder" is used of children, "turmoil of puberty" is ap-

indicated above, the eye block in itself does not prevent progress to higher levels of functioning; the type of schizophrenia is determined by other usual factors of character formation.

Characteristics and Symptoms

Reich has found that the problem in schizophrenia is a disruption of unitary biophysical functioning, a distortion in the perception of this disruption, and the individual's reactions to both. Some of the symptoms are direct expressions of the biophysical disturbance; these, for example, are the faraway look, the trance, *cerea flexibilitas*, catalepsy, retardation, and automatisms. Other symptoms are secondary reactions to this disturbance; they can include disorientation, loss of power of association, loss of the meaning of words; and the withdrawal of interests. Symptoms such as grimaces and stereotypy are actually attempts at self-cure. The later general deterioration is due to the chronic shrinking of the organism.

The classical symptoms of schizophrenia in its various types are well known and are presented in any text on psychiatry.[4] Here, I will concern myself only with basic characteristics which are not so well known, but which are essential for a proper diagnosis. Four of the five listed below are symptoms resulting from ocular blocking.

First, perception and sensation are split apart. Both perception and sensation are acute and are preserved to a very high degree, whereas they are both dulled in other character types. However, because of the split, although sensation may be unimpaired its true origin is not properly perceived. That is, misinterpretation occurs.

Perception of the self depends on contact between the excitation and the subjective feeling of the excitation; that contact is a source of consciousness, which is a function of self-perception. When self-perception deteriorates, consciousness also deteriorates. With consciousness go all of its functions, such as orientation,

---

plied to adolescents, and so forth. It is not until puberty that the character is finally fixed to a point where more precise diagnostic terms are informative.

[4] Especially good is "Schizophrenia," by Arieti, *American Handbook of Psychiatry*, 1959, Vol. 1, pp. 455–502.

speech, and association. When the ability to perceive recedes to the point where, however acute, it becomes detached from bodily functioning, projection occurs. If, on the other hand, self-perception is not disturbed but merely reflects a rigid organism, as in affect block, then consciousness and intellect will simply be rigid and mechanical, not confused or disoriented as in the schizophrenic.

In paranoid schizophrenia, self-perception is severely disturbed and thus association and speech become disjointed. In the catatonic stupor, the organism is acutely and severely contracted and immobilized and speech and emotional reactions are usually altogether absent. In the hebephrenic, a slow deterioration and dulling of all the biophysical functions occurs, and here, perception and consciousness become increasingly dulled.

Schizophrenics are terrified of most people because they are acutely aware of the hate they see and feel constantly threatened. They do not see that most of this hate is safely caged in armor. Perception is, again, acute, but it seems as if the schizophrenic looks into the depths and reacts to what he sees there, rather than to what the other person actually will or can do—in view of his armoring and social restrictions.

Because they preserve perception and sensation to such a high degree, schizophrenics are quite alive and much in touch with health in a distorted way. They understand cosmic longing, but bring in considerable mysticism. Any increase in sensation causes them to go off in the eyes and lose contact with the environment. The eyes frequently have a vacant expression, as if staring into space. The distortion in interpreting sensation brings in delusional material, which is their version of what they feel.

The second of the five symptoms mentioned above is that the chest is soft but does not move perceptibly in breathing. The greater the eye block, the less armor is present in any part of the body except the ocular segment (especially the base of the brain). Usually the more armor present, the better the prognosis, especially if there is armor in the pelvis. This means more activity is allowed into the brain and there is less contraction there. This can be seen especially in catatonics, where armor may be quite complete and severe. In cases with a bad prognosis the musculature has a stringy quality. Muscles are especially stringy in long-standing cases.

Thirdly, the schizophrenic does not breathe. This is, of course, not literally true but in watching them one gets that impression. Certainly, air excursion is at a bare minimum. Frequently they cannot themselves even distinguish between expiration and inspiration. One wonders how they survive. The bare breathing may account in part for the underdevelopment found in many organs in the schizophrenic.

There is a fourth characteristic not so apparent but nevertheless present that accounts for some features. The energy field is extremely extensive and widespread and seems to have no boundaries. The schizophrenic does not distinguish between his body and his field reactions; in fact, he lives in his field rather than inside his skin surface. (See the ocular segment discussion in Chapter 4.)

The schizophrenic's perception, apparently functioning from any part of his field, enables him at times to see his body as if he were looking at it from various places in his environment. His field is diffuse and weak because his organism is unable to hold it together with his low energy level. (In analogy, one may say that Mars has a thin atmosphere because it has less gravity to hold gas molecules than Earth has.) For these reasons, the schizophrenic has a tendency to spread himself out on the couch, presenting a general lack of cohesiveness.

Finally, there is a very severe throat block, second only in importance to the eye block. It produces a low, soft voice, and greatly restricts ability for expression. Schizophrenics are thus shy, timid, and retiring, withdrawing quickly from any signs of attack or aggression around them.

Genesis

The ocular zone is the first developmental level. It is the first contact with the world and the first zone traumatized, probably mostly by hateful eyes and expressions in the environment, causing withdrawal in the eyes. Developmental restrictions in this zone are a severe handicap, because without its full growth no adequate perspective of the environment or even of the self is ever attained.

The schizophrenic lives in a world without perspective, literally in a world that speaks another language and sees other shapes. Withdrawal of energy from the eyes leads to insecure or absent binocular vision and a vacant expression in the eyes, and causes a contraction at the base of the brain. The patient may complain that his brain is dead or rotting away, or like a stone. The contraction that holds energy from the eyes is the major armoring of the schizophrenic. It lowers stimuli from the vegetative centers in this area, from the hypothalmic and pituitary functions and particularly from the respiratory center. Thus breathing is minimal.

Minimal breathing keeps the energy level low and reduces sensations and stimuli, so that muscular armoring is largely unnecessary. Armoring binds anxiety, blunts emotions and perceptions; since this does not occur in the schizophrenic he remains very alive and acutely aware of his environment. However, the awareness is distorted by lack of perspective (the split due to failure to develop binocular vision). Add to this the oral blocking from repression at the oral level and one has the typical picture of a shy, anxiety-laden individual who lives in a world full of distortions.

Therapy

The schizophrenic is characteristically shy and easily frightened. He must be handled cautiously. Get the patient to open his eyes. This leads to panic from movement of energy and from a flood of sensations. The panic starts breathing. Too much sensation will cause him to go off in his eyes and become psychotic. The eye segment is mobilized by having him roll his eyes and move his forehead. He must be desensitized to stimuli from the eye segment. This can be done by having him repeatedly go away in the eyes and bring himself back.

The prognosis is best in catatonia, where armoring is present. Remission may occasionally occur spontaneously when armoring breaks down and excitation bursts out. The paranoid has the next best prognosis because of the phallic aggression present. The hebephrenic has a poor prognosis because he combines hysterical anxiety with the shyness and withdrawal from the ocular block. During therapy, as the ocular segment is mobilized, muscular armoring will take its place and must in turn be broken down.[5]

Essential Epilepsy (Ocular Repression with Release in Musculature)

There are types of epileptic seizures whose origin is known, such as those due to scar tissue in the brain or meninges, trauma, pressure, or disease. Epileptic-type seizures are found in hysteria and, rarely, in schizophrenia. All of these are basically different from idiopathic or essential epilepsy, which is the only type I wish to discuss. The cause of essential epilepsy has been argued for decades. There are those who hold to a physical or chemical cause, pointing out the changes in the electroencephalogram, in the brain, and in the chemistry of the body. Others argue for an emotional basis, emphasizing the irritability and emotional problems found in these cases and the fact that epileptic fits have been cured by psychoanalytical treatment. It is well known that emotional distress will produce physical and chemical changes and endocrine imbalance. Further details can be found in any good textbook on psychiatry.

Reich discovered the eye block in epilepsy which seems to ally it closely to schizophrenia, to which it is antithetical, however. He also pointed out that the epileptic fit was an extragenital orgasm. In schizophrenia, opening the eyes wide or rolling them up produces panic and splitting. The same procedure in epilepsy causes the fit. It has been observed that epilepsy and schizophrenia are rarely found in the same individual and that when a schizophrenic developed epilepsy, the schizophrenia improved. This observation in fact led to the treatment of

[5] It may be worth noting that in the orgasm the eyes roll up, binocular vision is lost, and the organism withdraws from the world and merges with the cosmos. Great men may become psychotic by merging with the cosmos and finding it too painful to return to an unappreciative world lacking in understanding. The schizophrenic also merges with the cosmos by going off in his eyes.

schizophrenia by artificially inducing convulsions in shock therapy.

It seems that in the epileptic, unlike the schizophrenic, increase of energy is discharged into the musculature and provides release (extra-genital orgasm). The catatonic excitement apparently is an intermediate link and is closely allied to epileptic furor.

Epilepsy, like schizophrenia, seems to occur in any character type; but three-fourths of my epileptic cases were phallics. Muscular armor is present but not well advanced and in some cases is lacking. In such cases, the patient rearmors during therapy, as the ocular block is released.

Characteristics and Symptoms

The child, even as a pre-epileptic, is sensitive, stubborn, and given to tantrums and rages when reprimanded. He demands that things be done his way and refuses to participate unless he can be the leader. He is inclined to be moody, morose, distrustful, asocial, and unable to conform. Daydreaming is pronounced, especially when he is irritated or restrained. As the child grows older these symptoms become accentuated and he becomes irritable, selfish, egotistic, impulsive, asocial, and rigid, with evidence of cruelty and sadism.

Although epileptic seizures may appear in childhood, they usually occur at puberty or later, as do most symptoms of other character disorders. Classical epilepsy is divided into grand mal and petit mal seizures, but so-called epileptic equivalents and even such reactions as syncope, migraine, narcolepsy, and cataplexy must be considered variants. Occasionally a grand mal attack may make clear the meaning of former minor symptoms such as myoclonic, local muscle spasm, "Absences," and dreamy states.

The grand mal seizure[6] is the most dramatic of the epileptic manifestations. From a moment to several seconds before loss of consciousness about one-half of such cases have an aura or warning that a seizure is imminent. The aura may consist of numb-

[6] After Noyes.

ness, tingling, uncomfortable sensations, and a feeling of distress in the epigastrium, or it may consist of a hallucination of the special senses, such as flashes of light, certain noises, or olfactory hallucinations. The aura is usually affectively unpleasant. Sometimes it is motor in nature consisting of a twitching or stiffness in a certain group of muscles preceding the loss of consciousness.

Loss of consciousness is sudden and complete. At the same time the patient falls and may sustain serious injury. Interestingly, it is rare that an epileptic has a seizure when he is in a particularly dangerous situation. As he falls, the entire voluntary musculature goes into a tetanic contraction, often producing a peculiar sound as air is forcibly expelled from the lungs—the epileptic cry. At first the face is pale but soon becomes cyanotic. The pupils are dilated and do not react to light; the corneal reflex is absent. The bladder and even the bowels are often emptied. After ten to twenty seconds this stage is followed by clonic convulsions and respiration returns. The saliva which could not be swallowed becomes mixed with air and appears as foam. After this stage, the patient may show a period of confusion or automatism but finally becomes sleepy or stuporous. Convulsions may occur during sleep, and in some patients always do. Occasionally, one seizure may follow another in rapid succession, a serious condition known as status epilepticus.

Petit mal usually consists of momentary loss of consciousness with the individual rarely falling, though he may drop whatever he is holding. In some cases, sudden and extreme but seemingly motiveless excitement may occur during which impulsive, even violent and brutal acts are committed. This is known as epileptic furor.

Genesis

I do not know why the eye block in epilepsy allows the overflow of energy to escape into the musculature while in schizophrenia this does not occur. It may.be a matter of degree or, again, of the time at which blocking occurs. Whereas the schizophrenic avoids buildups of energy by severe blocking in the vegetative centers of the brain, the epileptic discharges such buildups into the musculature, thus producing the epileptic fit.

Therapy

The patient is desensitized to convulsions by having him initiate the convulsion by rolling the eyes upward and stopping it before it actually comes on by bringing the eyes back to contact. When the eye is mobilized, the various character disorders are treated as in previously described character structures. One will find a great deal of heartbreaking longing for mother love; the mother usually showed cruel and sadistic behavior.

A thirty-five-year-old male, who had been an epileptic for over twenty years and had been hospitalized for several years, reached a point in therapy where he no longer had seizures and they could not be induced during the session. At this point he began to have temper tantrums and finally reached for me.

He said he wanted to throw his arms around me, sobbing bitterly, and crying "Mama." He wanted his mother. He developed serious anxiety over his feeling for his mother and thought about her the whole following week, but each time he imagined her he would see her beating him with a tennis racket. When he returned for the next session, he continued reaching for me and, in the end, climbed into my lap and relaxed. For several sessions he felt intense longing and wanted to be held, a thing his mother had never done. When this situation had come out in therapy, he felt more alive, could breathe through, and felt at ease.

Voyeurism (The Ocular Unsatisfied Character)

There are probably few men who would not avail themselves of a good opportunity to look at women in various degrees of undress if it presented itself. This, however, cannot be considered voyeurism in the strict sense of the term. Two further characteristics are necessary; that the looking be unobserved (especially the woman must feel that she is unobserved), and that the looking largely or wholly replace genital sexuality. One patient of mine who had ample opportunity to observe his wife would steal out of the house at night and climb to the second story window to watch his wife in the bathroom preparing for bed. This neurosis is confined exclusively to males.[7]

Characteristics and Symptoms

My findings are based on the study of only two cases of voyeurism so that it is difficult to be certain what circumstances and symptoms are specific for this condition. As in all neuroses, symptoms are usually first apparent at puberty. The home and upbringing have been strict with much discipline from the father. The mother has been soft and seductive but completely dominated by her husband. She allows privileges to her son which excite but never satisfy. Siblings seem to be mostly girls.

At first voyeurs struggle considerably to fight off the impulse to look. It starts with observing the mother and sisters, later girl friends, and finally any women they can find. They run great risks in their voyeurism and are frequently caught by the police. This creates tremendous feelings of shame; in fact, in their early experience at home the family shames rather than upbraids them.

They seem to be highly intelligent and capable, but their aggression is inhibited; they are submissive and the work function is greatly interfered with because of an almost constant contemplation of sex that seeks satisfaction only in voyeurism. With women they are shy, timid, and ill at ease.

They complain of sensations in their brains similar to those of schizophrenics, describing the brain as dead, or feeling as if there were a stone in it. This may be a very prominent symptom and may be accompanied by a feeling of disability with pain, numbness, and weakness. The disability is felt in the right arm and leg if the "stone" is felt in the left side of the head, and vice versa. The eyes have a peculiar hungry expression.

Genesis

The mother is acquiescent and seductive. She stimulates looking but inhibits other modes of satisfaction. The father is strict

[7] Some authors include women whose curiosity is aimed at witnessing catastrophes, accidents, war scenes, and the like, where such curiosity represents active sadistic castration tendencies reduced from action to observation. I have had no experience with such cases but it would seem rather they were poorly sublimated forms of sadism.

and is determined to instill manly qualities in his son. He succeeds only in intimidating him. The household presents a "don't touch it" attitude that allows outlet only in looking. The boy reaches the phallic level with strong unsatisfied curiosity and much inhibition and submission. He identifies with the frustrating mother in his ego and with the father in his superego and retreats to the ocular voyeuristic level. Puberty revives the struggle, but the submission (to the intimidating father) causes regression to the level of voyeurism. Shame over this impulse requires that he be unobserved, and curiosity as to what the female does when she is unobserved adds the other ingredient of voyeurism. Castration anxiety and fear of the female genital are prominent factors in this character type. In the deepest sense, the voyeur is looking for the penis on the "castrated" female genital.

Therapy

The therapist mobilizes the eye segment. The submission contains great buried hostility, which must be released. The patient is encouraged to become aggressive. He must control his voyeurism and depend on therapy for outlet.

13 · The Socio-Political Character Types

THE PREVIOUS DISCUSSION of character types dealt with the world's sickness from the point of view of the individual, the manner in which his own life is molded from birth by an unhealthy environment. The following description of character types pertains rather to the individual's attempt to mold society (his environment) to fit his own irrational needs.

The individual character neurotic, crushed as he is by society, suffers from crippling himself; he does not usually inflict this damage on others. Therefore, one has a great deal of sympathy and compassion for him. The socio-political character also is sick, but insists on inflicting the effects of his illness on his environment by restricting and regimenting it. One understands his condition but has little tolerance for its destructiveness when it prevents others from leading satisfying lives and, in certain instances, has caused mass murders and the destruction of entire nations.

The three social characters may comprise any of the individual character types, but, in addition, possess certain specific conditions in their structure. The characteristic common to all three is that, unlike the symptoms of the previous characters, their symptoms are not felt as ego-alien so they are defended strongly and emotionally. Their social attitudes have always been with us and have been accurately depicted in literature, but they have not been understood characterologically until Reich showed the way to understand character. The three types are not just different ways of viewing the world and our civilization; they are necessary characterological expressions emerging from a specific structure and its defenses.

The first socio-political pattern is what Reich termed the emotional plague. It is the necessity of certain individuals, instead of working out their own problems, to set themselves up as the standards of normality and to make their environment, and everyone in it, conform to their own inadequacy. The plague character as such develops where a high energy level is combined with an insuperable pelvic block. However, most people have some emotional plague in them; we are familiar enough with the unfeeling mother who cannot stand healthy functioning and proceeds to mold her infant in her own image. Cruelty, criminality, nasty gossip, resentment of other's good fortune, all are examples of plague behavior, behavior not just unhealthy but destructive of the health of others. We can say that to the degree that an individual tries to tear down other people or control their lives, he is functioning as a plague character.

The other two social character types can and perhaps should be viewed in relation to the emotional plague, because the core of healthy social or political behavior is the ability to maintain a life-positive attitude for oneself, but barrng that, the ability at least to allow others to live satisfying lives.

Defense against feeling may be one of two types, although both may occur in the same individual: 1) muscular contraction, where contact with the core is not lost, but sensations from it are diminished or distorted, and 2) an intellectual defense.[1] where the individual largely or wholly succeeds in losing contact with the core, enabling him to live primarily in the superficial layer of his structure. It must be remembered that this is not primarily a matter of intellectual capacity or intelligence, but rather the use of such capacity as a defense in meeting the anxieties of life. This is a later or more sophisticated means of

---

[1] Cf. Character Analysis, *op. cit.*, p. 112.

defense than muscular armoring. Except for the few healthy individuals, mankind may be roughly divided into these two types; that is, those who live an intellectual rather than a feeling life, and those who still maintain contact, whether true or distorted, with their basic feelings and are to a great extent ruled by them. Few are pure examples, but the vast majority belong predominantly to one group or the other. I call the two types the liberal and the conservative. In their simplest form, both are legitimate attitudes toward the world and, when represented by equal numbers, they offer a good balance in social and governmental progress. Exaggerations and distortions of either attitude bring social and political chaos.

The basic characteristics of the liberal are a tendency to intellectualism, mechanistic explanations of natural phenomena, and a collectivistic attitude toward social living.

The conservative, on the other hand, tends toward a feeling attitude toward life, a mystical explanation of natural phenomena, and a selectivistic attitude toward social living.

Schematically, we can say that these are armored attitudes sitting to the right and left of the healthy or natural way of functioning. The closer to center, the nearer they approach rationality. The further they deviate, the more irrational they become, bringing in bias and distortion to defend themselves against natural living and functioning, which terrifies them. Exaggerations of the liberal are what I term the modern liberal, socialist, and communist, while exaggerations of the conservative are the extreme conservative, reactionary, and fascist.

The diagram on the following page attempts to illustrate schematically the extent of functioning of the various types in the three layers of character. The liberal characters live largely in the superficial layer while conservative characters function primarily in the core and middle layers. The ideally healthy person lives only in the core and reacts from it in all circumstances. His intellect and feeling are in harmony, not at odds.

The more the core or primary drives are blocked from expression, the more the middle layer builds up its harshness and brutality in secondary drives. These in turn must be held back by muscular contraction or intellectual censorship until the

SOCIO–POLITICAL CHARACTERS

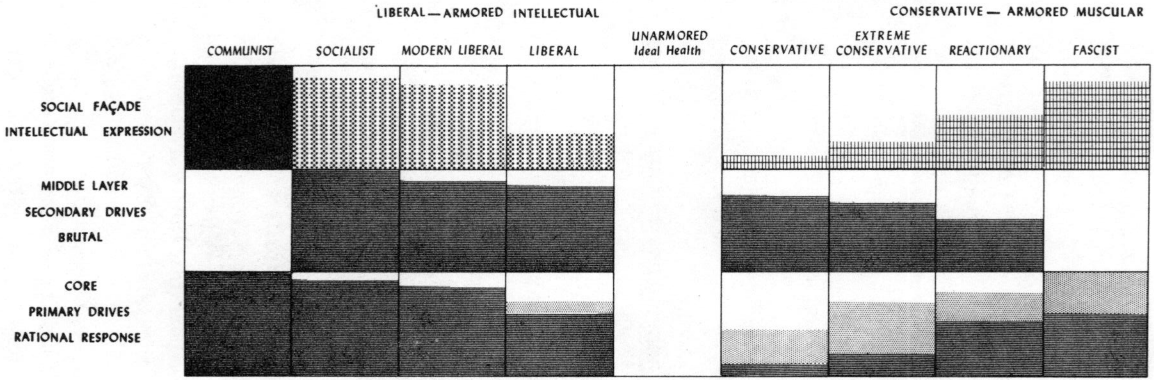

	LIBERAL — ARMORED INTELLECTUAL				UNARMORED	CONSERVATIVE — ARMORED MUSCULAR			
	COMMUNIST	SOCIALIST	MODERN LIBERAL	LIBERAL	Ideal Health	CONSERVATIVE	EXTREME CONSERVATIVE	REACTIONARY	FASCIST

Row labels (left side):
- SOCIAL FAÇADE / INTELLECTUAL EXPRESSION
- MIDDLE LAYER / SECONDARY DRIVES / BRUTAL
- CORE / PRIMARY DRIVES / RATIONAL RESPONSE

COMMUNIST: Ideology replaces religion and is all important. Individual only a tool. Beaurocratic Dictatorship. Freedom not tolerated. Justice by decree. Dialectic materialism. Machiavellianism. Sex physiological. Don't believe in love. Ruthless.

SOCIALIST: Individual unimportant compared to State. State owns all property. Non religious philosophical. Peace all important even at sacrifice of freedom and liberty. Mechanistic philosophy. Central Govt. responsible for welfare of all people. Initiative ignored. Ideological defense.

MODERN LIBERAL: Egalitarianism. Religion not important, tends to be philosophical. Peace more important than justice. Freedom and liberty less important. Education and Economics cure all ills of world. Govt responsible for education and economic security. Individual responsibility unimportant. Ideological defense. Sex-promiscuous. Revolutionary.

LIBERAL: Trend toward equalization, non-emotional religious. Justice and peace more important than freedom and liberty. Sex less discriminate. Obligations of Federal Govt. emphasized.

UNARMORED Ideal Health: Core and intellect in harmony. Contact with self environment and cosmos thus—Independent, responsible, secure. Freedom. Liberty. Justice. Peace for all. Local Govt. Work Democracy. Sex expression of love.

CONSERVATIVE: Decent. Religion replaces cosmic contact. Responsibility emphasized. Individual important. Central Govt restricted. Local responsibility for problems. Initiative rewarded. Freedom. Liberty. Justice. Peace in that order. Sex restricted. Social consciousness. Sex expression of love but virginity expected until marriage. Evolutionary changes.

EXTREME CONSERVATIVE: More fundamental religions. Country all important. Intensely patriotic. Freedom and liberty emphasized. Deserving individuals important. Local responsibility important. Initiative rewarded. Moralistic attitude toward Sex.

REACTIONARY: Status quo. White supremacy. Fundamental and evangelistic religions. Select individuals important. States rights. Sex morralistic and restricted. Ascetic. Sex considered animalistic. Brutality used to preserve concepts.

FASCIST: Racial dominance, religions distorted. Dictatorship. Race and Dictator important. Privilege and advantage for select groups. Brutal. Sex-sadistic. Absolute Authoritarianism.

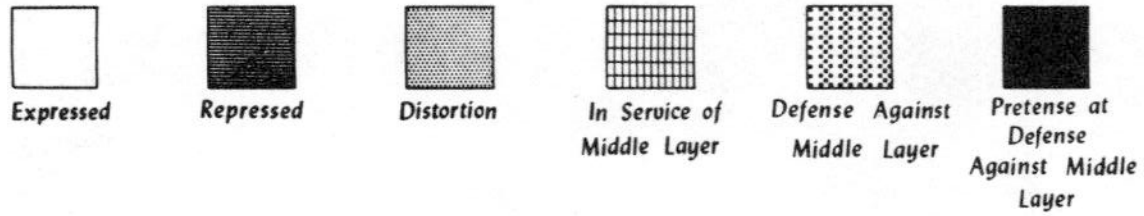

This chart is representative only and makes no pretense at being exact.

Legend:
- Expressed
- Repressed
- Distortion
- In Service of Middle Layer
- Defense Against Middle Layer
- Pretense at Defense Against Middle Layer

pressure becomes too great to maintain an equilibrium. On the conservative side of the spectrum, the individual maintains some contact with the core, even if distorted, which allows for fuller self-expression and tolerance of aggression. When equilibrium is disturbed, he begins to express his brutality; he rationalizes it mystically as necessary and in the best interest of the select groups involved. On the liberal side, where core contact has been lost, the individual must defend himself more urgently against any breakthrough of aggression. He brings in the intellect as his bulwark of defense, developing an ideology of humanitarianism (a reaction formation) and a desire for more and more central control to protect him from his own catastrophe. At the same time, the liberal becomes increasingly immobilized functionally until he lacks any aggression; he tries to substitute talk for action and reacts to aggression with appeasement. Finally, this defense also fails and the middle layer does break through, giving rise to the communist (red fascist). But even here the intellectual defense, no longer effective, continues outwardly to pretend that nothing has happened, denying the brutality and insisting on the humanitarian goals.

It must be remembered that all of these characters are convinced of the moral superiority of their particular mode of expression. Politics, like sex and religion, is indeed a sacred cow. Furthermore, people are not accustomed to having their philosophies subjected to clinical appraisal. Therefore, insight is conspicuously lacking, and, unlike symptoms of their personal character structure, these symptoms are successfully rationalized; that is, they are not ego-alien. This is partly because the individual has the security of millions of others who share his views, and he does not have to stand alone. But even more important, they do not threaten or interfere with his personal life, rather they protect and support it. When he is isolated in therapy and rationalization is no longer effective, strong emotional reactions, panic, and pure venom often ensue. Thus in discussing the social character types, I expect to be accused of bias, stupidity, ignorance, and so forth, just as I am accused of such things by the individual patient when his defenses are exposed. I do not presume to have the last word in understanding the socio-political character, but I believe this is at least a start.

An individual may take on socio-political ideas from his environment and education that are not in keeping with his structure. Such individuals change their ideation upon presentation of facts. For example, the majority of Americans have a basically conservative structure but from environment and education their political ideas may become liberal.

The healthy character maintains full contact. Contact with the self gives him independence, with his environment, responsibility, and with the cosmos, a feeling of belonging or security. He does not have to defend himself from his urges and so can behave rationally. He sincerely believes in freedom, liberty, justice, and peace for all. He lives in accordance with these values and does not need to proclaim his sincerity or concern for others, as his actions speak for themselves. He is self-respecting and self-reliant and would rather provide for his own welfare than accept government security. He spontaneously wishes to do his share for his community and nation and for the world as a whole, but he does not expect easy solutions to difficult problems and he will not give up his own identity for the sake of others. This attitude, if generally held, would probably result in some form of "work democracy" as outlined by Reich.[1]

The Emotional Plague Character[2]

Emotional plague reactions are due to sexual repression resulting in stasis; therefore no one is immune and anyone may experience a plague reaction at some time or another. There is, however, a type with specific structure who functions essentially as an emotional plague character. He may belong to any of the usual character types, with the addition of a particular type of pelvic block in a person of high energy.

The genital character is free flowing, direct, and life-positive.

[1] Wilhelm Reich, *The Mass Psychology of Fascism* (New York, Orgone Institute Press, 1946), Ch. X., "Work Democracy."

[2] For a more complete understanding of the emotional plague reaction see Reich, *The Murder of Christ, op. cit.*

The neurotic has been repressed by society so that although he longs for life he cannot live it and survives by flight, contactlessness, or reaction formations. The person suffering from the emotional plague is close enough to genitality so that he does not have these mechanisms available to any extent, but instead, handles his stasis by excluding natural excitation from his environment. He finds it necessary, therefore, to control the mores and attitudes of our culture and is life-negative. He cannot stand natural expression, because it creates a longing in him that is intolerable; that is why he tries to kill natural expression wherever he sees it. In this, he is actively aggressive and extremely competent. He rationalizes his behavior so well that it is accepted for the common good and tends to become organized in social institutions. His effectiveness is enhanced in that it finds response in the emotional plague existing in people generally.

Like character neuroses, the emotional plague is maintained by secondary drives. Plague is a function of character and is thus strongly defended; but unlike neurotic symptoms, the emotional plague is not experienced as ego-alien. It is rationalized to a very high degree and insight is lacking. However, as soon as the real motives behind the plague reaction are exposed, anxiety and anger inevitably develop. Everyone afflicted with the emotional plague is orgastically impotent, either chronically or shortly before the attack.

Characteristics and Symptoms[3]

The emotional plague is expressed in many forms: vicious gossip and defamation of character, pornography, bureaucracy, destructive mysticism, striving for authority over others, usury, race hatred, sadistic treatment of children, criminal anti-social behavior, all these are indications of the emotional plague character.

People with plague make the rules for children's behavior, put the taboo on sex, write the divorce laws, and make people conform to laws *they* can tolerate. They are the ones who report nude bathing or young lovers to the police and tell us what we can read and see. Occasionally the plague breaks out into a

3 For a more extensive discussion read *Character Analysis, op. cit.*

pandemic form, such as the Catholic Inquisition of the Middle Ages or the fascism—red or black—of this century.

It is an essential characteristic of the emotional plague that action and the reason given for it are never congruent. The real motive behind his action is always hidden and replaced by a more socially acceptable motive. For example, the plague-ridden mother who cannot enjoy any sexual pleasure, indeed, finds it "dirty," will not allow her children sexual expression under the guise of morality.

The emotional plague individual has no ability to accept change or difference of any kind. He differs from the healthy individual in that he must put restrictions not only on himself but even more importantly on those in his environment so that they conform more exactly to his way of thinking. These restrictions extend even to those who have no contact with his life at all. The mere existence of different ways of living provokes his antagonism. (This is why communism [red fascism] must conquer the world.) He can tolerate no belief which threatens his armoring or which might disclose his irrational motives. The genital frustration from which he suffers is the source of the energy (undischarged) which nourishes the emotional plague. This is the same stasis of energy found in other biopathies.

In those persons who are unable to experience natural orgastic gratification secondary impulses always develop; especially sadistic impulses. In fact, sadism is always present in fully developed cases of emotional plague. Fortunately for his victims, the person who suffers from the emotional plague has to give way temporarily when his motives are exposed and he is confronted, clearly and uncompromisingly with rational thinking. He is like a school-yard bully—protecting the smaller children from him doesn't help or change him.

The characteristic which most clearly distinguishes the emotional plague character from a neurotic character is the life destructive social activity of the former. Since his emotions are confused or irrational his concepts also become confused and irrational. His thinking is blurred. He always arrives at a conclusion before thinking it through; his opinion is set prior to the investigation. The thinking does not serve, as it does with rational minds, to lead toward a correct conclusion; rather it serves to confirm an already existing irrational conclusion and to rationalize it. This is commonly known as "prejudice." The emotional plague is intolerant of rational thinking that might expose it. Consequently it is inaccessible to argument. The given motive of an action is never the actual motive. This is true whether the hidden motive is conscious or unconscious. Such a person seriously and honestly believes his stated goal is correct and rational. But he is acting under a structural compulsion and cannot act except in this manner.

Such a character has no insight at all into the destructiveness or unfairness of his actions. He tries constantly to change his environment so that his manner of living is not interfered with. Everything that he encounters that is contrary to his mode of living or thinking provokes his anger and his opposition. His opposition, however, is so well camouflaged by socially accepted mores that it is difficult to refute or even to detect.

A good example is the attitude of doctors and hospitals toward newborn babies. A very charming and alive young couple of whom I am very fond recently had a baby. Before its birth they attended classes, at the hospital, on care of the newborn baby. During the course the instructress emphasized, "Remember, babies like to be wrapped tightly, even in hot weather. Be sure to wrap them up tightly." At the hospital the baby was separated from the mother except for feedings and under no other circumstances was the baby allowed to be with the mother. Also a great deal of pressure was put upon the parents to have the baby circumcised. Many reasons were given for the necessity of this procedure and the doctor became very angry when they refused, finally threatening, "Don't you know he will get cancer if you don't have him circumcised?"

The given motive in all three instances was for the benefit of the baby or mother: (1) "They like to be wrapped tightly." (2) The baby should be removed from the mother to allow her to rest and not be disturbed. (3) Circumcision is done for cleanliness and to prevent difficulties that may present because of the prepuce. It may be long and have a very narrow opening which can interfere with free urination or it may get pulled back over the glans and from restriction cause swelling and pain. Circumcision is also done to reduce the frequency of masturbation, to help prevent the possibility of venereal infection, and lastly to prevent the development of cancer of the penis. These are the given motives, accepted almost universally as reasonable and right.

In the first place, anyone who has seen a baby kicking and waving his arms about, gurgling with joy, cannot possibly believe, "the baby likes to be wrapped tightly."

In the second instance, a new mother and her baby need each other so both can relax and expand in each other's loving contact. When separated the mother worries and the baby is alone and suddenly bereft of the intimate contact he has had for nine months and still needs. He is brought to the mother only for feeding and this determined by the clock instead of his individual needs. This is easier for the hospital routine.

As to circumcision: The first sensation the baby feels from his penis is pain. I have seen babies cry and sob for hours after circumcision, in spite of the belief that they feel no pain from this operation. How incredible that this belief should have become so widespread. There is no doubt a baby feels pain if you accidentally stick him with a diaper pin. The four reasons given are true to some extent but in a negative sense. Today cleanliness is not an issue as it was in the past before daily bathing became common; any difficulties from a narrow opening in a long foreskin can be easily overcome by gentle dilatation; it does indeed reduce masturbation because pleasure is reduced as is his sexual satisfaction; circumcision *may* help avoid venereal infection—I doubt it. If it does it is probably more from his inhibited sexuality than from the loss of his foreskin; the incidence of cancer of the penis is extremely small and is usually found only in derelicts who have lived in filth. Whether circumcision would have prevented cancer in these cases I do not know but research has found that more babies die from circumcisions than there are deaths from cancer of the penis.[4]

What are the real motives? They are to stifle and kill the

[4] Douglas Gairdner, "The Fate of the Foreskin," *British Medical Journal* (Dec. 24, 1949), p. 1443.

natural flowing movements of the living because the plague cannot tolerate it. Bundle the baby so he cannot move, take the baby away from the mother so they cannot thrill in each other's presence, and circumcise the penis so it will retract and remain deadened. The plague believes it is sincere and righteous and is very convincing.

The sex life of the plague character, whether actually or vicariously expressed, is always sadistic and pornographic. Because of his structure he cannot help being pornographically lascivious and sadistically moralistic at one and the same time. This is the core of the character structure of the emotional plague. Even if he could develop insight and understanding he could not change this core. He develops intense hatred against any course of conduct which arouses in him orgastic longing and concomitant orgasm anxiety. To remove such arousal from his environment he demands puritanical moralism of those around him and directs sadistic rage against those enjoying a natural love life.

There is, unfortunately for society, a strong tendency among plague individuals to form organizations which are centers of public opinion whose main characteristic is an intense intolerance for natural love life. These organizations are found everywhere and under the ostensible motive of "culture" and "morals" they harshly condemn any manifestation of a natural love life. They are particularly skillful in character defamation from which they receive a kind of perverse satisfaction of a sexual nature. This is one way of experiencing sexual pleasure outside of the natural genital function. Perversions particularly are often met with in these circles. Their sadistic persecution is directed against the natural rather than against the perverse sexuality of others. And most especially is it directed against the natural sexuality of children and adolescents. They seem to be violently opposed to natural sexuality and completely blind toward any kind of perversion in themselves and others.

The emotional plague frequently hates work, particularly creative work, for to him it is a burden and a responsibility which he cannot tolerate. He flees responsibility especially from work which demands patient persistence. He may dream of doing important research, writing a book, of excelling in some chosen field but since he is incapable of enjoying creative work he cannot accomplish the organic development necessary to success in an endeavor. This inability gives him a tendency to engage in activities which do not require patient persistence and organic development. He may become a politician, a prophet, or a crusader for various causes or even an unemployed drifter. At the same time he feels others should work. In fact the less capable he is of working and the less self-confidence he has the more he is likely to boss others and tell them how to work.

Genesis

The emotional plague character is an individual endowed with a high energy, native intelligence, and ability, but with a pelvic block that does not allow discharge of excess energy. Instead of developing neurotic symptom formation to handle this energy, his defense is an active attempt to control his environment in order to prevent excitation, which would create intolerable orgastic longing and force him to sadistic fury. He is essentially an organism ready to burst, and must prevent excitation that would cause such bursting.

Therapy

Plague reactions in the average person usually respond when they are adequately exposed or stasis is relieved. This may even stop the attack in an emotional plague character but it does not change him. Theoretically he could be helped, but practically his high energy held by his particular structure and muscular armor render this impossible with our present knowledge. Furthermore, he seldom seeks help since his symptoms, consisting of a life-destructive social activity, are not ego-alien as are symptoms in the simple neurotic. They are rationalized so effectively that he feels no pain nor is he aware of being irrational and thus has no desire at all to change himself. Besides they give him his only means of satisfaction—a brutal, sadistic pleasure. This destructiveness shows the degree of force necessary for his energy to break through the armor. It emerges in the form of harsh secondary drives no matter how acceptably it may have started. The emotional plague longs for life but cannot live it, he longs for love but is incapable of it, and when he meets it he is driven to sadistic fury regardless of his best intentions.

The emotional plague can be eliminated from the world only through prevention by allowing or reestablishing a natural love life in children, adolescents, and adults.

The Liberal Character

The liberal side of the socio-political spectrum lies to the left or intellectual side of the natural or healthy attitude toward life and social living. Liberalism developed in an attempt to break away from the chains of repression and mysticism that held mankind in bondage for thousands of years. Seeking knowledge as the solution, man began to demand more and more freedom from his masters and from his gods. However, being biophysically unprepared to accept and handle that freedom, it caused increasing anxiety and guilt from which he found it necessary to defend himself; that is, from expression of his primary and secondary drives. Thus, his intellect, as well as being an outlet for expression, began to take on a defensive function against emotional release. In essence, the intellect having produced greater emotional freedom, it is now called upon to defend man against its effects. The brain takes on the defensive function of control, preventing emotional release, and becomes the sole outlet for expression. Energy is drawn up from the body, particularly from the pelvis, and contact with the core is at least partly, if not wholly, lost. Liberalism itself may be defined as the chronicity of this state.

Cut off from real feeling, he found himself in an intellectual world of words and ideas that offered very little organismic satisfaction. The intellectual path cannot lead to health, however much the "principles" may seem to coincide. He thus developed an urgency to find solutions that drove him on forever to constant change. But the solution is always out of reach because he can seek it only with his mind, which is itself preventing emotional expression and release. When contact with the core is given up, the feeling of personal responsibility and pride in one's accomplishments is lost. Thus the individual, feeling lost and anxious, looks not to himself but to an outside source to provide him with security. Eventually, with his own body controlled by his armored brain, he demands central control for his surroundings. Having lost touch with himself, the liberal tries to compensate by mass association and irrational ideas of brotherhood with people he has never met. He runs from solving his own problems to solving those of all mankind.

Vaguely aware of his situation and contactlessness, today's liberal attempts to regain contact through mass association and supports collectivism and urban living. His intolerance of feeling forces him to explain nature mechanistically and to overemphasize mental pursuits at the expense of actual living. It is understandable, with the liberal's emphasis on the intellect, that he should prescribe education and economic security as cure-alls for the world's evils. He has a misplaced optimism, misplaced because it comes from the brain and is not something he feels naturally, about man's perfectibility and believes with naive trust that his concepts of education and economic security will make man free.

Since nature creates feeling and cosmic longing which he cannot tolerate, he proceeds to destroy it by cutting down forests, blotting out scenic wonders with unnecessary dams, building expressways through irreplaceable redwood forests, or building huge, monstrous developments, all of which he insists are necessary for the "good" of the people. Art, music, and architecture become drab, mechanical, and ugly.

With suppression of emotional drives, he becomes increasingly immobilized and unable to tolerate aggression, except in abstract causes and verbalization. He thus finds himself moving further and further to the left from true liberalism to exaggerations and distortions of his original goal. His increasing emphasis on leveling eventually produces the socialist with his stifling and repressive society that eventually breaks through to the plague-ridden communist.

In America the changes of this century have been accompanied by a general shift in attitude toward the left side of the sociopolitical spectrum. The change to an urban industrial economy has brought with it greater dependency upon centralized, depersonalized authority and removal from direct contact with the land and its creatures and the expansiveness of agrarian life. Two world wars have increased our contact with the world and demolished the former sense of security; Darwin and Freud have played havoc with the set ideas of our forefathers; there is increasing leisure, and easy travel, and communication have made the world small.

The liberal's demand for greater freedom has in part been answered. However, that freedom has come about largely through technical and scientific, that is, intellectual advances, not through bioemotional readiness. Mankind is little more ready than it has ever been to handle freedom rationally and responsibly and thus what should have been true freedom is actually just license and confusion.

In a great many cases, the conservative has yielded to the temptation of the new freedom flourishing around him and has taken on a liberal outlook not in keeping with his structure and as a result he is now adrift, confused, and alienated.

From the outset, the liberal tends to belong to an academic, literary, scientific, or artistic milieu, although any career is acceptable so long as it emphasizes brainwork over physical. For example, it is not the union members, the toiling masses, and so forth who provide the bulwark of liberal attitudes but the leaders and organizers of working people, "the brains at the top," and this has historically been true of communism itself as well as Fabianism.

The liberal is, to a far greater degree than the conservative, obsessed by guilt.[5] In part, this is due to the liberal's lack of re-

[5] James Burnham describes this guilt well in *Suicide of the West*, pp. 195–197, published by John Day Co., New York, 1964. He says, "The guilt of the liberal causes him to feel obligated to try to *do something* about any and every social problem, to cure every social evil . . . even if he has no knowledge of the suitable medicine, or for that matter, of the nature of the disease; he must *do something* about the social problems even when there is no objective reason to believe that what he does can solve the problem—when, in fact, it may well aggravate the problem instead of solving it. . . . The real and motivating problem, for the liberals, is not to cure the poverty or injustice or what not in the objective world but to appease the guilt in their own breasts; and what that requires is *some* program, some solution, some activity, whether or not it is the correct program, solution and activity. The

course to religion to handle the guilt. In part, it is due to the lack of a definite idea of right and wrong, so that he always feels wrong. In part, it is due to subversive rebelliousness against the parent, in contrast to the open competitiveness of the conservative. Also, however, the tremendous display of guilt derives from loss of core contact as such, and substitution of intellectual for direct emotional response. He feels, rightly, an element of unreality or insincerity in voicing this concern for others, and to the extent that he is not deceived himself by the image he presents, he feels he is deceiving others. He is therefore driven to prove his sincerity by showing even more concern. Thus begins an endless self-perpetuating process, which can be halted only if he will stop trying to escape from his own problems to those of others.

Characteristics and Symptoms

The Liberal. The liberal is generally a verbal type, optimistic, intelligent, and prone to intellectualism. He is outwardly sophisticated, emotionally superficial. The energy concentrated in the head gives him buoyancy and general lightness, having nothing to do with actual weight; his feet are not quite on the ground. He is prone to anxiety and concomitant impatience. His outlook is mechanistic so he usually likes urban life. His acute intellect often makes him sensitive and perceptive, but intellectualization also prevents great depth of feeling. His emphasis is as much on style as on content. Violence is abhorrent to him, aggression disturbs him; he would not choose a career in the military, police, or FBI. The liberal's concentration of energy in the brain allows for fuller development of mental talents, but at the expense of contact with his core. His values are thus less in keeping with nature, more superficial. Thus his character is less stable than the conservative's and more prone to degenerate into exaggeration and destructive social attitudes.

---

good intention . . . plus plenty of action is assumed to guarantee the goodness of the program."

This may well explain the recent immolations that have entered the American scene. Unable to force their solutions on the public and thus atone for their guilt, these people become so frustrated and overcome with guilt their only relief is to sacrifice themselves by fire, which offers a symbolic purification.

Socially, the liberal is a moderate who stands, both rationally and out of guilt, for extensive improvement for the lot of the common man. Pushed to impatience by anxiety, and disillusioned with the slowness and inefficiency of social progress, he calls upon a central government to innovate and force changes. Believing in the common man and identified with him, he is sure he will respond to these changes by assuming the necessary responsibility to handle them. He calls for more education, an easing of moral restrictions, and less repressive religions, all of which are unquestionably commendable goals. Having maintained some contact with his core, he has feeling, but his intellect is dominant in trying to solve the problems of humanity. He does not understand the structure of man, with its sexual repression and guilt, and cannot see that this structure will not allow man to respond to freedom, nor to accept it. Thus bewildered, the liberal believes that ever more and more change is necessary, so he must continue his Herculean task forever onward. His outlook is constructive, but hampered by insufficient insight and by his own guilt and anxiety. Certainly he effects much good, and when his ideas are well balanced with the conservative philosophy, the result is a very satisfactory solution to social progress.

The true liberal is open to reason and facts, is accessible and naturally polite. He can openly show his disturbance at facts and reasons that shake his prior beliefs and is capable of change. If he becomes emotional, he may express appropriate anger at abuses or frustrations, but he never becomes hysterically derisive like the modern liberal, because he has no need to defend his beliefs by a dogma. His liberalism seldom comes up as an issue in therapy.

The Modern Liberal (Collectivist). Strictly speaking, although he calls himself one, the modern liberal is not a liberal at all, but a collectivist. He is strongly defended by a dogma and when this is attacked he becomes contemptuous, derisive, and replies with verbal formulas and sarcasm.[6] He has an unshakable, unrealistic conviction of his own infallibility and intellectual

[6] For an excellent exposition of modern liberalism as an elaborate system of dogma read, James Burnham, *Suicide of the West* (New York, Day, 1964).

superiority. This attitude becomes a crucial one in therapy.[7]
Nietzsche has described such a modern liberal as follows:[8]

> There is a very narrow, imprisoned, enchained sort of thinker who
> wants approximately the opposite of our intentions and instincts. . . .
> They belong, to make it short and sad, among the *levelers*, these falsely
> named "free-thinkers." They are glib-tongued and scribble-mad slaves
> of democratic taste and its "modern ideas"; all of them are men with-
> out solitude, without solitude of their own; what they would like to
> strive for with all their power is the universal green pasture-happiness
> of the herd: security, lack of danger, comfort and alleviation of life
> for everyone. Their most frequently repeated songs and doctrines are
> "equal rights" and "compassion for all that suffers." Suffering is taken
> by them as something that must be abolished.

Characterologically this liberalism represents a misfired solution to the problem of guilt and anxiety: the anxiety gets bound
up in political attitudes and ties, fixed to a specific and characteristic ideology. These "self-evident" truths the modern liberal
sees as unshakable and unarguable, since any attempt to challenge
them shakes the very core of his defenses and stirs up intolerable
anxiety. The modern liberal retains the essential character structure of the true liberal, but in an exaggerated form; he is further
from genital primacy and less capable of rational functioning.
He expounds all the ideas of the true liberal, not any longer for
their own sake, but because they give him the feeling of righteousness and purpose. His humanitarianism is largely rationalization.
His concern for others is not at all sincere, as in reality he is
quite venomous, and his sympathy for the underdog is merely a
reaction formation. The modern liberal lives almost entirely in
his intellect. His brain is his substitute for genital potency; it

[7] Although modern liberals are actually few in number compared to true
liberals or environmental liberals, their influence is felt out of proportion
to their number because their anxiety presses them to force acceptance of
their needs and since, by nature, they are clever, vociferous, and exceptionally
articulate. They are the policy-makers behind the scenes in government or
the writers of articles of opinion in intellectual magazines and other media
of communication. It is because their dangerous ability to influence the
thinking of people not only in this country but throughout the world is so
great at the present time that I devote so much time to a description of their
character structure.

[8] From *Beyond Good and Evil*, Friedrich Nietzsche, H. Regnery Co.,
Chicago, 1955, paragraph 44.

gives him a basis for feeling superior, much as the phallic character uses his erect penis to feel superior. The liberal pierces everyone around him with his sharp brain. In place of phallic contempt, the liberal uses intellectual contempt, arrogance, and clever verbal castration. His wit is barbed, amusing at the expense of others. He is void of kind or gentle feelings, except superficially in his causes, and that of course stops all argument, since anyone who "feels so deeply" about the injustices of the world must be above reproach.

This intellectualism is his chief defense against feeling, especially his guilt and anxiety which color and pervade all his attitudes. His anxiety makes immediate fulfillment of his needs imperative, so he tends to favor revolutionary rather than evolutionary tactics. Since his real problem lies elsewhere, he is never satisfied, but needs to advocate constant change and expediency rather than long-range goals. Behind his guilt lies the unresolved Oedipal conflict with the father, whom he fears. Characteristically, he is secretly rebellious against the father[9] whereas the conservative is openly competitive. Because he cannot compete with the father, he hates both the competition and the father and identifies always with the underdog, the unsuccessful and the indolent. Subversively defiant, he dare not show any open aggression, so great is the fear of the father and so intense the guilt. Moreover, his biosystem cannot stand it.[10] He can allow himself to be aggressive only in causes and abstractions. Any other aggression fills him with intense anxiety and leads him to pacify, compromise, appease. For this reason he is unable to assume responsible leadership whether it be in government or in raising a child. Privilege he wants as a right and not something that must be earned competitively.

The liberal's intellectualism, guilt, and fear of the father leads directly to his egalitarianism. He feels guilt at his own success or advantages and is thus opposed to differences in social structure. Basically he needs to feel that all people are the same. They are

[9] Although this is literally true in many cases it is meant rather as an expression of rebellion against the father image or heritage. The same is true in the case of the conservative's identification with the father.

[10] See "Genesis," p. 183, for further discussion.

brothers and should fraternize freely. Because of his anxiety he cannot wait for evolutionary change and therefore advocates governmental social and economic planning, at a federal rather than local level. He wants the government to remove all differences among people (leveling). From this he gets a sense of belonging which dilutes his guilt. No one (the father) is better than he, no one (the criminal) is worse. The liberal is essentially a socially oriented being, a part of the herd, and depends on the herd for security and the expression of his needs. Security, then, becomes more important than freedom and independence and even genuine justice.

In his secret rebellion against the father he identifies with the underdog. An extreme form of this is his sympathetic indulgence of the criminal with whom he identifies through guilt.[11] This indulgence of the criminal the liberal calls his "enlightened" or "modern" attitude of "understanding" the criminal. Punishing the criminal activates his own guilt and interferes with his ability to suppress criminality and juvenile delinquency. The criminal, the delinquent, and the law-abiding citizen all become "equal." At the same time, liberals view the entire military with contempt, as they do the police, because (1) their purpose is to protect society, not rebel against it, and (2) these are not intellectual careers but active, aggressive ones, and what the liberal cannot accept, he derides. This is of course, an emotional plague reaction. That the military and police provide for his personal safety and well-being, and this at great peril to themselves, evokes no feeling of gratitude or admiration.

11 In a letter to the New York *Times*, October 4, 1964, Daniel Gutman, Dean of the New York Law School and former President Justice of the Municipal Court of the City of New York, said in part: "Every day in the week lawyers engaged in defending criminals argue that it is better for '100' or '500' or '1000' guilty men to go free than have one innocent person punished. This interpretation of the ancient biblical axiom means that it is better to let loose an army of inhuman felons on society than to risk erroneous conviction of an innocent person. The possibility of error cannot be entirely eradicated. . . . We are virtually encouraging criminals. . . . Every safeguard must be provided to protect the innocent [but] every proper means should be invoked to enable us to combat . . . the evil, destructive acts of the wanton criminal. . . . In many of these cases where the convictions have not been permitted to stand, the guilt of the accused has been established beyond any doubt . . ."

The liberal's need to identify with the underdog is most passionately expressed in his stand on the racial question. In this, as in all his causes, the liberal is hysterically impatient. His anxiety will not allow him calmly to consider what is best for the Negro or for the whole country in the long run. Thus the Negro must have all rights and privileges immediately; some liberals even advocate giving the Negro preferential treatment to compensate for past wrongs, which would only result in reverse bias. The liberal fails to see that one may oppose segregation without calling for enforced integration. He tries to correct social wrongs by legislation, but the real problem goes back to biophysical readiness, which means responsibility. This requires change of structure, reorientation, and education, through gradual rather than sudden processes, for both Negroes and whites. Because the liberal has little feeling for true responsibility, he also ignores the Negroes' share of responsibility for their behavior and situation in life.[12] He rationalizes and excuses Negro lawlessness and rioting as expected behavior from their long suppression. At the same time he agitates that the Negro be given a responsible say in the affairs of the country.

One must also mention the degree to which the collectivist attitude is built into the civil rights movement. The liberal does not speak about this or that particular Negro whom he knows personally, he talks about "The Negro." To him the Negro is not an individual, self-respecting person, but just a representative of "Negroness." All Negroes are thus one and the same, their color is the only significant thing about them . . . an extremely insulting idea. There is an underlying attitude of insincerity and

[12] A Negro clergyman in Harlem, Bishop James P. Roberts, had the courage to say of conditions there, "Instead of hurting the children and talking of bussing, let's get down to the main trouble in Harlem schools, the indifference of the Negro parents and the lawlessness of their children. . . . But first we must show that we can be responsible in our own community; this is not a question of poverty but one of morality." New York *Times*, February 14, 1964. A few other Negro leaders have similarly pointed out the need for responsibility. This is not a modern liberal attitude.

The Interfaith Health Association in Queens, Long Island is another good example of responsibility in the community. This association has already won a small victory in eliminating both slum and slum psychology and at the same time promoted true integration rather than a paternalistic one.

superiority at work here, creating an artificial barrier between the white and the Negro which the latter quite rightly resents. One finds a New Yorker traveling to Alabama to join the cause, while he gives little if any thought to the living conditions of the Negro maid who has worked for his family for twenty-five years.

Many injustices are committed on the altar of social consciousness.[13] I do not mean to imply that a sense of social justice is pathological. One has to look at the source. In the liberal the express motives are not the real motives. There is a great difference between a stock altruism based on hidden guilt and a genuine feeling for the golden rule, reality based. This stock altruism is not open to argument, because the liberal does not argue rationally, rather he uses sarcasm to imply that any intelligent and reasonable person would think as he does. He supports his premise by rhetoric rather than logic.[14] He mentions reason often in his arguments—and even enthrones it as a panacea[15]— but seldom is he open to it.

Through his intellectualization he has withdrawn energy from

13 Cf. Wilhelm Reich, *The Murder of Christ, op. cit.,* pp. 217–218. Reich says "Liberals will tell you that the plague has a right to free speech, too. Yes, but in the open fresh air only, not in the dark corner of my backyard, in the middle of the night with a knife in the fist ready to strike me in the back. The help rendered to the plague by the liberal soul is enormous. The new leader will have to surmount the defense of the plague by the liberal soul. . . . He will have a hard time convincing the liberal soul that liars and murderers and gossipers and defilers of honor are criminals against the security of freedom and happiness of men, women and children. . . . Here the liberal, meek souls become truly dangerous. Weak in their guts with no prospect ahead of themselves, resting only on a once valid great doctrine of humanism they delivered the German society to the Nazis and they may succeed in delivering the American society to the habitual spies of the reactionary Russian empire. Such liberals are deeply impressed, though they may not feel or know it, by the skill and show of power on the part of the generals of the organized plague; they succumb to the temptation like virgins weakened in the virtue of abstinence submit to the knight in shining armor. Beware of the soul which always appears meek and softspoken and which never raises its voice in anger or revolt against evil. . . . They are the more dangerous in that they use the most peaceful and innocent dreams of people for their evil doings."

14 Cf. Sydney Hook's discussion of the ritualistic liberal who relies on rhetoric rather than logic, slogans rather than analysis of problems. *Political Power and Personal Freedom* (New York, Criterion Books, Inc., 1959).

15 Just as the French revolutionaries proclaimed "The Age of Reason."

his pelvis. He has largely or wholly lost contact with his core, that is, with his natural feelings, and substituted a superficial social façade of concern for all mankind. He likes to think of himself as a world citizen and has contempt for nationalism, a defensive repudiation of his country (father) and its success. His concern for the peoples of the world is purely verbal, especially in those who approach the extreme left of the spectrum. It is based on security of the herd needs rather than humanitarianism. It is also a reactive defense against his real contempt for people. He has no loyalty to home, community, or country.

His intellectualism makes the modern liberal mechanistic rather than mystical. Religion is taken lightly if not discarded altogether for a purely mechanistic philosophy or dialectic. Having no recourse to religion to solve or handle his guilt, he is driven relentlessly to solve all problems of humanity with an overpowering immediacy, regardless of the rationality of his means or solutions. He is unaware that neither mechanistic nor mystical philosophy can really solve problems which must be approached functionally.[16] He thus advocates with firm conviction the efficacy of the "universal dialogue." He does not say discussion and this is interesting and correct. He does not believe in discussion but merely in words. He talks and writes voluminously but never gets to the point.

Sex, like religion, the liberal also takes lightly. As supporter of "modern" sex concepts, he calls for sexual freedom, as he does for all other freedoms, but does not want the responsibility that goes with it. Thus what he really supports is license and promiscuity.[17] Cut off from real feeling, he writes books on sex—glib, unrestrained, and irresponsible as to what they urge on the public. He misleadingly depicts "different kinds of orgasm," that is, pregenital orgasms in adults, as the goal of genital union and is totally ignorant of the nature and function of genital orgasm. He equates fornication with genuine sexual love or else denies that sex and love have any connection. His excessive concern over the minutest details of pregenital play, his mechanical and

---

[16] Wilhelm Reich, *Ether, God and Devil, op. cit.*, pp. 62–96.
[17] One can understand his interest in pornography, which is essentially an intellectualized sexual outlet. He frequently calls this art.

studied approach, are in direct proportion to his personal orgastic frustration and impotence. Glutting oneself with secondary compensations of sex is comparable to the chronic overeating of the orally blocked character.

Another facet of the liberal approach, particularly in keeping with his intellectualism, is in his promotion of progressive education. This is a misinterpretation and distortion of the teachings of the liberal philosopher and educator John Dewey and his followers. The emphasis is placed on social adjustment, group activities, group thinking, and social studies rather than on learning *per se*. Discipline is given minimal consideration if any, and students are promoted automatically regardless of marks. Competition is considered bad for the child, and it is felt that examinations should be eliminated. Since World War II there has been a trend orienting the child toward thinking of himself as a world citizen, downgrading patriotism, loyalty to country, and respect for America's past heroes.

Or, the modern liberal may attempt to follow the teachings of A. S. Neill of Summerhill. He claims to be "on the side of the child" but fails to understand either Neill or the child.[18] The result is a guilt-distorted, mechanical application of "freedom-oriented" and "sex-affirmative" techniques in which "all the right things" are rammed down the child's throat, creating confusion, resentment, frustration, brattiness, beatnikism. What is ignored is the child's emotional capacity to accept such teachings or to assume the responsibility for their correct application.

The liberal's attitude toward personal freedom is accurately reflected in his attitude toward political freedom. There is a great hue and cry for the independence of underdeveloped countries (the underdog again) and against the tyranny of colonial rule (overthrow of the father). The fact that these countries are frequently unprepared to govern themselves responsibly, that freedom means only license to them, that horrifyingly barbaric behavior, war, and chaos result, these things the liberal cannot allow himself to see. Rather he continues to insist that not only

---

[18] This does not apply to all schools that follow Neill. The Fifteenth Street School in New York City, for example, is seriously interested in the welfare of the child and has a true understanding of freedom.

must they be independent but have an equal voice in world government with the major powers. He reacts to the poor results of his liberal policies with only increased doses of liberalism. He is not really concerned about freedom, as is obvious from the fact that he has shown little concern for the billion people who since 1945 have been enslaved by communism. Freedom is only the expressed motive, not the real one.

The same is true in the matter of civil liberties. Everyone must have equal rights regardless of motive or responsibility. Thus, for example, the liberal supports the rights of communists even though their purpose is to take away those same rights. He claims that his emphasis on what he interprets as constitutional not only guarantees, preserves, and defends democracy, but actually immunizes us against communism. Therefore, he reasons, we can permit communists the same freedom and accessibility to impressionable minds as we do any other group. This is comparable to saying that the criminal has as much right to mold youthful minds as the honest man, or that exposure to a mortal disease is a good test of health. In this he is not only dangerously foolish but insincere as well, for he shows no interest in defending the rights of conservatives, let alone reactionaries or fascists, all of whom terrify him, because, whether directly or distortedly, they make contact with the deeper characterological layers. It is not surprising then, that a Caryl Chessman and the Rosenbergs could have stirred up their greatest reactions, whereas the imprisonment and persecution of Wilhelm Reich caused not a ripple in their passion for "justice" and "civil rights." Indeed, they themselves, in both their scholarly journals as well as their smutty periodicals, have contributed and still do to the defamation of Reich and his work which deals with emotions they cannot tolerate.[19]

The liberal does not set out specifically to foster communism, he sets out only to protect his own defenses. Yet liberalism is every day steering civilization toward communism and away from free-flowing life. In becoming emancipated from old repressions and restrictions, the human being must be that much more ade-

[19] Such articles have appeared in *New Republic, The Menninger Bulletin, Commentary,* The New York *Times* Magazine, The New York *Post, True, Real, Time, Nugget,* etc. etc.

quate and capable of accepting the greater responsibility which goes with greater freedom. Never having understood himself and his feelings, however, and never having been capable of behaving rationally, he was not prepared for any new freedom. He has reacted to it by increased fear of life, and, as a result, by trying to reduce the size of life to the size of his own brain. Every day contact with himself and his true feelings becomes that much more difficult and that much more to be feared. In his effort to keep control, he has become not only more irrational, like the ordinary neurotic, but has moved increasingly toward controlling other people, like the emotional plague. Total mechanistic control over everyone is what communism is, and as the liberal moves steadily and quickly to the left, the point will occur where liberalism turns into communism. The process is evident in the fact that the liberal is today less interested in opposing communism than in opposing conservatism. The liberal considers that the enemy is to the right; communism is "not so bad."[20] In place of the old self-control imposed by repression and taboos, there is now to be the "improvement" of mass control by bureaucracy. In place of a sex-negative attitude imposed upon a basically healthy feeling of life, there is now to be sexual "freedom" with the loss of the capacity for love. The latter is by far more life-negating. Contact with nature has been given up, without which man has no feeling of belonging, no real home, without which life is no longer life but only a worthless imitation.

It is this core of total devitalization in the liberal which is responsible for his attitude of "peace at any price." Functionally, to be at peace is to be bioenergetically unblocked, to flow and stream, consonant with a deep, inner feeling of well-being. That

[20] Malcolm Muggeridge, British critic, in his review of *The Liberal Establishment*, by M. Stanton Evans in *Esquire*, September 1965, makes the following statement: "We liberals are so made that . . . anyone foolish enough to be on our side is a villain. We despise a Tshombe who, by and large, would seem to be well disposed toward us, and venerate a Nkrumah, who hates our guts and never hesitates to say so. . . . Liberalism will be seen historically as the great destructive force of our time; much more so than communism, fascism, nazism or any of the other lunatic creeds which make such immediate havoc. . . . As mankind goes to their last incinerated extinction, the voice of the liberal will be heard proclaiming the realization at last of life, liberty, and the pursuit of happiness."

is, there is no such thing as peace without true inner freedom. Those whose devotion to peace is real know full well that there is a time for tranquility and a time for fighting.[21] The pacifistic liberal of today is seeking rather to arrange his environment so that there is the least disturbance to his crippled energy system. His assumption that the communistic plague can be appeased, educated by example, or blackmailed by world opinion is, from the functional energetic viewpoint, an untenable illusion. It is an acute political myopia; he cannot look clearly at the political situation because it is a product of his own structure, which he cannot afford to view objectively. The pacifist is using his intellect to rationalize his real motive, which is fear of genuine movement. He can propose only one solution. Talk. But no matter how prolific or eloquent he is with words, he is, very simply, unable to get to the point. The pacifists and ban-the-bomb groups call for peace at any price. To this end they are for unilateral disarmament of the non-communist world: "Better

21 Paul Mathews points out: "The tragedy is that as each error is compounded, a strong assertion on our part does seem to become more portentous and cataclysmic. What is forgotten is the liberal pattern of concession and appeasement over the years which led to this predicament. The liberals continuously validate present concessions and appeasement on the basis of unfortunate situations created by past concessions, and become more and more righteous in the process. Like the communists, the liberals, too, are driven into a desperate system of rationales for their constantly compounded errors and refuse even more doggedly to acknowledge them. It is an endless cycle. If it is frightening now to think of invading Cuba, for example, it is because certain concessions based upon the liberal attitude should not have been made at Yalta, Korea, China and the Bay of Pigs in the first place. One must remember that the liberals since 1945 allowed one billion people to be swallowed up into slavery under communism and forgot them—at the same time crying for the independence of nations not yet ready. It is also because the liberal attitude on the internal situation encouraged the series of espionage fiascos which expedited the communist acquisition of the A-bomb. We must go back to the basic sources of historical perspective to understand the pernicious consequences of character attitudes upon our lives. We must wonder now whether the risk of a dramatic assertion of force in Cuba or in South Vietnam or formerly in Korea would not, in the long run, be considerably less precarious than the continuous appeasement which eats away little by little." *Functional-Energetic Thought and Contemporary Social Phenomena* (unpublished).

Robert Murphy in *Diplomat Among Warriors* clearly expounds the pattern of liberal-motivated appeasements which led to our present dilemma.

Red than Dead." They equate Russia morally with the U.S.A. and sometimes imply that its motives are loftier.

The modern liberals play up our guilt over Hiroshima and Nagasaki and say that only the U.S.A. has been inhumane enough to use the bomb. They ignore the fact that the bomb was deemed militarily necessary at the time and may have saved many more lives than it destroyed. This guilt over our use of the bomb is intended to suppress even necessary aggression by psychic de-vitalization.[22] Behind the liberal exhortation is a crippled energy system which cannot tolerate movement or healthy aggression.

The modern liberal is contemptuous of capitalism. The ex-pressed reason is that capitalism is cruel and heartless: the real reason is that capitalism is cruel to *him*, because it is a system in which individuals must compete on their own, which he cannot tolerate. The liberal thus favors governmental control over a free market and federal rather than local control. This effectively removes the element of his personal responsibility, either for his own welfare or for his social projects. The expressed motive is to help those unable to succeed; the real motive is to eliminate success, so that he will not have to feel anxious and inferior. Otherwise said, his wish is to castrate the successful (father) and to eliminate the means by which people become successful (what might be called castration of the nation, i.e. the fatherland). The stated motive is never the real one, which is why I call his rebellion subversive. The liberal's opposition to all differences in social structure, is, likewise, an expression of his need to pull down the mighty (father).

The Socialist.   The socialist emphasizes what he feels are the economic evils of capitalism. His aim is the complete abolition of class (individual distinction) whether through confiscation of property or taxation. The socialists maintain that conditions of the modern world demand varying degrees of collectivism and the individual is unimportant compared to the state. The present and past generations of the "haves" are guilty of and responsible

[22] See Sydney Hook's book *The Fail-Safe Fallacy*, Stein and Day Co., New York, 1964, for an excellent exposition of the dangers to freedom induced by liberal "peace-mongering" and exploitation, in distorted ways, of natural fears of atomic disaster.

for the deprivation and miseries of the "have nots." Only the state can, with justice, direct and protect the interests and activities of the people and guarantee economic security. The latter they consider the right of all individuals and the major cure of the world's ills. They believe that capitalism has failed and leads to imperialism and totalitarianism. What they refuse to see is that capitalism is not synonomous with either fascism or militarism and has especially proven itself more capable of providing a higher standard of living than socialism, although it may not be the ideal system. It did not create world misery and because of its vital and individualistic nature is less prone to deteriorate into totalitarianism than socialism.[23] The socialist state may be compared to a zoo where all the needs are cared for but the animal is not allowed to express his own capacities for survival. It is therefore stifling. The trend toward a socialistic society is both a manifestation and perpetuator of the crippled life force in humanity. This does not mean we should abandon the poor and helpless. It does mean that if we fail to encourage individual freedom and initiative, we shall leave our children crippled and paralyzed by our own sickness and inadequacies.

The Communist. The communist or red fascist is a political plague character at the extreme left and approaches in many respects the Nazi (black fascist) of the extreme right.[24] Here we must distinguish the true hard core communist character from the naive, idealistic follower or sympathizer, who is usually a leftist liberal or socialist. Communism is the greatest external political threat in the world today[25]—for more than any other brand of political fascism that ever existed, it has mastered su-

23 Freidrich A. Hayek, *The Road to Serfdom* (Chicago, Univ. of Chicago Press, 1962).

24 Reich in his "Basic Tenets on Red Fascism," has stated that the abuse, misuse, and discarding of truth is "typical of all politics" but that ". . . Red Fascism differs from other political disrespect for fact and truth in that it eliminates all checks and controls of the abuse of power and drives the nuisance politician to his utmost power." *People in Trouble* (New York, Orgone Institute Press, 1953), p. 159.

25 Burnham, in *The Managerial Revolution* (New York, John Day Co., 1941), prefers to look upon the situation in Russia as a rule by managers (bureaucrats) as was the case with Nazi Germany and he points out that the U.S. is well on the same road. These "managers" are the organized emotional plague.

premely the art of anchoring itself to the unfulfillable yearnings of mankind while providing just the opposite of those yearnings. It thus spares its victims both the terrors of truth and the responsibilities of self-determination. It is the political graveyard of those who are most desperate about not being able to face up to the enormity of the human task. It is the political illusion beyond illusion of those who fear the truth and would rather destroy the world than face it. Reich has stated that, "Fascist rebelliousness always occurs where fear of the truth turns a revolutionary emotion into illusions."

Characterologically the basic characteristics are hiding for its own sake not to achieve rational ends, and the need for power. This leads directly to subversion. The prodromal symptoms of the communist are restlessness, angry dogmatism, indiscriminate attachment to any causes that sow discord, generalized rebelliousness. Machiavellianism, all of which lead finally to the embrace of arch dogma. He is absolutely closed to argument or fact and will promise anything to obtain his ends. This with no thought of carrying out his promises and no guilt over his duplicity,[26] for everything is just what furthers his ideology and protects his position from his own awareness.[27]

The terror of being forced back into reality by the unworkability of the system drives him to the most desperate measures of brutality and deception. The most meaningful writers on communism (Reich, Djilas) understand it as far more than an ordinary socio-political system with despotic elements; rather they get to the mechanistic and bioenergetic nature of this phenomenon.

[26] One has only to examine the number of agreements with the United States that Russia has broken.

[27] Milovan Djilas, the idealistic Yugoslav communist who rose to one of the highest ranks of communism before realizing what it was, has this to say: ". . . there is an integral feature of contemporary Communism which distinguishes its methods from other political movements. At first sight this feature might seem similar to features of some churches in the past. It stems from the idealistic aims which Communists will use any means to further. These means have become increasingly reckless as the aims become unrealizable. Their use brands those who use them as unscrupulous and merciless power wielders. . . . Indeed these methods are just now achieving their full measure of inhumanity." *The New Class* (New York, Praeger, 1958), p. 149.

Red fascism cynically exploits liberal attitudes to elaborate its dogmas. Its affinity to liberalism lies in its intellectualism and subversion; the expressed motives are not the real motives. It is therefore more cunning, insidious, and difficult to spot or see through than black fascism of the extreme right with its open display of brutality and inhumanity. For example, the whole world was shocked at the six million Jews murdered by the Nazis, but scant notice was paid to the thirty million Russians and Chinese destroyed by communism.

Genesis

Reich has given the clue to the bioenergetic nature of liberalism. He states, "In the ethical and social ideals of liberalism we recognize the representation of the superficial layer of the character, self-control and tolerance. The ethics of this liberalism serve to keep down the 'beast' in man, the second layer, our secondary impulses, the Freudian 'unconscious.' The natural sociality of the deepest nuclear layer is alien to the liberal. He deplores the perversion of human character and fights it with ethical norms, but the social catastrophes of this century show the inadequacy of this approach."[28]

The liberal, thus, is ever in the position of defending himself against a breakdown into secondary impulses. He organizes his life and his thinking (his intellectuality) in the service of his defense. His fear of aggression is rooted in the fear of a collapse of his defenses that might result from an energic push, particularly if the aggression is directed against something that would expose the nature of his character. He cannot tolerate movement and tries to avoid excitation of his biosystem. From this may be derived the ideas concerning adjustment, equality, peace, etc. This is the character type who swells the ranks of the so-called peace movements, civil rights groups, and "friendship with the enemy" societies. Their frequent show of anti-American feelings, whether open or disguised, is a reaction against the amount of healthy aggression still prevalent in American institutions. It is also a reflection of their unresolved Oedipal situation of rebellion against

28 *The Mass Psychology of Fascism*, Preface to the Third Edition (New York, Orgone Institute Press, 1946), p. viii.

the father, a rebellion that is always subversive, never open (the role of Oedipal guilt is discussed above under "Characteristics and Symptoms"). They magnify and dramatize a basically rational fear of atomic disaster as a projection of their own personal fear of bioenergetic disintegration. They use their intellectual resources and media to create a mass hysteria that is paralyzing to a defense effort. They are more willing to see the necessity of direct action against a Nazi threat than against communists, since an exposure of the communists is a partial exposure of themselves.

As noted above, the use of intellect as a defense is particularly characteristic. Reich has suggested that the brain may have become so large and complex that it acts essentially as a parasite, sucking up energy from the body, particularly from the pelvis. This may account for the frequent eye block problem of intellectuals and the so-called "intellectual look" of the "egghead." In fact loss of contact by withdrawal or blocking in the eyes is, I believe, a prerequisite for the use of intellectualism as a defense. The resulting fear of disintegration explains the inordinate need among liberal types to "belong." They find in the mass protest groups of society the support, compensatory aggression, and extra strength for their defenses as well as revenge against their alleged tormentors. They tend to be either hysterically energetic or passively intellectual (superior). Neither type of expression is of course indicative of natural healthy energy regulation or genitality. They are quick to support any group which provides them safely with the belonging, revenge, and defenses they seek—to fill the gap between their longings and their poor capacity for fulfillment. They have lost contact with their core and must defend themselves from any impulses that come from it.

Communism represents an even more desperate flight and may be said to be mankind's most desperate flight from itself in history. In communism, man flees from unattainable god within himself (the bioenergetic core) and from historical theism—which he rejects intellectually and cannot tolerate emotionally —to the attainable and tolerable *illusion* of God to which in final desperation he surrenders with complete faith everything that is basically human. For communism offers him salvation by computer and robot, the political promised land where anything is possible since no genuine feelings are necessary. The communist has guilt too, but it is directed toward the state. The guilt is created by destroying religion and replacing God by the state so that only offenses against the state arouse guilt. This immobilizes the people, allowing the state to call on them for any sacrifice or obligation. It explains why those brought before tribunals for crimes against the state confess so fully and flagellate themselves. Thus they expiate their sins almost with relief.

As Reich has pointed out, the communist, like the liberal, tries to live in the superficial, intellectual layer—the social façade (appearance) of concern for freedom and humanity. He thus keeps one foot in the superficial layer but has the other in the middle brutal layer of secondary drives. The latter he expresses in a more concealed, intellectualized manner than the Nazi, who functions wholly in this middle layer. Not that the sadism of the communist is any less brutal, in fact it maybe even more effective because of the intellectual and psychological cunning of its administration. The underlying terror from which the communist so desperately flees is his fear of disintegration. He desires omnipotence in the vain hope that he will be able to control this terror, or ward it off. Rejecting the concept of an unconscious mind and a cosmic life force in favor of a mechanistic Pavlovian conditioned reflex theory, he attributes his terrors and fears to the deliberate conscious acts of scapegoats such as the "capitalist-imperialist"—and must destroy him at all costs in order to evade the truth—"the shaft of light that leads directly to the genitals."[29] Since he is basically an emotional plague character, all that applies to the emotional plague syndrome applies to him as well.

Treatment

The liberal is intellectually oriented and uses the intellect as his chief defense. This must be stopped. Thus the liberal is not allowed to talk; if he does he will outargue the therapist and insist on everyone being what he terms "reasonable," although he himself is not open to genuine reason. In this respect he feels on safe ground, since one cannot argue against his high ideals even

[29] Wilhelm Reich, *The Murder of Christ, op. cit.,* pp. 197–198.

though his methods, motives, and general attitude toward these are irrational. Even this would not be so crucial if he succeeded in attaining his goal. He never does. Rather he creates new problems more difficult to solve than the old. If he is permitted to talk he will successfully evade his problems. He needs a great deal of character analysis—particularly of the defensive function of his intellect—and must learn to face and tolerate his anxiety and guilt. His contempt, hatred, and subversive tendencies must be exposed, his aggression mobilized, and tolerance to energy movement developed. It is also helpful if he will learn to do some work with his hands.

One is constantly struck by the absolute terror evinced by the liberal when his defenses are successfully attacked. He becomes frantic and irrational. After years of watching liberals spontaneously become more and more conservative as they improved in therapy, I now feel that I have missed something crucial if they do not give up their leftist attitudes.

The communist, like all plague characters, is not amenable to therapy.

The Conservative Character

The conservative side of the socio-political spectrum is a product and perpetuator of the patriarchal system. At his best he probably comes closest to health, at least in his social behavior, of any group in our sick society. At his worst, that is, the reactionary and fascist, he has been responsible for many of the horrors of the past: for example, the Catholic Inquisition. He has persecuted or murdered nearly every great man who tried to help him, from Socrates and Christ to Freud. The conservative is as destructive to nature as the liberal but he does not rationalize it as being for the public good. He does it out of ignorance, financial gain, or "sport," an example of the last being the slaughter of sixty million buffalo during the nineteenth century. The real motive is an expression of his underlying brutal aggression.

Steeped in and following the tradition of his forefathers, the conservative tends to maintain what he insists are the tried and true attitudes toward social and political life. He is thus cautious and slow to promote innovation and prefers evolutionary development to the liberal's rebellious, revolutionary change. Having maintained contact with his core, whether true or distorted, he tends to identify with the father, rather than rebel against him, and thus follows in his footsteps, making slow and gradual change in his way of life. In fact, he does not adjust well to sudden change.

Reich touches upon the core contact of the conservative when he says, "The freedom peddler . . . believes that he defends the truth if he is righteous. The conservative, who, out of an instinctive knowledge of the great difficulties connected with the pursuit of truth, defends the status quo in social living, is by far more honest. He has, at least, a chance of remaining decent. The freedom peddler *must,* if he wishes to get along, sign his soul over to the devil."[30]

He has generally grown up close to the earth and tends to work with his hands, in contrast to the urban intellectualism of the liberal. He has maintained a feeling for nature and the universe which he tries to understand and express through his religion. It is interesting to note that the U.S.S.R has had its greatest difficulties in socialization with the farmer, a man who works with his hands and lives close to the soil. One notes, in this regard, that physicians in private practice are usually conservative, while psychiatrists and psychoanalysts, being far more intellectual and verbal, are generally liberal; this may account for the increasing trend in psychiatry to deemphasize feelings and Freud's libido theory, which deals with the core, in favor of a more neutrally charged, desexualized ego psychology. Thus, too, psychiatry's repudiation of orgonomy, which functions almost wholly in the emotional realm and directly aims at reaching the core of natural sexuality.[31] This is in keeping with Reich's observation of the prevalent tolerance of pornography (intellectualized sexual outlet) and, at the same time, the bitter reaction toward healthy sexuality. That is especially true of the liberal

[30] *Ibid.,* p. 173.

[31] Reich repeatedly warned that the liberal intellectuals would take over orgonomy and emasculate it as they did psychoanalysis.

and plague characters. Conservatives, of course, may be severely repressed sexually (and usually are) but they are even more strongly opposed to pornography and unhealthy sexuality than they are to healthy sexuality.

Having contact with his core, the conservative is aware of himself as a distinct and independent being; he feels his individuality. Contact also gives him a sense of individual responsibility and self-confidence and consequently he is much more concerned about his rights and freedoms than about security. He wishes to be free to plan his own life and grants others the same right. He wants the maximum amount of political freedom consistent with social order, which makes him opposed to centralized social and economic planning. He feels that an individual's freedom is only an illusion if he depends on the state for his economic needs, and this attitude is in accordance with health. Dependency on government help will change even an industrious, self-reliant person into a weak, dependent creature without his being aware of it. This character damage cannot be avoided. To be free one must have the personal responsibility of caring for one's own material needs.[32]

The conservative is often accused by the liberal of being selfish and insensitive to the needs of others. Actually his concern for others is just manifested in a different way. He sympathizes with the helpless and handicapped as well as with the capable and industrious, but unlike the liberal, has little tolerance for those whom he thinks are not trying to help themselves. The true conservative is generous and progressive toward those for whom he is directly responsible. This is the basic difference in social attitude between the liberal and conservative. The liberal wants to help people in the mass; the conservative concentrates on a few people whom he has first come to know and respect. The con-

[32] Everyone is familiar with the effect on animals and birds if they are fed rather than left to seek their own sustenance. Alexis de Tocqueville, in *Democracy in America*, Vol. 2, Bk. 4, Ch. 6, p. 320, says, "It is vain to summon a people, which has been rendered so dependent on a central power, to choose from time to time the representatives of that power; this rare and brief exercise of their free choice, however important it may be, will not prevent them from gradually losing the faculties of thinking, feeling and acting for themselves, and thus gradually falling below the level of humanity."

servative rejects the tenet that all men are equal and reserves the right to choose his associates. He is thus opposed to the leveling attitude of the liberal, which penalizes the industrious and capable and encourages inefficiency through various welfare and socialistic programs. He has, in fact, very little sympathy with the latter.

The conservative, in simplest form, is rational, well-intentioned, independent, self-confident, socially conscious, and quite progressive. He may be repressed and mystical himself, but he does not inflict his inadequacy on others; it remains personal. As he extends further and further to the right, he becomes increasingly rigid, repressed, and finally plague ridden. His interests become more restricted and rest increasingly on those of his own class or group, until in a reactionary environment others are ostracized and hated, and in fascism they are cruelly persecuted and murdered. Sadism is rationalized on mystical grounds as being righteous and necessary.

Because he has maintained contact with the core, even if distorted, the conservative is more tolerant of feeling than the liberal and thus has a better prognosis in therapy, other things being equal. Breaking down his mysticism can be a problem; the religious Catholic and Orthodox Jew are particularly difficult. The fascist, like all emotional plague characters, is not amenable to therapy.

Characteristics and Symptoms

The Conservative.[33]   One may say that the basic philosophy of the conservative is "live and let live." Characteristically he is an individualist: decent, open, rather naive, and trusting. He is tolerant of others as long as they do not interfere with him and even inclined to put up with such interference unless pushed too far. He does not wish to direct the lives of others nor allow others to direct his life. This does not mean that he is indifferent to the needs of others, rather he is usually quite concerned for the welfare of those for whom he is directly responsible. He has a great deal of feeling for life and healthy attitudes and, even

[33] The character Levin in Leo Tolstoy's *Anna Karenina* is typical of the conservative.

though repressed, is the closest to health of the socio-political characters. He has less social façade and reacts with feeling rather than intellectualization. He is thus more direct and honest.

His defenses tend toward muscular armoring rather than intellectualism, so that he is reasonable in an argument. He is less inclined to go to extremes in making promises, and feels more commitment because he has more feeling. He is always concerned with the responsibility of the individual.

He identifies with the father and the successful rather than with the underdog, as does the liberal. This does not mean that he is necessarily satisfied with the father. In fact, he often feels the need to do better than the father did in working his way up. That is, he competes rather than rebels. Where there is rebellion it is open, never subversive.

His sympathies go out to the helpless and handicapped but he has little tolerance of the lazy and indolent. He deems privilege as something to be deserved, not as a right to be taken for granted. He is content to work his way up and believes others should do the same. Each man is, and should be, responsible for his own development both spiritually and materially.

The conservative believes not only in equal rights and equal opportunities but also in the freedom to make of these what one can so that the gifted, energetic, and thrifty may rise above the masses. He feels that permanent equality can be had only under dictatorship and the surrender of liberty.

He has maintained contact with feeling, but since he is blocked from full contact, he is inclined toward mysticism and is usually religious. He emphasizes constantly the spiritual values and looks to a higher Being for guidance. This he takes seriously because he feels it. Religion helps him handle his guilt, so that he does not have to atone for it constantly as does the liberal.

Sex he likewise takes seriously and knows that it is an expression of love. He believes that its expression should be reserved for his mate in marriage. This is his ideal. He emphasizes the importance of chastity but usually practices the double standard. This is because his is a representative of the patriarchal system and still is inclined to view the female as inferior. The liberal tends to eliminate differences in attitude toward the sexes. The

conservative is relatively tolerant of others' ideas and more inclined to control his "passions" than to control others. Since he
considers pornography and perversions sinful, he is inclined to
treat them as crimes.

He does not believe that education is necessary or of equal
value to all. He is interested in meeting the needs of the most
talented and ambitious students and does not like to see them
held down to the level of the slower ones. Education should not
be directed at teaching the child to adjust to his environment,
but rather to overcoming its obstacles and mastering it. Typically, he favors competition, and his school readers carry a moral
for developing character. Schools are to educate the individual,
not society. Everywhere he is concerned for his personal freedom
and independence.

Because of the sense of personal responsibility felt by the
conservative he takes a consistent position on all contemporary
problems and feels they should be solved as far as possible locally
rather than by a central government.[34] He believes accumulation
of power in a single authority always restricts freedom whether
from a central government or trade union. It inevitably becomes
corrupt and ceases to function in the interests of the people,
until eventually it serves only to perpetuate and extend itself.
Thus he believes the best governed are the least governed and
power should always be restricted clearly to the specific reason
the power was conferred. He is opposed to the central government's enlarging its interests into activities that should be left
to the states or individuals. He is also opposed to the unions engaging in activities outside their specific purpose, such as politics.
He believes that membership in unions should be voluntary and
that the union should confine its activity to collective bargaining
conducted with the employer of the workers concerned. A union
with the power to enforce uniform conditions of employment

---

34 Richard Cornuelle of San Mateo, California seems to have made real
strides in such a program in enlisting private enterprise, private institutions
and the people themselves to take the initiative in solving the problems of
our society instead of expecting the government to do it. See "A New Conservative Manifesto," *Look* magazine December 29, 1964. Also, his book, *Re-
claiming the American Dream* (New York, Random House, 1965).

throughout the nation and to coerce its membership into voting patterns has the power of a dictatorship.

In the present racial question the conservative does not believe in enforced segregation, but he is equally opposed to enforced integration.[35] Like all social and cultural problems, this problem, he feels, is best handled by the people directly concerned. Consequently, he believes, however desirable such changes may be, they should not be effected by national power. Problems are only increased when solutions are arbitrarily forced upon individuals before they are prepared to accept them responsibly. The conservative is aware of the Negro's responsibility to the present situation and feels that the Negro leaders should emphasize this,[36] as some of them have done, rather than just make demands. Where the Negro has assumed responsibility, he has had little difficulty in integration except with the more extreme right. The conservative is concerned that Americans will lose basic rights, such as freedom of association and private property rights if the Negro is granted privileges without assuming the responsibility that goes with these privileges. He feels that little by little basic rights may be whittled away through apparently good causes until the nation is enslaved by bureaucracy and totalitarianism, so that everyone has lost.

The conservative is quite aware of the danger of communism (red fascism) and fears it because it is so alien to his feeling and functioning. He is especially fearful because of its interest in

[35] Joseph F. Albright, Negro patriot, in *This Way Out,* says, "All racial integration carries with it the inference that there is nothing worth while to be attained until and unless I am permitted to 'mix' with the white folks . . . any such philosophy is a direct insult to my racial pride.

Dr. Frances L. Ilg and Dr. Louise Bates Ames, directors of the Gesell Institute of Child Development, observe that, "we belittle colored children when we assume that they will be benefitted by sitting beside any white child in school."

[36] One greatly overlooked problem of the Negro is parental attitude toward the child. This is frequently severe, brutal, and negligent, rendering him incapable of rationally accepting and asserting his rights and responsibilities. All of my Negro patients have given this history and from my studies it seems to be the general situation especially among the less affluent. Children of the poor are severely crippled by lack of contact. I understand the native African is equally brutal to his children except for a few tribes such as pygmies and Bushmen.

world domination, which would deprive him and other free people of their freedoms. He is therefore active in expressing his opposition to communism and fighting it. Here the liberal has a blind spot since he approximates the communist structurally and characterologically, depending on how left of center he is.

At this point I wish to clarify one type of liberal that seems paradoxical in this context. This is what I call the environmental liberal. Actually he is structurally not a liberal at all but is a conservative with liberal ideas. He is anti-communist, moderate in his views, and sincere and one can sense his conservative structure almost immediately. His liberalism changes spontaneously in therapy and outside of therapy with presentation of facts or his own evolution. He grew up in a liberal environment but liberalism never became a part of his structure. It is therefore easily given up. This type of liberal remains open to education and facts, but albeit is rather naive to political persuasion. He probably constitutes the greatest number of liberals.

The conservative, feeling self-sufficient, tends toward isolationism, rather than internationalism. Although he sees the necessity for international relations, he bases these on what is best for his country and the principles for which it stands. He has no pressing need to be part of the herd. He is proud of his country and sincerely patriotic. The American conservative believes in the Constitution and wishes to be governed by it. The liberal is more inclined to advocate that it be changed. The conservative is loyal to his friends. The liberal seems more concerned with placating his enemies, except on the right, than in holding his friends. The conservative sincerely believes in peace, but not at the expense of freedom. For example, he would never suggest unilateral disarmament or concessions to the reds without equal concessions from them.

Interestingly, the conscious goals of the conservative and liberal are identical but reversed in order of importance. Moreover, the methods of obtaining these goals are entirely different for each character. As Burnham has pointed out,[37] the goals for the conservative are freedom, liberty, justice, and peace, in that order, and he will fight and even die if necessary for freedom and

[37] Burnham, *Suicide of the West*, p. 159.

liberty. For the liberal the order of importance is exactly reversed: peace, justice, liberty, freedom. The liberal demonstrates for justice and peace and is willing to make many concessions to freedom for the sake of peace.

Typically, the conservative is a farmer, a small (independent) businessman, or a craftsman who works with his hands.

The Extreme Conservative.   His ideas and beliefs differ little from those of the conservative, but he is somewhat more militant in obtaining and preserving them. One could say he is an avid conservative awakened to a crusade. He is somewhat more rigid and therefore more defended characterologically than the conservative. He believes in fundamental religions, expresses a great deal of mysticism, and is inclined to interpret the Bible quite literally. His religion takes on more of an emotional character in an effort to express his restricted core feelings. (This is also demonstrated by his love of pomp and display.) At the same time, religion must be more devout to counteract the increased hate from his acutely rigid armor.

His country is extremely important to him, and with his zealous patriotism he is willing and eager to protect and defend it at all cost. This is true of his liberty as well as his freedom. He is one who like Patrick Henry would say, "Give me liberty or give me death." He has utter contempt for the appeasement attitude of the liberal.

He has a moralistic attitude toward sex, believing that any sexual experience outside of marriage is morally wrong. Marriage is sacred and the family precious. He is still in contact with his core, but unable to express it naturally because of his rigidity. Instead, he expresses it compulsively through taboos against unnatural expression. A healthy person would find such taboos unnecessary since unnatural sexual behavior would not interest or threaten him. There must always be desire behind a taboo.

The extreme conservative is the rugged individualist who was largely responsible for making America great and he is heartsick at observing its trend toward socialism and appeasement of its enemies. He favors the military, the police, and pioneering pursuits as careers. He is ambitious, aggressive, and determined, with unfaltering faith in his ideals. He still defends himself fairly successfully from his secondary drives, but at the cost of being rigid and militant.

The Reactionary. The reactionary finds himself far to the right and resists change. Having found his place in life, he wishes to defend it at all costs, even with violence if necessary. He is less concerned for the rights of others, less rational, less stable in his defenses, and less capable of experiencing satisfaction in life. He tries to remain static to support his failing defenses.

Sexually he is very moralistic and restricted, which is the basis for his sadism and mysticism. He is inclined to be ascetic with sex taking on a mystical quality requiring the maintenance of purity of his race. He therefore condemns miscegenation. At the same time sexual desire is looked upon as animalistic, even brutal, so he feels free to express hate through sexual contact with an "inferior" race.

The white reactionary is not interested in civil rights for Negroes and would maintain segregation, believing the Negro to be an inherently inferior human being. Behind this attitude lies deeply rooted primary process thinking in keeping with his mystical tendency. Thus, to the reactionary, the Negro takes on a symbolic value stemming from his most salient attribute, the simple fact that the Negro is black. Psychologically, we shun black and associate it with evil, death, depression, and gloom.[38] Shakespeare conveys this idea vividly. "Black is the badge of hell, the hue of dungeons, and the suit of night." According to legend, Negroes are descended from Cain and carry his mark, a black skin for a black deed. The reactionary with his tendency toward mysticism and symbolism is particularly prone to this kind of distortion. The Negro himself prefers to be called brown, a warm color.

Correspondingly, the black reactionary, such as the Black Muslim, believes the white man to be an inferior human being and goes to great lengths to prove that a black skin is to be preferred.

The reactionary's mysticism is marked and not subject to rea-

[38] We may have to learn, through a fundamental emotional reeducation, that black is not necessarily bad. Reich thought the prejudice against the Negro was largely because he was considered sexual (animalistic). In dreams the Negro appears to denote forbidden desires, particularly incest.

son or proof. He takes the Bible literally, believing in fundamental and evangelistic religions, in a personal God, and the
reality of hell.

He is a militant states-righter and intensely resents outside
interference in his way of life. He would like to build a wall
around himself and enjoy isolation from all pressures foreign to
his particular milieu. To this end he may employ military dictatorship. Communism is an urgent threat to him. He exaggerates
its danger and sees communistic activities everywhere.

His structure contains a great deal of brutality, frequently
overtly expressed or thinly disguised, and always rationalized as
justifiable and necessary. Existing simultaneously with this is the
reaction formation of a reputation for unexcelled hospitality
and graciousness.

The Fascist.[39]   The fascist is at the extreme right of the socio-
political spectrum. He represents the ultimate in rebelliousness
with reactionary ideas. He is an emotional plague character and
stands for absolute authoritarianism. He is the little man who
grew up so inhibited and restricted and so dependent upon the
father that he requires a father figure or the fatherland to continue to dictate his life and give him permission to express the
brutality and hate he can no longer control. Characterologically
this type lives and acts almost entirely in the secondary (brutal)
layer. Race ideology, top-sergeant mentality, mysticism, and
automatism are all biopathic character symptoms stemming from
his orgastic impotence.

Rigidly armored, he still senses the motility of life within himself but cannot experience it directly. Tantalized, as Reich says,
by intolerable longing, he lashes out brutally and with murderous intent toward the living. This is rationalized through his
extreme mysticism as necessary and just, to maintain the purity
of his race and bring it to dominance over other inferior or con-
taminated races. He is thus an extreme nationalist and an abject
slave to his leader and his country.

Both the fascist and the communist strive for absolute power,
but while the communist craves power for its own sake, the

[39] For a detailed study of fascism see Wilhelm Reich, *The Mass Psychology
of Fascism, op. cit.*

fascist rationalizes it into a mystical cause as necessary to maintain his purity and the purity of his race (a religious concept). To this end, he fanatically stops at nothing in eliminating all who threaten him and his race. The communists "liquidate" cynically and practically (in a Machiavellian fashion). Thus, an absolutely authoritarian and mystical religion is to the fascist what ideology is to the communist. To the fascist, religion and sexuality are functionally identical, often with a strong trend toward paganism. Thus sadism, brutality, and perversion are the rule, usually directed at races other than his own and rationalized as a pious duty.[40]

Education and history are slanted at preserving and justifying his actions and beliefs. This the communist also does to the extent that he rewrites history.

The fascist is active in fighting the communist since he sees him as a rival for the omnipotence they both seek and as a threat to his essential mysticism (distorted core contact). The communist (red fascist) on the other hand has an essentially mechanistic structure (lack of core contact).

Genesis

The conservative maintains his contact with health and naturalness because he has contact with his core or healthy layer. (Identification with the father helps to maintain his core contact.) His attitude is, therefore, closer to the criteria of the genital character than the liberal's, for he maintains considerable healthy aggression and ideals. Because of his solid foundation, he is less apt to deteriorate toward the right than is the liberal to the left, which may account for the prevalence of communism today, as opposed to black fascism. Schematically, we can say that the conservative on deteriorating moves up from the core into the fascistic secondary layer; the deteriorating liberal moves down from the surface social façade also into the secondary layer, while keeping one foot still in the social layer. Thus when the conservative breaks down into the fascist, he smashes through to freedom with reckless force giving rise to sheer brutality. Like the com-

40 Sexual expression of the middle layer.

munist he needs a scapegoat to fight, as for example, Hitler's use of the Jews and Slavs. But by contrast the liberal breakdown into communism is much more subversive and insidious, since the resulting brutality is cynically veiled in humanitarian rationalizations. More important, the brutality itself is carried out much more on the psychological, emotional level rather than just in physical torture or direct humiliation, and thus it is harder to perceive or combat. In the same way, parents who *do* all the "correct" things, can be worse for children than those who are openly cruel.

Treatment

The conservative usually requires less character work than the liberal but more active work on his muscular defenses. Since he is not an intellectualizer, he can safely be allowed to talk for catharsis, and is more open to exposure of his defenses. His mystical tendencies must be broken through to allow him to experience full contact. This may be very difficult, or even impossible in the more devout, such as the orthodox Jew and the Roman Catholic.

The fascist is not a candidate for therapy.

14 · Common Somatic Biopathies

SOMATIC BIOPATHIES are organic diseases that owe their existence to the orgastic impotence of man. They may be looked upon as complications of the character neuroses. Orgasm anxiety creates chronic sympatheticatonia; this in turn creates orgastic impotence and this, in a vicious circle, maintains the sympatheticatonia. In the somatic biopathies the contraction thus caused has progressed to the stage of physical change producing organic disease. Therefore, all biopathies, whether they appear in people as neuroses or as somatic manifestations, are caused by a disturbance in the autonomic nervous system resulting in a disturbance in the biological function of pulsation through the total organism.

A limitation on full expiration and a chronic inspiratory expansion of the chest are basic to sympatheticatonia. The function of this inspiratory attitude is to prevent the rise of those affects and bodily sensations which would appear with normal respiration. To aid in this suppressing, other muscles of the body contract and chronic armor forms.[1] Somatic biopathies may occur

[1] Reich, through later research, believed that the biopathies result not only from chronic contraction but also from a resultant accumulation of a toxic energy which the organism is unable to metabolize adequately. Cf. Wilhelm Reich, "Re-Emergence of Freud's 'Death Instinct' as 'DOR' Energy," *Orgonomic Medicine*, II, 1, April 1956.

in any character type and are not due to the specific character but rather to the specific armoring. One cannot expect permanently to cure the disease medically unless the emotional problems behind it are also solved.

Therapy is conducted according to the character type present, except that special caution is used and emphasis is placed on releasing the segment in which the somatic condition occurs; for example, the chest segment where there is asthma or a heart condition, or the diaphragmatic segment where there is an ulcer, gall bladder disease, or diabetes. In allergies, the major block generally seems to be in the eye segment. Since the contraction has resulted in physical disease, therapy is more difficult and more dangerous and the condition may have reached an irreversible stage. Therapy should be carried out in conjunction with standard medical procedures by an appropriate specialist.

Following are some of the results of the chronic attitude of anxiety and resultant armoring. The list is by no means complete. It cannot approach completion until all diseases have been thoroughly studied from a bioenergetic viewpoint. I have treated patients suffering from each of the diseases discussed below, with the exception of leukemia.

Skin and Special Senses

Myopia

Certain types of myopia are biopathic. Where they are due to chronic contraction and anxiety, the pupils are dilated. Where the pupils are normal, myopia is usually not functional and cannot be expected to be cleared up during therapy. On the other hand, not all cases with dilated pupils are functional; the dilation may be separate from the myopia. Most schizophrenics are myopic.

Skin Disease

Many skin diseases, such as hives or eczema, are functional. In these conditions there seems to be a push of energy through the contraction at the skin surface. Many of these tend to occur during certain phases of therapy when energy breaks through to the skin.

The Locomotor System

Muscular Rheumatism

After a period of years, chronic contraction of the muscles leads to the formation of rheumatic nodules following the deposit of solid substances in the muscle bundles. It affects especially those muscle groups which play a prominent role in the suppression of affects and bodily sensations. For example, in the musculature of the neck ("Stiff-necked"[2] or "headstrong"), and in that between the shoulder blades where the muscle action is that of pulling back the shoulders ("self-control" and "holding back"), disorders are apt to develop. Similarly affected are the two sternocleide mastoids which suppress anger (the "spite muscles"). Also the masseters, whose chronic hypertension gives the lower half of the face a stubborn and bitter expression.

In the lower part of the body, those muscles that retract the pelvis are particularly often affected. Retraction of the pelvis suppresses genital excitation, and chronic retraction produces a lordosis that leads to lumbago. Lumbago is also found very frequently in those who keep the muscles of their buttocks contracted in order to suppress anal sensations. Another muscle group affected is the superficial and deep adductors of the thigh which keep the legs pressed together. Their function, when chronically contracted, is to suppress genital sensation (the "morality muscles"). The flexors of the knee suppress sensations in the pelvic floor.

The chronic inspiratory attitude of the chest maintains chronic contraction of the pectorals, which often results in intercostal neuralgias which disappear with the disappearance of muscular hypertension of the thorax.

Arthritis

Calcium deposits in the spine and joints occur from chronic sympathetic contraction. Sympatheticatonia causes an acid im-

[2] All similar, common expressions are biophysically accurate.

balance in the organism which stimulates calcium deposition. There is always a great deal of repressed rage present in these cases.

The Internal Organs of the Chest

Cardio-Vascular Hypertension

Chronic contraction of peripheral blood vessels limits their amplitude of expansion and contraction. The heart has always an unusually heavy job because it must move the blood through rigid vessels. The feeling of oppression in the chest results. Tachycardia, high blood pressure, or even full cardiac anxiety are also symptoms of hypertension as well as hyperthyroidism. One seems justified in questioning how far disturbance of the thyroid is itself only a secondary symptom of sympatheticatonia.

Arteriosclerosis with calcification of the blood vessels is the end result of long-standing functional hypertension. The body acid produced by constant anxiety allows Ca ions to depoist calcium in the tissues. Some valvular heart diseases, coronary heart disease, angina pectoris, and paroxysmal tachycardia are also results of chronic sympatheticatonia. In these heart conditions, even years before physical disease results, one consistently finds a triad of extremely painful points—one below the left nipple, a second above the nipple, and the third in the left axilla. Relief of the spasm at these points relieves the heart symptoms. In paroxysmal tachycardia where the patient is taking quinidine relief cannot be obtained by this means.

Pulmonary Emphysema

Pulmonary emphysema with its barrel chest is a result of an extreme chronic inspiratory attitude of the thorax. Any chronic spasm impairs the elasticity of the tissues, and in emphysema the elastic fibers of the bronchii are damaged.

Asthma

Asthma is due to a parasympathetic overstimulation in an attempt to overcome the underlying chronic anxiety. This causes contraction of the bronchioles and interferes with expiration. There is always a great deal of repressed rage in asthmatics, and when it is expressed the attack is relieved.

The Internal Organs of the Diaphragmatic Region

Peptic Ulcer

Chronic sympatheticatonia causes a tendency to acidity which is reflected in excessive gastric acidity. With diaphragmatic blocking, the mucous membrane of the stomach itself is contracted and the blood supply is interfered with. Also, in a state of contraction it is more vulnerable to the effect of the acid. The typical localization of the ulcer is on the lesser curvature of the stomach or in the first portion of the duodenum, just in front of the pancreas and the solar plexus. It seems that the vegetative nerves here retract and thus reduce the resistance of the mucous membrane to attack by the acid. Toxic substances which have been isolated are probably a result rather than a cause of the ulcer. If definite improvement is not obtained in twelve to eighteen months, operation should be considered. Scar tissue is probably interfering with healing. Ulcers are found in persons with a strong drive, a deep sense of responsibility, an underlying anxiety, and strong dependency longings.

Gall Bladder Disease and Diabetes

These diseases seem also to be biopathies resulting from diaphragmatic blocking and contraction of the solar plexus. In diabetes there is undoubtedly also an inherited influence. I saw one case with symptoms typical of gall bladder disease, including painful obstruction, tenderness and spasm in the right hypochrondrium, indigestion, sense of fullness in the epigastrium, flatulence, and jaundice; the whole complex of symptoms was completely relieved by massage of the pylorus. When the pyloric spasm gave, gurgling could be heard and the symptoms disappeared. I presume the spasm included the sphincter of Odi and thus produced an obstruction to the flow of bile and caused jaundice. At the same time as the spasm was released, the patient brought out a great deal of bitterness she felt toward her husband.

Hyperinsulinism

This condition appears to be due to blocking in the diaphragmatic segment, but it probably is the result of a block less severe than diabetics have. The contraction is sufficient to cause stimulation of the pancreas and other organs in the area (such as the liver), but not severe enough to produce destruction. I have seen the hypoglycaemia improve when tension was released in the diaphragmatic segment.

Cardio Spasm and Pylorospasm

These disorders result from contraction of the annular muscles of the cardia and pylorus. (See gall bladder disease.)

The Internal Organs of the Abdomen

Spastic Colitis

The mechanism that produces spastic colitis is similar to that appearing in asthma, that is, a parasympathetic overstimulation in an attempt to overcome anxiety. This condition is found in persons who must present an outward calm and bravery in spite of deep underlying anxiety.

Chronic Constipation

Chronic constipation is a result of the diminution or cessation of the peristalsis in the intestines. Chronic sympatheticatonia allows dilation of the intestinal walls while at the same time producing a spasm of the anal sphincter. Hemorrhoids usually develop eventually. The relief following evacuation is due to the movement of energy started by the activity, and not to the removal of intoxication. The relief occurs too soon after evacuation to be due to the latter.

The Internal Organs of the Pelvis

Vaginismus

Vaginismus is a result of contraction of the annular muscula-ture of the vagina. Underlying it, there is a deep rejection of the penis.

Hemorrhoids

Hemorrhoids develop as a result of a chronic spasm of the anal sphincter. The blood in the peripheral veins around the anus is mechanically dammed up and the vessel walls undergo dilation. In the last analysis, the condition can be traced back to toilet training, unless it is a result of physical pressure, such as that which may be produced by tumor growths in the pelvis.

Fibroids and Ovarian Cysts

These are the result of an expansive push of energy against the contraction of the uterus and ovaries causing a ballooning of the tissues. In such cases, the pelvis has a high energy charge but is blocked from adequate sexual expression. The contraction has occurred to prevent sexual energy from making itself felt as vaginal sensation. During menstruation, this proceeds to severe spasms which are felt as menstrual cramps. The emotionally healthy woman has no menstrual pain.

General and Miscellaneous Conditions

Allergy

Allergy, including hay fever, seems to require three factors for development: a foreign protein, sensitivity to that protein, and an emotional condition. All three must be present to promote the allergic reaction. It seems that the foreign protein produces an excessive (allergic) excitation of energy in the organism, causing an expansion which the organism cannot tolerate. Counter-con-traction occurs and blocks the energy's escape. Then, the energy caught between the push and the block balloons the tissues.

Itching or pain results from pleasure sensations beyond the tolerance level when energy reaches the skin surface.

Phobia also appears to be an allergic condition, but one restricted to the emotional realm. Here, too, there are present an exciting factor resulting in excessive excitation and a counter-contraction, causing an intense anxiety. I believe the mechanisms in both allergy and phobia are very similar, and I have seen cases who developed a phobia when the allergic condition cleared up. I also saw one case in which the reverse occurred. That is, the patient developed an allergy when the phobia disappeared. In some cases both may be present. Individuals who suffer from these conditions seem to be unduly sensitive, that is, "thin-skinned" or ectodermic in type. They are overly sensitive to their environment, which is very threatening to them. They tend to withdraw, especially in the eyes. An explosive, destructive rage builds up directed at the object selected as dangerous, usually symbolic of incest fears. The sensitivity of the skin and genital which is part of the skin reactivates the Oedipus problem. Withdrawal in the eyes probably allows the projection of the fear onto a symbol.

Cancer, Leukemia, and Poliomyelitis

These three disease pictures are presented together, not because they are considered similar but rather because the origins of all three are still a subject of controversy from the standpoint of classical medicine. More and more often suggestions are made as to their emotional origin; that is, that they may be disturbances of the biophysical functioning of the organism. Trueta and Hodes, reporting in *Lancet* (May 15, 1954), state that they produced a disease picture essentially that of paralytic poliomyelitis in experimental animals by injecting irritants, Formol or croton oil, into the limbs of these animals, without using any kind of virus. In reference to this report, R. J. Dittrich, in a letter to the *Journal of the American Medical Association* (March 11, 1961, p. 925), observes that if these results can be verified on a larger scale it may become necessary to revise our present concepts of the cause of this disease and direct our present efforts toward a search for other factors that may be operative in the genesis of paralytic poliomyelitis.

Greene[3] has for several years studied the emotional factors present in leukemia and found the common denominator in all case histories of leukemia was the separation from a significant object or goal with concomitant emotional distress.[4] The American Cancer Society in their 1959 report lists emotional stress as a possible cause of leukemia.

It is fairly well recognized now that resignation is a prominent finding in cancer cases and that the prognosis largely depends on the amount of aggression still present in the individual. Psychological factors in cancer have been investigated by several workers.[5] Gengerelli and Kirkner report sexual inhibition as a cause of cancer, particularly in persons who are unable to discharge anger. Persons with a serious conflict of impulses who are trained to inhibit their real emotions are particularly susceptible to rapid growth of cancer. The "nice" person fails to respond to treatment. The aggressive person has a better outlook.

Reich did considerable careful and painstaking research in all three diseases. Much of the work I observed personally. He concluded that all three were in fact due primarily to emotional disturbances and were thus properly biopathies.

Poliomyelitis, as Reich observed, occurs in young persons with a high energy level and a severe pelvic block. The increased push of spring and summer's reawakening is counteracted by a

[3] Cf. William A. Greene *et al,* Department of Medicine and Psychiatry, University of Rochester School of Medicine, *Psychosomatic Medicine, Psychological Factors and Reticulo-endothelial Disease:* (i) "Preliminary Observations on a Group of Males with Lymphomas and Leukemias," Vol. 16 (1954), p. 220; (ii) "Observations on a Group of Women with Lymphomas and Leukemias," Vol. 18 (1956), p. 284; and (iii) "Observations on a Group of Children and Adolescents with Leukemia; An Interpretation of Disease Development in Terms of the Mother-Child Unit," Vol. 20 (1958), p. 124.

[4] The press recently reported the case of a homesick girl suffering from leukemia who had a spontaneous remission when she returned to her family in Ireland.

[5] Blumberg *et al,* "Possible Relationship Between Psychological Factors and Human Cancer," *Psychosomatic Medicine,* Vol. 16 (1954), p. 278. Also see J. A. Gengerelli and F. J. Kirkner, eds., *Psychological Variables in Human Cancer* (University of California Press, 1953).

withdrawal of energy from the limbs.[6] It seems probable that the success of the Kenny method of treatment with hot packs and massage is due to the induction of this flow of energy. In paralysis of the upper limbs, oral frustration seems also to be present.

Leukemia occurs in the same type of individual as poliomyelitis and one can theorize that it is an alternate reaction. One wonders, therefore, whether leukemia will increase correspondingly if poliomyelitis is prevented. Classical medicine still looks upon this disease as a form of cancer; it is true that there are many features to warrant this conclusion, but there is also an important difference which can be observed and understood only if one is familiar with the energy concept of functioning. The difference is that, in leukemia, the red cells are tremendously overcharged bioenergetically, while in cancer the red cells have a low charge and some degree of anemia is always present. At the same time, the red cells in leukemia are very fragile and disintegrate readily. They are sick cells. Leukemia seems to be primarily a disease of the red and not of the white cells. The leucocytic increase is apparently to handle the toxic process from the disintegration of red cells. This theory receives some support from the fact that cases have been reported of a-leucocytic leukemia (that is, leukemia cases in which there is no increase in the white cells). Radiation is also a causative factor in leukemia in present circumstances: it causes an intense excitation of energy in the red cells and, in fact, in the whole organism (increasing, by the way, the push on a blocked pelvis).

Cancer, according to Reich, is basically living putrefaction of the tissue. Whereas in stasis neurosis the push of energy outward continues and the impulses remain strong under the armor, in cancer, in some cases, the very impulses cease. That condition starts with an overbalance of contraction and a plasmatic inhibition of expansion. As impulses toward pleasurable expansion gradually become more rare, the flow of energy in the organism

[6] Cf. Trueta and Hodes, *Lancet,* May 15, 1954 (see pp. 998–1001). One seems justified in assuming that the paralysis in the experimental animals resulted from withdrawal of energy from the limbs as a reaction to the shock from the irritant injected. This would be entirely in keeping with Reich's theory.

decreases. That is, in cancer cases, the organism has given up trying to circulate its energy. This is manifested as emotional resignation, which may precede the appearance of the cancer tumor by several years. Given the ending of attempts to push energy outward and expand the organism, cancer may develop because the tissues are literally starved of pleasure. The local cancer derived from tissues denied expansion is caused by chronic shrinking of the organism and an inadequate sex economy.

The connecting link between sex economy and the cancerous affection lies in the fact that poor respiration leads to poor internal (cellular) respiration in the tissues, followed by greater carbon dioxide content and anoxia. Orgonotic charge and discharge in the autonomic system, particularly in the genitals, automatically become disturbed as respiration fails. Chronic spasms of the musculature logically follow, and finally chronic orgastic impotence is established. The cancer is most apt to appear in the specific areas where the individual concentrates his defense against excitation by contracting the musculature. (That is, cancer appears in the heavily armored areas—women develop it in breast and uterus most frequently.) Contraction of annular musculature is especially efficient in damming up energy, and cancer is particularly frequent in annularly muscled areas such as the throat, anus, stomach, etc. The general result of biopathic shrinking is putrefaction in the blood and tissues; the cancer tumor is only one of the symptoms of this putrefaction. The cancer cell is a result and not the cause of the disease. The tumor should be removed surgically; treatment to alleviate the causative emotional condition is also indicated.

What happens in all three diseases is that as the tissue cells break down they degenerate through various stages and eventually form T. Bacilli (*Tod* or death bacilli) which accentuates the disease picture. T. Bacilli, which Reich has demonstrated originate within the organism, are undoubtedly the same as classical medicine terms virus and micro-plasma. Once formed these can be transferred to other living beings and act as a toxic agent causing breakdown of cells and producing the same disease in a susceptible individual. The cancer cell arises as a pathological independent cell from the breakdown and detachment of normal cells from the tissues. It is capable of proliferating by the usual cell division.

I believe Reich's estimate of these disease pictures should be seriously considered and studied as a basis for further research. Those interested beyond this mere mention of these diseases should see Reich's reports on his work.[8]

[8] Cf. Wilhelm Reich, *The Cancer Biopathy* (New York, Orgone Institute Press, 1948), *The Oranur Experiment* (New York, Orgone Institute Press, 1951), and "The Leukemia Problem, An Approach," *Orgone Energy Bulletin*, Vol. 3 (April 1951), p. 2.

PART III

.

CHARACTER MANAGEMENT:

The Removal of Armoring

15 · The Initial Examination

History

THE HISTORY OF A PATIENT should be short enough to be readily usuable; long histories are discouraging, tiring to refer to, and contain a great deal of material that is never used. No question should be asked unless the answer is directly pertinent to the therapist's understanding of the case. In other words, the object is not a great mass of information, but just those facts diagnostically necessary.

Briefly, three facts are necessary: a therapist must know what the patient is complaining of, how he has functioned in the past, and how he is functioning in the present.

That information is sufficient to provide a general picture of the seriousness of the patient's problem and of the capacity he has shown. A comparison of his capacity with his present handicap gives some idea of what can be accomplished. For example, if the patient has never been able to function very well, less accomplishment can be expected than if he has demonstrated good capacity in the past and is presently crippled by neurotic symptoms. Also, if his symptoms are severe and he is nevertheless making a reasonable adjustment, he is better material to work with than if he is wholly incapacitated by what would be considered a mild neurosis.

There are three factors in the outlook for any case: the skill of the therapist, the neurosis present, and the individual who has the neurosis. The last is by far the most important for the prognosis. If the individual is made of good material, has "guts" and determination, the outlook can be good even in the most severe cases. On the other hand, those who give up easily and have to be carried warrant a conservative prognosis.

Complaints

Complaints are best given spontaneously by the patient in his own words. I usually ask, "Why did you come?" The manner in which he answers the question as well as the complaints themselves is quite revealing. The compulsive will often have his reasons all written out and will want to read them to you, or he will simply hand them over. The phallic may make some sarcastic quip like, "That is your problem," or "That's for you to find out." The schizophrenic will not know and his complaints will be vague. "I am not doing well," he may say, "I don't feel I am getting anywhere," or "Things just aren't right," or even, "I feel strange and things about me seem strange." The depressive will respond laconically, "I need help," and his appearance will tell the rest.

I do not accept any patient who does not feel personally that he needs help to change. Those who come merely because their families have persuaded them and feel no need in themselves would be unsuitable candidates for therapy. Even though they seem to need therapy, they can be reminded that they have a right to their own opinions and sent away. Frequently the family has felt that once they got their problem to a therapist he would do the rest, and in such cases they are apt to be disgusted, understandably enough.

The individual's own pain from his condition and his desire to change is the best aid to therapy. Without it, the task is more or less hopeless. That is why it is a mistake to try to "sell" therapy or paint rosy pictures. Personally, I much prefer to let a patient persuade me that I should accept him in spite of discouragement on my part.

Age

Usually, the older the patient is the less pliable he is, but this is a very individual matter. Some people are more rigid at twenty than others at fifty.

General Level of Functioning

Other things being equal, more can be expected from a college graduate than from someone who stopped in the first year of high school. But there may have been some compelling reason to stop school that has nothing to do with the patient's ability, so the circumstances should be understood. Whether schooling was easy or pursued with difficulty is also significant. A man who has slogged his way through high school after work at night deserves at least as much respect as one who squeaked out of a four-year residential college with a minimum average.

Some idea of the patient's potential can be obtained by comparing his background and education with his job. A college graduate doing a laborer's work or an eighth-grader holding a responsible position do not always merit the same kind of attention from a therapeutic point of view.

To find how far a patient has been able to carry through in adult adjustment, a therapist needs to understand how he relates to people, whether he is seclusive with few contacts or quite social, if he is married and how old he was when it happened, and whether there are children. It is helpful to know whether children were wanted and why. Here again, a comparison of present ability with past attainments is revealing.

Bodily Functions

A patient's attitude toward eating can be normal, but it is likely that he either enjoys food too much or does not get enough pleasure from it, and that his eating is excessive or deficient. If excessive it may be from unsatisfied oral strivings or from a need to fill the emptiness in his stomach, and if deficient it indicates a probable oral repressive with concomitant depressive tendencies.

His sleep may be normal if he is tired when he retires and refreshed when he awakes, or it may follow one of two disturbed patterns. If he is tired both when he goes to sleep and when he wakes up, low energy and general exhaustion are indicated and the condition is serious. If he is refreshed at bedtime and tired in the morning, it indicates that he has been avoiding contact during the day and struggling against relaxation and the loosening of his armor during his sleep. This situation is commonly complained of by neurotics, and it occurs when armor is in the process of breaking down or when it is not adequate to bind anxiety.

A patient's dreams often reveal his trend before it becomes evident in actual living. His functioning improves in dreams before he can achieve the improvement in reality.

The patient's habits of evacuation are also significant. Constipation is determined according to consistency rather than actual frequency. One patient will complain of constipation if he does not have one or two movements a day, while another will feel he is normal at once a week. In the character with a spastic colon, there will be stools of small diameter because of anxiety (contraction) about expansion which leads to spasm and absence of motility. In such cases, parasympathetic overreaction to overcome sympathetic contraction is operative as it is in asthma. When stools are large and hard, the anal holding type is indicated; this condition is related to toilet training and involves a sympathetic contraction without the parasympathetic overreaction. Diarrhea indicates extreme anxiety in which the sympathetic system is paralyzed and parasympathetic action forces out the bowel contents. In urination, a frequency similar to diarrhea may be present, or with neurotic conditioning the patient may be unable to urinate when anyone else is in the room or if he is in a strange place.

Among women, menses are rarely completely normal in the absence of emotional health. It may be too frequent or too rare, too profuse or too scanty, painful or depressing. All of these are evidence of pelvic block. Sometimes there is a neurotic disgust or resentment directed toward menstruation.

The therapist must also have some idea of the patient's sexual functioning in childhood, during puberty, and after it. Pre-puberty activity is usually confined to masturbation and sexual play. Information about puberty should include whether or not there was masturbation and its method and associated guilt, the pleasure and guilt of any homosexual experiences, and of hetero-sexual experiences. The first homosexual experience occurs quite regularly at sixteen years.[1] For the post puberty period there is no narrow range. A comparison of past and present sexual func-tioning, if any, helps. It also helps to know the degree of satisfaction attained with the current partner and how it com-pares with the past and with other partners. An idea of how many partners the patient has sought and whether sex is a duty instead of a pleasure is useful; some patients find masturbation preferable to dealing with a sexual partner. He may be dis-turbed by anxiety or by fantasies or even find fantasy necessary to his sexual performance.

Much judgment is needed in asking questions on sexual mat-ters, especially in dealing with hysterics, and it is a mistake to get involved in discussion at too deep a level too early. Indeed, one may postpone such questions until therapy has been in progress for some time, since many of the answers can be inferred closely enough from the rest of a patient's behavior.

It is, however, vital that a therapist know about any physical illnesses, including asthma, skin conditions, and allergies, so that he may take them into account in his treatment.

Examination

The examination of a patient actually starts during his first telephone call or with his letter asking for an appointment. There are many patients whom I decide against seeing at this time—and others whom I decide to see immediately if they seem serious and urgent. Even with those who appear indifferent, reluctant, or merely curious, one must remember that they are somehow asking for help but are not quite ready to accept it.

[1] See page 89.

After some experience one knows pretty well what to expect even before seeing the patient—from his tone of voice, his ability to put his request across, and his clarity or confusion in saying why he wants to see you.

The picture is further revealed the moment the patient enters the room. He presents one or more of the following attitudes. He may be natural, poised, courteous, and serious; in which case one may on rare occasion have a pleasant opportunity to tell him he does not need treatment. More likely, he will be anxious, suspicious, aggressive, confused and out of contact, depressed, or shy. If he is aggressive, he may either be hostile, ridiculing the appointments of the room, your appearance, and so forth, or friendly, shaking your hand almost off your wrist, calling you "Doc," putting his feet on the desk, and more or less settling down for the day.

The Façade

The façade is the most superficial of the three basic layers of the personality; it is the surface the individual presents to the world. A patient's façade may appear quite different on the couch than it was when he was sitting at the desk. The difference is due, of course, to the fact that he has fewer defenses available when he is lying on the couch. Suspicion becomes more evident or may appear where it was not noticed before. The anxious and shy lie near the edge of the couch away from the therapist. Where anxiety is acute, the skin is cold and moist and the pupils are dilated. The aggressive patient is warm, flushed, and defiant; he has the "don't touch me" attitude and holds back with clenched fists, arched back, and so forth. The holding back may be limited to certain areas or the patient may curl up in a ball, as the hysteric frequently does. The schizophrenic seems to be spread out all over the couch and gives an impression of being diffuse; occasionally the schizophrenic may look like a case of simple stasis the first time he is interviewed. Both weaknesses and defenses are more apparent on the couch than when the patient is sitting up, and the expression of the eyes and face needs to be carefully noted. Also, the basic character trait should be isolated as early as possible.

The Couch

Timing in putting the patient on the couch is quite important. The anxious patient ought to be reassured first, while the aggressive patient should be put on the couch as soon as possible because his position there makes him easier to control. If a patient is suspicious, it is best to work through enough of the suspicion so that he attains a degree of conscious trust, but if a patient is confused the sooner the therapist takes charge and starts work on the eyes to relieve the confusion, the better. History is painful to a depressed patient and it is preferable to leave as much as possible out and start work immediately. The servile patient can be put on the couch whenever the preliminary interview is over. On the other hand, some rapport needs to be established with a shy patient first. With hysterics, it is necessary to be cautious; it is effective to let her persuade her therapist that it is all right to put her on the couch.

Initial Approach

Once the patient is on the couch, a rapport can be made by asking questions like, "Are you frightened," or "Do you understand the necessity of being on the couch?"

If the patient breathes through his mouth for a bit, the process will eliminate conscious holding in the jaw. Then if he is excited enough to eliminate conscious holding in the rest of his body, for instance, if he is poked in the ribs, his involuntary responses will show up his defenses clearly. A poked hysteric will shrink away, but a phallic gets angry and fights back. The compulsive will probably look amused and put on a knowing smile, while a depressive just puts up with it. The schizophrenic withdraws or becomes fearful or shows no response.

During the first session better responses can be obtained than during later ones when the patient is better prepared and more familiar with his surroundings. He may appear healthier than he is during the first session and a final diagnosis should be put off for two or three sessions. It is important to learn as much as possible during the first session while doing as little as possible to learn it. Much action on the part of the therapist may make the patient overreach himself and he will be frightened away, or it may even cause an acute exaggeration of symptoms, especially in schizophrenics. Before diagnosis, all seven segments should be examined for degree of functioning or restriction.

General Physical and Laboratory Examinations

Such examinations should be done routinely, and in certain cases they are imperative. Not all symptoms are emotional and there is a danger of overlooking physical disease. This is important throughout therapy and when in doubt suitable specialists should be consulted. I have frequently had to insist with patients, convinced that everything is emotional, to have the specialist confirm an ovarian cyst, fibroid, peptic ulcer, and other conditions. One of my great concerns is not to miss urgent organic disease.

Principles of Dealing with Various Attitudes

Very briefly, the following general procedures are indicated for each type of façade presented.

After reassuring an anxious patient, the therapist should get him to express his anxiety by looking frightened and by screaming. Later, aggression can be elicited with hitting and rage on the patient's part. In anxiety, movement in the organism has been from periphery to center, and this movement must be reversed.

The suspicious patient's attitude needs to be kept in the open, constantly pointed out and discussed.

An aggressive patient must be made to stop the aggressive behavior, which is a cover for anxiety.

Confused patients should have their eyes mobilized immediately and depressed patients need to be set into almost any sort of motion. As discussed earlier, it is advisable to mobilize the chest in depression so that the organism will have greater available energy and the shrinking process will be arrested. Mobilization of the chest should release some of the rage the patient has turned inward to depression.

A servile patient needs to be provoked into the anger his attitude is covering up; confronting him with that servility is effective.

16 · General Therapeutic Principles

I HAVE EMPHASIZED that this book is not designed to show therapeutic technique but to convey understanding of character rather than how to treat it. Using this technique is a complicated process requiring extensive training. Here I wish only to point out the more obvious therapeutic principles in the treatment of human problems.

Requirements of the Therapist

The therapist should be adequately trained and know what he is doing. His first consideration always should be to help the patient in his problem, that is, to help him find a rational solution and enable him to face life and himself more unafraid. The goal is always to establish genital potency. It may or may not be attained but should never be forgotten. Therapy must be functional and there is no rule that is always valid. A general rule to follow is that unless one knows exactly what to do in a particular instance, it is best to do nothing until the answer becomes clear.

Object of Therapy

No matter what secret reason the patient may have for coming to therapy, both he and the therapist must be clear on the point that there is only one objective—therapeutic help enabling him to gain independence even of the therapist. The patient is not coming to become dependent on the therapist and the therapist who encourages the patient to run to him with every small problem is not handling the case well. The patient is not coming to have the therapist support him in a family feud, or to attain certain other ends, such as holding the wife (or husband). Nor should the patient become involved in the therapist's problems or ambitions.

The Therapeutic Situation

A therapist must not be hesitant to look at the patient and find out what is there and what he is up against. If the patient expects help, the therapist is entitled to know everything necessary to his effort. Since anything about him may be significant, modesty and shyness on the part of the therapist work counter to the goal. The orgonomist has the advantage of being able to probe both psychologically and physically, while the psychoanalyst has to content himself with the former and "doesn't touch." The mechanistic psychiatrist bothers little with either, depending on machines and drugs to do the work—and he, also, "doesn't touch." The orgonomist uses words and may use drugs if necessary, but he looks at his patient and is not afraid to touch him. He has had to overcome his own fear of orgastic streamings and of natural sounds and movements, so that literally nothing human is alien to him. The more he knows the better he can help.

The patient will never tell the whole truth until the end of therapy, and will constantly try to seduce the therapist away from making him reveal himself. But the therapist is in charge and the patient expects direction; it is not only his right but his duty to tackle every problem. But it is possible to get lost in symptoms, so character attitudes must be constantly kept in mind. The therapist must tell the truth, but only so much of it as the patient can accept. Showing off impressive knowledge doesn't help—it frequently comes down to "the less said the better." Also, it is unwise to promise salvation in any form.

Finally, no therapist should attempt to treat patients who have problems he has not been able to handle in himself nor should he expect a patient to do things he cannot do and has not been able to do.

The Selection of Patients

Not all patients should be treated; some can only have their defenses broken down and have no ability for synthesis. Others will develop serious physical disease if therapy is vigorously attacked. One must approach human life and human problems with respect and caution. It is best that a therapist select the patients he can understand and refer the others on. On the other hand, once a patient has been selected as a suitable candidate for therapy, considerable daring and risks are necessary.

The patient should be encouraged to continue normal life activities as much as possible, to make decisions and stick to them even if he risks failure. He, too, has to become daring and take chances. Life requires it if he is to do anything at all. Failure is not important; only giving up is. Patients who pay their own way have a better prognosis because they are better material than those who have to depend on parents or relatives to support them. Besides, therapy will be more meaningful to them if they are paying for it.

Understanding the Patient

The simple, basic aim in therapy is to enable the patient to use his organism to its whole extent. This requires mobilization and direction of his aggression. Where he is restricted in this respect it must be corrected. Only his illness is treated; the health in him needs only support. He cannot do what is against his principles or what he is unprepared for. But what he is prepared for does not have to be urged on him. He does, however, need support and encouragement.

On the other hand, it may be necessary to command him to stop many things he does. However, there must always be some good reason for such a command; it must never be based merely on dislike or disapproval of what he is doing.[1] When he begins to be aware of his armor, it means he is rejecting it and the outlook is good.

If a therapist cannot understand a patient in six or eight sessions, he probably never will and the patient should be sent on to someone who may understand him. No therapist can understand everyone and should not expect to; no disgrace is involved and the next therapist should not feel superior if he does understand the patient. His character may be different enough to allow him to see different things.

Some patients should not be touched; others have to "ripen" for six months to two or three years before they can accept treatment. Sometimes a patient cannot complete therapy, but later returns and therapy can be finished.

Legal Aspects of Therapy

It is essential that any therapist know the law as it applies to him. There should be permission from guardians before treatment is undertaken for a patient under twenty-one. Such a patient should not be allowed to do things that may entangle him with the law or lead him into legal difficulties unless there are very compelling and specific reasons known to him and his guardians.

Patients who insist on leading a life of crime are not candidates for therapy—except for cases such as kleptomaniacs, sexual deviates, and drug addicts. These types are not criminals but merely sick, in the medical sense. Here, one must be convinced of the patient's sincerity and determination to be helped. Homosexuals usually are not good candidates—not because they cannot be helped, but because their reasons for coming are usually not good. They seldom feel pain from their condition; only the social or legal stigma affects them.

[1] Patients often display emotions merely to please; what may look like a breakthrough may be meaningless.

Handling Serious Problems

The psychotic, the suicidal patient, the impulsive, and those patients whose emotional condition causes particular concern require great skill and good transference. Here, the situation must be discussed openly and freely, and the patient must be understanding and willing to cooperate fully. It is best to have an understanding with the patient that if the situation becomes acute he will contact the therapist and abide by his decision. I have had psychotic patients hallucinating in two fields (auditory and visual), who carried on their regular work with no one suspecting their condition.

If a suicidal patient will promise to contact his therapist before he makes any suicidal attempt, he can be handled. It is necessary to understand the suicidal threat thoroughly. Any threat should be taken seriously, but where spite is clearly evident one can often make the patient aware of his spiteful attitude by saying, "Thank you for calling; I will cancel your next appointment." Before saying anything like this, one must *know* what he is doing. This method of handling the suicidal threat can only be employed when the therapist is completely sure the patient makes the threat out of spite and does not intend to carry it out. If the patient is seriously contemplating suicide he will become desperate from lack of understanding and will proceed to carry out his threat.

Patients who show impulsive behavior that risks the lives of others are even more nerve-wracking but, fortunately, more rare. The same promise is necessary, and if possible there should be full knowledge of the problem by responsible members of the family.

Dreams

Dreams are unimportant in therapy until one reaches the pelvis, although they can be useful to indicate the progress and trend of therapy. Dreams prior to opening the pelvic segment should be interpreted from the ego side rather than from the side of the libido. Dreams, and communications too, may reveal deep complexes involving the Oedipus situation early in therapy but it is a mistake to make deep interpretations too early. Such deep material is presented merely to cover up more superficial but at the moment more painful problems. When dealing with the pelvic segment and genitality, dreams may be interpreted from the libido side and are then acceptable and meaningful to the patient. Just before genital anxiety breaks through dreams of falling and dreams of incest may occur.

For example, early in therapy a patient who suffered from vaginismus brought the following dream:

I was standing on the porch of my house with my pet cat. A bird flew near and the cat grabbed it and started to kill it. I rescued the bird which lay on the step almost dead. Finally it flew into the air and the cat grabbed for it, so I hit the cat and killed it. (In real life she was devoted to the cat.)

From the libidinal level, the bird represents the phallus and the cat the female genital. She kills her genital (vaginismus) which does not allow entry of the penis. This avoids the deep destructive hatred for the penis. If I had given this interpretation she might have understood intellectually, but it would have had no emotional significance. To interpret it thus would have prepared her defenses for later on. My interpretation was to point out that the cat was earth-bound while the bird was free; she was choosing freedom in preference to security and was accepting the goal of therapy. This she understood at once, as she had previously complained much that she didn't understand what we were trying to do and didn't know if she should continue.

A second patient who started therapy following his father's death brought the following dream: He dreamed he was having intercourse with his mother. Knowing psychology, the patient said, "I guess, Doctor, that is the Oedipus complex." I told him I was not concerned with whether it was or not, and asked him if he had become the head of the family when his father died. He looked surprised and asked how I knew, saying that, although he had an older brother this brother could not assume the responsibility. I said, "The head of the family sleeps with mother." (He had taken his father's place.)

A third patient who had been profuse in her praise of how I was helping her brought the following dream: I whispered in her ear a technical term which she did not understand. When she asked me to repeat it, I told her to blow on the side of my head. She immediately said, "That is a fellatio wish." I asked her, however, what was on the side of my head and she replied that it was my ear. "Now," I asked, "what would you blow into my ear?" Obviously, hot air, which meant that all she had been saying was hot air. I told her that this was a resistance dream and that she must tell me what she had against me which she had covered up with all her praise. She finally admitted that she had been resentful at having to pay my fees.

When one reaches the pelvis and streamings begin to appear in the genital the patient begins to react negatively toward sex and toward the therapist. The following is a rather typical dream of such a stage. The dreamer, a young man, was in Africa. A group of Nazis and Arabs were plotting to blow up the world. He, an observer, was frightened. A drunken American soldier turned a cannon on them and killed them. Then an actor dressed as an Arab came and touched him on the arm. The scene shifted and he was in South America registering at a hotel, the name of which was the Inhospitable Hotel.

The first part of the dream represents his struggle to maintain the status quo and prevent surrender (the sensation of bursting or blowing up). I am the actor. His associations to an Arab were that they are sly, cunning and cannot be trusted, and also dirty. I touch him on the arm, which is therapy. He admitted he had begun to think of me as a charlatan and only interested in sex. The hotel he said was furnished like my office. Prior to the dream he had had strong genital sensations which were new to him (strange country).

Occasionally dreams can awaken us out of a complacent attitude and make us aware of something we are missing. A young man who seemed to be progressing well in therapy said that his work function was excellent, he had an increasingly good relationship with his girl friend and people in general. He felt very well. He began to bring dreams of rather marked ability such as driving his car superbly and taking corners at high speed, writing examinations with ease, and beating competitors in running. Among these was a dream I failed to see clearly because of his glowing reports. He was driving his car up a mountain when he ran into a flood and had to abandon the car and continue on foot. As he climbed the water turned to ice but he climbed to the top with the usual success. I was uneasy about dreams of such facility but merely commented that he seemed to do everything so beautifully in his dreams. I watched him and waited until the following dream made the situation clear. He was driving along a mountain highway with his girl friend when glancing back he saw a flood approaching. Others on the road seemed to pay no attention to it but he knew immediately that he must get to higher ground. Fortunately his car was powerful and he started up the mountain on a side road. The road soon forked and he took the left fork as he saw houses that way. He was fortunate as he found later the right fork came to a dead end. Eventually he got to the houses and safety and relaxed. (The *right* road would have let the flood overtake him.) He was very familiar with psychology so I said to him, "You know what water stands for don't you?"

He said, "Yes, feeling."

Then I asked, "What are you doing with all your success?" He looked very surprised and then said, "You spoil everything." He had been successfully running away from feeling and at the same time lulling me to sleep.

Events in the following week further clarified the situation. He reported that after the last session he had become completely impotent for two days and when his erective potency returned sensations were markedly diminished. He brought the following dream: He was with his girl friend when they passed a man. He said to her, "There is so and so, you remember him." When he woke up he realized that she could not possibly remember the man as she had never known him and he had died before she had come there to live. The man had been an old friend of his parents. I asked, "Who would remember him?" Obviously his mother, which he immediately realized with a great deal of shock.

Handling Expressions of Affection

Handling expressions of affection and overtures on the part of women patients may be a frequent necessity. It is even more frequent when the therapist is young and attractive—and also less experienced. Early in therapy or prior to freeing the pelvic segment, the therapist should not be too flattered by overtures. These are a negative response from the standpoint of the goal and are designed to seduce the therapist away from painful subjects by changing the professional situation into an affair. If one could witness the scorn displayed by patients for therapists who fall for this and get entangled, one would need no further warning. They despise the therapist for sacrificing the professional situation and their patient's chance of health. No real love can be felt by the patient until the pelvic armoring is removed, in any case. The situation can usually be handled simply by accusing the patient of being in love with you. She will deny it vigorously, giving reasons why she would never think of such a thing. She may even become hostile. If she is truly in love she will merely admit it earnestly. Some of the feeling of love is stimulated by feelings of relief in therapy, and is simply gratitude and very temporary.

When pelvic armoring is removed, however, the patient may begin to feel love for the therapist. She becomes open and frank. The reality can be determined because the physician feels her sincerity and becomes emotional himself. It is conceivable that he may love in return since the health now being presented is a thing to love. She becomes soft, serious, and giving.

In such a case, the patient should be allowed to describe her desire thoroughly. It is necessary here to be very frank and honest and for both to keep their heads. The most important objective is still her health and nothing must interfere. She must not be sent abruptly away or her love will turn into hate through frustration and lack of attaining her goal of health. It must be worked through. One must remember that in most cases what feels like love is gratitude for help in therapy and rapidly resolves itself. Even love may be temporary, and can usually be transferred easily to a suitable mate. The therapist must not use his vantage point as bringer of relief to fix his patient's attraction to him; the object is rather to enable her to find a suitable partner on her own, and she may need much help and encouragement in this respect. On the other hand, the therapist should not refuse her offers of love by giving the impression that she is not desirable; she has lately come to health and is easily crushed. She should be made to feel desirable (as she really is) but that for her own welfare she must find love for herself.

Problems of the End Phase

The end phase presents the main danger in therapy. This is the time when the patient reaches out and cannot take it and then contracts. This is especially dangerous if the patient is hooked somewhere; he will break down at the hook. A persistent block is reason to give up therapy. The end phase begins with the full flow of energy into the pelvis, when all blocks have been dissolved and the totality of the organism begins to function.

Here in a typical way dangers begin to arise: If there is a hook, energy cannot get through the curve. It is not the expansion that creates the danger, but the sudden rise in energy level. Previously, the organism functioned by binding energy; the danger is the reaction of the organism to the high level to which it is unaccustomed.

Juvenile delinquency, for example, is a result of trying to function above the tolerance level. The child with low energy or the greatly repressed one is not a delinquent. But when energy cannot be handled rationally, urges of the moment are given in to with no evaluation of the consequences. When the last segment of armor is dissolved, a jump in energy occurs and wrong concepts of freedom, such as promiscuity, may be displayed.

Orgasm anxiety occurs at the end of the end phase and the organism must be prepared to accept the anxiety. At first the patient feels he is right back where he started. Symptoms reappear, sometimes stronger than before. Preparation for this should start at the beginning of therapy with the determination, in the first few sessions, of the point at which the patient will break down.

One sure source of danger in schizophrenia is a tenacious eye segment block where the patient cannot develop an ability to open his eyes. Clinging to a certain type of blocking shows where the block will occur in the end phase; for example in a rigid chest. If it is to be in the diaphragm, somatic symptoms and collapse must be watched for. The more tenacious the block, the more trouble is ahead. Anorgonia will reoccur in a most severe form when the pelvis is reached, and it is best not to rush toward the pelvis.

The main block plus orgasm anxiety may make the situation insoluble. Suicide, psychosis, murder, or criminal behavior can occur. These possibilities must be recognized early, and for that the physician should possess at least a minimum of orgonotic sensing of the genital streamings. One senses in one's own organism when, where, and how the patient pulls away from the pelvis. It is vital to know what frightens the patient away, and in order to know, the therapist must have orgonotic pelvic streamings.

The following symptoms precede orgasm anxiety. There is a retraction of the pelvis. Energy draws back from the pelvis and symptoms recur higher up. One must start from the head again and work down as before; this may have to be repeated several times. One must structuralize the patient's health and make him more capable of tolerating pelvic sensations. Also appearing will be a bursting feeling; falling anxiety; failing coordination of legs, and a feeling of falling apart; disorientation; feelings of emptiness and exhaustion; fear of dying (a bursting sensation from expansion against contraction which leads to fears of dying or feelings of dissolution); fear of losing control and becoming psychotic (at the point of emission the patient may block and feel a desire to choke; in life, murder is such a breakthrough); and absentmindedness will appear in the end phase and the patient appear ament.

These symptoms originate at the end phase at the point of breakthrough into the pelvis. Organic symptoms may also appear and require operation. Such symptoms may include appendicitis, ovarian cyst, etc. Cancer could also develop. At this point, blocks are felt as coming from outside; orgasm anxiety is always felt as something done to you, from outside. The final problem is to structuralize the patient's health; that is, to keep him under observation and assist him until he is secure against regressing.

A Special Problem of Puberty

Children between the ages of eight and sixteen years should be treated with caution and should usually be subjected only to emergency measures with no thought of complete removal of the armor. During this age period the increase in energy that will come with the push of puberty renders removal of the armor unsafe. The child cannot handle the double increase of energy resulting from puberty and loss of armor. They *need* their armor.

Freedom and License

One of the greatest difficulties for patients, parents, and even therapists is to distinguish between license and freedom. The moment the patient grasps that the therapy stands for freedom he conjures the picture, "Now I can do anything I want to." This attitude is applied toward the therapist as well as toward the world in general and must be clarified very promptly.

To do anything one wishes is license; it assumes no responsibility. Freedom, on the other hand, always assumes responsibility and does not interfere with the rights of others or endanger the patient's own life. Freedom, so far as therapy is concerned, is most important in regard to natural needs, not social needs. That is, it really matters little what social customs are required of us as long as we are allowed freedom to express our emotions and satisfy our natural needs.

17 · Orgonomic Biopsychiatric Therapy

THE FOLLOWING CASE PRESENTATIONS are given to illustrate the practical application of Reich's theory of character. It is true that this selection is not representative of the average case met with in practice, for each of these cases presents some particular complication which renders therapy more difficult than usual, if not impossible. These cases were in fact selected for that very reason; they demonstrate the effectiveness of the technique in forcing the individual toward functioning even, as the second case illustrates, where the patient cannot tolerate such functioning. The basic problem in therapy is the organism's ability to tolerate the rise in energy level obtained through dissolving the mechanism of binding energy. This is especially a problem when the final pelvic armoring is removed and a sudden jump in energy occurs. The organism has to be gradually prepared for this jump from the start of therapy.

Therapy is not simply a matter of "working" on muscle spasm or producing dramatic emotional outbursts. The efforts of the organism to express itself must be carefully watched and the organism must be assisted in that expression by overcoming the obstacles which present themselves. Resistances are recognized and eliminated by releasing muscle spasm, increasing push through it, revealing character defenses, overcoming ignorance, and presenting problems in understandable perspective. Thus the organism gradually unburdens itself of its restrictions and expresses its buried emotions from superficial to deep, until basic repressions that involve the Oedipus conflict are met and overcome. Sexual impulses become acceptable and the organism can then function as an integrated whole. However, the newly acquired health must be structuralized and the patient is not secure until he can overcome by himself any tendencies to revert to his former neurotic traits and inhibitions. Neurotic tendencies are deeply ingrained after years of irrational training and neurotic living and are easy to fall back into until the patient has learned to live spontaneously the new freedom he has found.

The average case can be greatly relieved. One has reasonable hope of removing all major symptoms. Still too few, however, reach that approximation of health we term orgastic potency. This goal is ever kept in mind and worked for and, although it cannot be wholly attained in the majority of cases, one can approach close enough to allow the patient a satisfying life, closer to health in many instances than the so-called "normal" in our society. Where stasis can be prevented or overcome and the environment adjusted satisfactorily, one can expect the patient to continue to improve for years after therapy has been discontinued.

Reich felt strongly that the medical orgonomist should make a point of seeing a patient for not more than two hundred sessions to avoid a laissez faire attitude resulting in prolonged treatments, such as one frequently encounters in psychoanalysis. I must confess that my early cases seemed to require much less time than they have as the years passed; they usually took less than one hundred sessions. Reich said this is usual; one gradually sees more to correct and becomes more particular, and at the same time less inclined to push as vigorously. Perhaps increasing age and declining necessity to work miracles are factors.[1] I am not convinced, however, that this is necessarily an advantage to the patient. Some of my early, short therapies have done as well as more thorough and more prolonged later successes. One case

[1] I am convinced that the pollution of our atmosphere is a factor which should be considered. This tends to immobilize people and render therapy difficult.

consisting of only twenty-two sessions has remained well for eighteen years. The important factor is the ability to attain and maintain a satisfying sexual life regardless of the length or thoroughness of therapy.

I reviewed the first one hundred patients terminated during my first five years of practice as a medical orgonomist. All these cases can be looked at for a period of at least ten years since they discontinued therapy. Of this hundred, nine stopped early because of negative reactions to therapy, two remained unimproved at the time of their discharge after two years of therapy (one of these, a paranoid schizophrenic, later became actively psychotic and was hospitalized).

About a quarter of the cases stopped when they had been relieved of their misery but before I felt that I had done all that I could do for them. Four of these later relapsed to the point where I would have to consider them unimproved. Another patient, a schizophrenic, subsequently developed a psychosis and was hospitalized. I would thus consider that the sixteen cases so far mentioned did not profit from treatment.

One woman was discontinued because I felt that recovery could not be obtained without a broken marriage which she would not be able to accept. She had by that time become comfortable and has apparently continued to adjust. I discontinued another because I felt we were not progressing satisfactorily; she went to another orgonomist. One marriage was dissolved; but, on the other hand, one marriage was saved and most were placed on a firmer basis, particularly where both parties were treated. Nine patients have continued to see me on an occasional visit to prevent slipping back into old neurotic patterns; they probably would not have survived otherwise. Three of these had been hospitalized before I saw them—one for eight years, one for four years, and the other for one year. All of them have continued to make overtly good adjustments and have found some enjoyment in living.

Fifteen patients reached orgastic potency. These patients have made rather definite changes in their way of life and have maintained health. One was a paranoid schizophrenic who was psychotic at times during therapy.

The remaining forty patients were free of major symptoms at the time of their discharge from therapy and were making good adjustments in their environments, capable of pleasurable sexual experiences but short of full orgasm. Three of these returned for further treatment after ten or more years with recurrence of symptoms.[2] One of the three is described in the first case history below. Three others, I learned, returned for treatment elsewhere, two of them going to other orgonomists.

Of the remainder, I have no definite information on the present condition of about half; they were complaining of no problems when I last heard from them. The rest have continued to live satisfying lives.

Thus, about three-fourths of this hundred of my patients have apparently remained free of major or crippling symptoms since their therapy.

This résumé demonstrates, I am sure, that orgonomy does not pretend to be a cure-all. Too many people have developed a mystical attitude toward this therapy; they expect salvation through orgastic potency, and either expect us to bring it to them or else accuse us of claiming to. This situation does not arise from any claims the therapy has ever made, but rather it raises from the mystical character of the individuals themselves. Orgonomy is based on a great truth which the individual naturally reaches out to, but some reach out mystically instead of rationally. Thus we are accused either of failure or of being quacks. Occasionally, a disillusioned soul leaves in bitterness or in rage to continue his search for salvation elsewhere—in Yoga, Zen Buddhism, or astrology.

However, with all our limitations (and I am convinced the limitations are due to the human element, the patient and the therapist, not due to the therapy's theory), our results seem to make a reasonably good showing when they are compared with other therapies. The hundred cases mentioned were unselected. In those first years, I accepted practically everyone who came to me. Later I became more selective, not in the emotional problems involved, but rather in my estimation of the patient.

Looking back on my ten years of psychoanalytic work prior

[2] See "Stasis," p. 104.

to my familiarity with orgonomy, I estimate that only one of my patients reached orgastic potency.

Orgonomic technique is less dependent on verbal communication from the patient; it is more effective in attacking the neurotic structure; and it requires less time than various schools of psychoanalytic procedure. I believe it is worthy of serious study by all those who can overcome their own fear of life and movement. The primary goal, however, remains prevention, not cure of the already crippled. The hope of prevention lies in educating parents toward rearing children more and more in the ways of health. Even though members of this generation cannot attain health, they can at least learn to cease preventing their children from attaining a higher degree of emotional freedom.

A Case of Hysteria with Asthma

The patient in this case was an attractive twenty-two-year-old white woman. She had been married at seventeen during her last year of high school while in a rebound from a broken love affair. The older of two daughters, she was brought up by a severely neurotic mother who could not leave the house because of her fears. A maternal aunt had committed suicide and an uncle was institutionalized. The father was quiet, patient, and overly concerned about her welfare. The younger sister was indecisive.

Throughout her life she had been overprotected, warned against the wiles of men, encouraged to stay home with her mother, and watched over by her father when she did go out. Because of her good looks and gay vivacity she was sought after socially and was the life of the party She had many dates but no serious love affairs; boys never seemed to get serious, which worried her a great deal. In her early teens she had been employed as an artist's model after winning a beauty contest. She frequently had to pose in the nude, leaving finally when the artist made advances to her.

At the age of twelve, coincidental with the onset of menstruation, she had developed asthma, with frequent attacks up to the time I first saw her. Menstruation was painful and irregular.

Until the time of her marriage she had had no sexual contact and had never been sexually aroused. She married, not for love, but to spite another boy she imagined she was in love with. On the wedding night, she cried bitterly, and she cried during most of her honeymoon. The sexual embrace brought her no pleasure and she thought that it was just something she had to put up with in marriage. She longed for her parents. Becoming pregnant almost immediately, she submitted to an abortion because she did not feel capable of accepting a child. After a few months of marriage, she fell in love with a friend of her husband; but, feeling guilty, gave him up and decided she loved only her husband.

Her husband was drafted into the armed forces at about this time, and on his return told her about various affairs he had had in Europe. This shocked her and for months she could not bear to have him touch her. Eventually, she again became pregnant, and had a daughter two years old when I first saw her.

Following the birth of her daughter, she became sleepless and anxious, developed nightmares, and was disturbed finally by painful and distressing thoughts while awake. She felt depressed, thought of suicide constantly, could not be left alone, and grew afraid to leave the house. Fear of dying from a cerebral hemorrhage or a heart attack, or of killing her husband or her daughter, led her to return to her parents in a panic.

She began to think everything was death and felt that she was not responsible for her actions. Her dreams became pleasant ones about the good times of her past, but her days were filled with panic, fears of insanity, and of sudden death. She had to be escorted everywhere. Her legs felt automatous and she was afraid they would come up and hit her; palpitation was marked and she felt that something was pressing on her mind. Life brought no joy and she wanted to die yet shrank from it in terror. She was finally placed in a general hospital, with commitment considered.

When I first saw her, she was lying rigidly in bed, obviously in acute panic in spite of the heavy sedation she had been receiving. When I explained that I was a psychiatrist she was very much upset and was sure she was considered insane. After some reassurance she told me her story.

Quoting the physical studies done at the hospital, I assured her of her physical fitness and explained the emotional origin of her condition. The catharsis and assurances calmed her somewhat. The panic left her face; she held my hand for contact and smiled wanly, but her face remained stiff and mechanical. Her whole body made one think of a mannequin rather than of a living being. Biophysical examination showed a marked spasticity of the whole musculature: the chest was immobile, the masseters and sterno mastoids stood out in contraction and were hard and painful to touch. The abdomen was boardlike, thighs rigid and spastic, and the pelvis immobile. A stiff neck gave her a haughty, unbending expression.

I asked her to breathe through her mouth, manually compressed her chest, and encouraged her to scream, which she did in a stifled way. I dissolved some of the spasm in her throat and jaws and asked her to lie on her face and then to beat the couch as I was pressing the trapezii. The effort was tiring, but she was relaxed and said she felt much better. I advised against the necessity of commitment and suggested that she come to my office for therapy. Both she and her father felt it would be impossible since she was so afraid of going anywhere, so I urged her to return home.

Three days later, her father made an appointment and brought her to the office; she had developed sufficient confidence to attempt the trip. When she walked in she was a living automaton: body stiff, walk mechanical, arms held rigidly at the sides, face immobile with a sad expression, and anxiety in the eyes. Her head was held high and her neck rigid; she looked as though she were resigned to execution.

I asked her to lie on the couch with her knees flexed and to breathe through her mouth. She was overtly passive but remained rigid, thighs held tightly together, arms hugging her sides. She could take only shallow breaths; the chest was fixed in the inspiratory position and did not move. Setting about freeing her chest brought on an asthmatic attack, which was relieved by deep inspiration. Then I encouraged her to concentrate on expiration while I exerted considerable pressure on the sternum. There was some movement in her chest, but still with much wheezing in expiration.

The intense emotions buried in this girl were clearly evident; superficially she showed anxiety, crying was there, and rage is always present in asthma. The problem was to decide which emotion was to be released first. It seemed probably best that rage should be brought out if it could be reached, because the aggressive action would relieve the anxiety and the rigid contraction. I asked her to make a face and she looked angry. Pressing on her masseters, I asked her to continue looking angry, clench her fists, and snarl like an animal. Continuing this, I asked her to turn on her face, and told her to let herself go while I pressed on the dorsal muscles. She began to yell and strike the couch, becoming more and more angry until she stopped exhausted and cried. Her chest was moving easily and breathing was free with no wheezing.

She remarked that she felt peculiarly free and that a weight had been lifted from her chest, but she was ashamed of having let herself go, particularly when she had nothing to be angry about. I explained that she had never learned to express her feelings so that they had remained buried throughout the years and must be released if she were to get well. She felt much better and had only two minor attacks of asthma before the next session, but she continued to complain of a fear of impending insanity.

I continued to concentrate on her rage, paying no attention to the psychic complaints. This time she grew almost wild in her yelling and beating, screaming, "I hate you! I hate you! You did this to me!" When she was again exhausted, she explained that she had felt a sudden hatred for her mother, who had interfered with everything she had wanted to do and restricted her in keeping with her own neurosis. She could not understand how her father had put up with the marriage. Once again, her chest was free and her breathing easy.

However, that night she called me to say that she had had a severe attack of asthma for which her physician had given her adrenalin; she was sure that the wind had brought on the attack. On the way out for her next session, she developed another attack when she saw the leaves swaying in the breeze. She was positive that wind or trees brought it on, but I did not understand the significance of this until much later. I looked skeptical, which angered her, and she accused me of not under-standing (which was true). I was not prepared for the tre-mendous falling anxiety to come later.

For about twenty sessions I concentrated on her chest, jaws, and back, getting her to express rage and pointing out her haughty stiff-necked attitude. Her asthmatic attacks became milder and less frequent, until one day she came in highly elated because the wind had blown a gale without producing an attack. I smiled skeptically and told her that she could no longer be called a weather prophet. By now, her chest moved freely, she had no wheezes and felt very much encouraged. She said I was a magician to have cured a long-standing asthma where many physicians had failed. But her fear of insanity persisted; in fact, it grew worse. She developed distressing dreams of going out with many men when consciously she wanted only her husband.

I then proceeded to her abdomen, thighs, and pelvis. Im-mediately the wheezing started but was mild, and I continued. Her thighs began to tremble, she became anxious and restless, finally sat up and said that she wanted to go home; that she couldn't stand the treatment after all and doubted that I knew what I was doing. She was going crazy and I could not stop her; besides I had not cured her asthma after all; perhaps I was crazy myself. I again pointed out her stiff-necked attitude—she must be prim and proper at all costs. She burst into tears and felt considerably relieved, apologizing profusely for her attitude, begging me not to be angry or to throw her out because I was the only one who could help her. All that she wanted was to remain near so that she could feel safe.

After three or four more sessions she appeared with severe eczematous rash extending in a band around her lower abdomen and back, with intense itching. Her asthma was gone. Her fears were lessened but her days and nights were taken up with the intense itching. This continued for about six weeks, by which time her thighs and pelvis were soft. Breathing impulses now extended into her pelvis so I encouraged her to breathe through to establish the orgasm reflex, bringing her pelvis forward at the end of expiration. This immediately brought on an asthmatic attack and she said she felt like a tree bent in the wind. At last I understood her intense fear of pelvic movements and pelvic sensations: she was afraid of being bent as the trees were in the wind and could not tolerate movement. She had thus become board-(tree-)like.

I returned to her chest, bringing out more anger and sobbing which relieved her asthma. Then I concentrated on her eyes, inducing her to express anxiety and to look at me. She was never able to do this, and when I insisted she became very alarmed and sat up, saying that she would stand no more. I accused her of having thoughts about me and she confessed that she had an intense desire to throw her arms about me and to kiss me.

Reassuring her that such impulses were natural enough, I asked her if she trusted me. Was she afraid that I would take advantage of her? She was sure that she had no fears in that respect but she was afraid of her own impulses. Finally she became more comfortable, could look at me, and talked more freely. I continued pointing out her haughty attitude, her virgin purity as contrasted to her promiscuous dreams, and worked on her neck.

She grew dissatisfied with her husband, his coldness, and her emotionless sex life. I returned again to her pelvis, which was now freely movable. She was ashamed to breathe through, saying it was just like sex when one lets oneself go. Finally she began to report sexual dreams involving several men, during which she experienced genital sensations, and she even developed some feeling with her husband.

She felt quite free, started going out alone, and definitely began to look around for someone to love. She complained that I was married and wondered why that had to be—because I could take care of her and be an ideal husband. I pointed out her continued fear of sexuality and she bargained that if I would find a man for her she would leave her husband. I told her that this was in the social sphere and that she must learn to handle her own life. Therapy progressed smoothly; her fears subsided, she went about freely and presented no armor.

Her pelvic movements became smoother and occasionally spontaneous, but one day she came in with acute anxiety. She reported that she was back where she started; she could not even go down the steps or walk on the sidewalk because she was afraid that she would fall. Her knees would give way and she had no control of her legs; her fear of insanity became acute. I induced her to breathe through and encouraged her to accept her pleasurable sensations, and explained that she was suffering from falling anxiety, a fear of melting or of preorgastic pleasure sensations.

This continued for several sessions until her marital situation became more prominent. She could not tolerate her husband and left him to return to her own family, but finally went back to him because living with her mother was worse. I encouraged her to find a position and live by herself until she knew what she wanted, but she could not bring herself to take the step. I told her it was her life, and if she wanted to continue being miserable she could. I cut her visits to once a month. She constantly complained but would do nothing about it, so I advised her to discontinue therapy since the social aspect alone remained to be solved and this she must do.

Finally she did find an apartment by herself, obtained a position, and became self-supporting. She made many superficial contacts with men but was dissatisfied with them and maintained a weekend relationship with her husband. She did not love him, but felt only a fondness for him. Less than two years after she discontinued therapy, she returned to him and decided to make the best of the situation.

Although she had considerable genital feeling and found the sexual act pleasurable, she had not reached full orgastic potency. Biologically, she was capable, but it was unlikely that she could surrender sufficiently to her husband to reach this goal. Therapy had consisted of eighty-five sessions.

Four years passed, and she continued to make a good social adjustment with no return of asthma or other symptoms. The social aspect, however, prevented her from reaching the final goal of full health and she began to build up tension. She called, complaining of a lump in her throat and I saw her six times. She identified the lump as long and cylindrical and finally recognized it as a fantasied penis, upon which the symptom cleared up.

For eight years after that I did not hear of her, except to read of promotions she periodically received.

Twelve years after she first discontinued therapy, she called me in a panic. Her anxiety was so intense it was interfering with her work; she could not remain alone or go out by herself, being afraid she would do something foolish or become immobilized. At that point her mother was dying of cancer and she had been spending all her time caring for her. Even more upsetting from the standpoint of guilt was the fact that she had allowed herself to give in sexually to a married man with whom she had been in love for several years. She felt guilty when she thought of her husband and daughter.

When I saw her she was in an acute state of anxiety. I mobilized her generally and had her scream and express rage; she responded very well with all her effort and felt very much relieved and I continued to see her weekly. She took her mother's death quite well and made rapid gains in going places and feeling more and more assured. However, the problem of her love for a married man continued to be a central concern. He was willing to obtain a divorce and marry her if she would consent and also obtain a divorce. She did not, of course, love her husband, but could not think of hurting him. Further, she felt it would be hard on her sixteen-year-old daughter. But her sexual guilt diminished and she experienced a high degree of pleasure and relaxation in her occasional relations with her lover. With her husband, she was anaesthetic, submitting only for his sake. Life with him was dull and stifling, whereas she felt alive with the man she loved.

Finally she decided that the only rational course was to leave her husband and made definite plans to divorce and remarry.

As the time grew near, however, for her to actually take the step she became more and more indecisive and wondered whether she really wanted to marry her lover. I reminded her that I had suggested that she live by herself as a first step in deciding, and here I went further. I told her that she did not love either her husband or this other man because a third man was interfering.

I suggested she could not leave her husband until her father remarried. (He was planning to marry shortly, although she objected to the woman he had selected.) She agreed immediately, saying she felt it would hurt her father for her to leave now and she felt responsible for him since he had a bad heart, but, that if he were married she would feel free. I told her she felt this way because she wanted her father herself. She was very shocked but admitted she had always been very attached to him *as a father*. I said, "No, it is more than that." She became very upset and asked me if she should stay away from her father. I said, "By no means. Why not let yourself become aware of what you really feel for him?"

Prior to this she had endeavored to hide her unhappy marriage and extramarital interest from her father. Now she discussed it freely with him and discovered he had known it all along and wondered why she had not left her husband years ago. She decided her father could look after himself and did not need her. She had enough to look after in her own life. To continue living with her husband was unthinkable and although she wished he would fall in love with another woman, she was going to secure a divorce anyway.

Even with this resolve she again felt the difficulty of leaving and hurting her husband. I pointed out her need to look after the interests of others—her mother, father, husband, and daughter rather than herself, as though she had no right to her own wishes. She replied that was exactly how she felt. She did believe that now she was healthier than she had ever been before. She said that if she were going to lose her lover by her procrastinations she would cease to worry about others because she could not afford to lose him. She knew she would have a relapse if she gave him up and settled for remaining with her husband.

Once more, time will have to decide her future.

A Case of Intolerance of Vitality

One of the tasks of the medical orgonomist is to accustom the individual to tolerate functioning at higher energy levels. This may be a very trying and even disastrous undertaking in a patient of high charge and little or no ability to make the adjustment.

A case of this sort was that of a thirty-one-year-old housewife who complained of extreme nervousness and said she felt frightened about something; she could not define her fear but had been in that condition for six months. It had started a month after the birth of her fourth baby. At the onset of the condition she had felt something slowly creeping up the back of her neck and had thought she had developed tuberculosis. She had a feeling of pressure in her head and was afraid of losing her mind. Her legs were weak, particularly in the morning when she was especially nervous. She had had a constant ringing in her ears which disappeared before I saw her; also a palpitation of the heart, occasional headaches, and a variable appetite. Her bowels were constipated, her nights were sleepless, and she was afraid of harming her children, and worried constantly about her husband's safety. Finally, she had a paralyzing fear of thunderstorms.

She had consulted various physicians and had improved temporarily, but during the week before I saw her, the nervousness had increased to the point where she could not remain alone. Her husband had had to leave his work and stay with her; she felt much better when he was present. She had been married seven years and had known her husband for eight months before they married. He was her only love and she insisted that the marriage was entirely congenial. Both were Roman Catholic but she claimed that she was not very religious, while he was quite devout.

Sexually, she had been anaesthetic, particularly since the birth of her last baby. Prior to this she had had occasional genital sensation and prior to her marriage she had experienced some pleasure in the sexual act, but had never had a climax. She had had no genital contact with anyone but her husband. Within her memory, she had never been able to masturbate. The sexual act was not disgusting; she merely experienced no pleasure. Because of her worry over becoming pregnant for a fifth time, she had persuaded her husband to agree to contraception (that is, a diaphragm), although it was against his principles.

She had no complaints about her children, but admitted she

did not enjoy them as much as she had before her illness. Her father, to whom she was attached, had died suddenly of a heart attack when she was sixteen. He had been an alcoholic. Her mother, a cold and dominant woman was living and well.

Very much frightened about her condition and extremely anxious to be helped, she impressed me as being serious and honest and agreed readily to cooperate with any treatment necessary. She was a rather large, stately, well-proportioned, beautiful, businesslike-looking woman. On the couch, she presented a striking picture of rigidity. One felt that she could be lifted up by her head without bending. Her arms hugged her sides, shoulders were tight, legs crossed, and head held fixed by a very prominent spastic neck. Her jaws were tightly closed, her eyes were wide open and anxious to the point of panic, and she watched me constantly with a marked suspicion. Her pupils were widely dilated, pulse 96, her face was frozen and her neck and face flushed. Except for her thighs and legs, which were cool, her body was quite warm. Her chest was held high, not moving. Her spinal muscles were hard and spastic, pelvis immovable, and thighs, which she held tightly together, very spastic and tender. Everything about her indicated that she was holding in against great tension—she seemed ready to explode. She was quite bristly and ready to argue against any suggestion.

Finding herself on the couch was very embarrassing to her and she complained that she was not accustomed to lying in front of a man with so little clothing on.[3] I reminded her that I was a physician and recalled her four pregnancies. Just the same, she felt exposed and threatened, but denied any fear of me. Scoffing at any thoughts of a sexual attack, she said she understood the necessity of the examination. Finally, she admitted that her greatest concern was that her abdomen was "not flat" and that she had worried very much about her shape since the birth of her babies. She said she could not help being embarrassed but

[3] In this therapy where movement in the body is so important the therapist must be able to see the patient and also work on muscle holding. Therefore patients wear a minimum of clothing—either underclothing or a bathing suit. One might think it would be better if the patient were nude, but as Reich observed, man has covered his genital for thousands of years and who are we to uncover it.

wanted to cooperate and would do anything to get well; she added that she had heard a great deal about me and had complete confidence in me and wanted to continue. Her forehead and cheeks were stiff and she could scarcely move them, but when I asked her to make a face she showed the most murderous hate I have ever seen on the couch. However, she had no contact whatever with this expression, nor had she any with her suspicion; with the latter she never did acquire any contact.

I asked her to express rage; she stiffened even more and said, "I won't do that. It's foolish." I got the same reaction with every attempt at getting her to express any emotion or sound; I explained that some day she would have to respond to all of them if she were ever to get well and that if it seemed too much she was free to stop right then. She was determined to go on and pleaded that I just give her time and she would cooperate. Thus started my greatest battle against human defenses, calling for all my patience, determination, and ingenuity for 177 sessions; and I lost.

In the following sessions I explained her biophysical state in detail—her high energy, her defenses against its free-flowing sensations, our aim to break down her defenses to release energy. I told her that the released energy had to be drained off by emotional expression or it would only result in an increase of her panic, and that that was why she had to learn to give in to her feelings and express them. I reassured her about her anxiety, pointing out that, although it was distressing, it meant that she was very much alive but merely afraid of that life. Repeatedly, I tried to make her aware of her suspicion, but she denied any awareness of it or any mistrust of me. Her embarrassment continued and I may say that, except for short periods, it persisted with the suspicion to the bitter end. She seemed to understand very clearly when I explained, and I felt that at least I could depend on her best ability to help. Therefore I asked her to breathe as fully as she could, emphasizing breathing out, and to be embarrassed, if she must, but not to let it interfere with her cooperation.

She objected even to breathing, belittling the request and saying she thought it was silly and "what would it accomplish anyway?" I pointed out her defense, reminded her that I had explained all of this before and that I had no intention of arguing every point with her. Adding that her bristliness was covering up her fear and her suspicion of me, I asked her if she thought I just wanted her to appear foolish and if she thought I would ask her to do foolish things. She promised to cooperate and challenged me to continue, making feeble efforts at breathing but without moving her chest. When I applied light pressure on the chest she immediately became very upset and belligerent. She said she would not stand for such treatment. So I sat back and explained everything again and asked her if she wanted to stop. Again there were promises to cooperate and determination to continue. Each succeeding step followed a similar pattern until it became almost routine to say, "We have to take another machine gun nest."

Finally I mobilized her chest fairly well and got her to make sighing sounds, although she objected at first because it sounded "too sexual." She also objected that the position she assumed on the couch was too sexual. When I set about loosening her jaws, spinal muscles, and neck, it was a real problem. Her back and shoulders refused to give and I pointed out her stiff-necked attitude, her righteousness, her necessity to be strong, always blaming others and unable to accept the blame herself—she was a perfectionist. She admitted at length that she thought it was weak to show one's feelings. Reproaching me, she said that she wasn't an animal and that she was afraid I wanted to make one of her. I remarked that animals were more rational than humans and that if her beliefs would not allow her to be just a human animal I could not help her and she should stop therapy. She said health meant more to her than religion and we went on.

Then I tried to get her to express fear by screaming but ran into a complete block; she became very bristly, belittling, and said she would do no such thing. She asked me if I wanted people to think she was crazy. I told her I did not accept "won't" and if it were that she could stop; if, however, it was a matter of "can't" I could understand, and we would have to try to find out why. Finally and with great difficulty she did admit that she could not scream—no sound would come. She did not know how to go about it and the thought of screaming made her panicky.

We concentrated on mobilizing her forehead and eyes, particularly in looking anxiously from side to side, trying to make contact with her suspicion. I encouraged her to breathe in gasps and repeatedly tried to get her to scream. She simply could not. All I accomplished was to make her more upset without any release. When it was not frozen, her face continued to show the murderous hate, so I decided that it must be faced first, feeling that her panic was at least in part due to fear of her own murderous impulses. I tried to accustom her to this face; she made it several times and I imitated it but she claimed that she still did not feel it. In the end, I got her to make sounds with the hateful expression and encouraged her to hit the couch. She hit timidly. All of this was accomplished over the usual protests, belittling remarks, and "I won'ts."

To irritate her, I told her that she was too nice to hate, and that she must be strong and keep in her emotions, reminded her that she was no animal. At length she became explosively angry and hit me, harder and harder until I was quite bruised. I allowed her to keep on because here, at least, was some success and I did not want to discourage it. For several sessions she beat me, twisted my arm, beat the couch, and bit a towel; she preferred beating me. Each outburst was followed by trembling which embarrassed her. During one session, she suddenly recalled that as a little girl of eight or nine, she was once sitting alone in a room when she suddenly saw a man's face at the window. She became very frightened and then she recognized it as the face she had been making. But she continued to make the murderous face and still she raged, hurling epithets at me. She seemed to enjoy it. She said that I didn't understand her, that I was trying to make an animal out of her, and so forth.

Finally I suspected that this could go on forever if it were allowed and that her continued expression of hate was covering up something deeper. She raged and screamed but still her neck and shoulders remained rigid as ever. Her pupils, however, were no longer dilated and her pulse remained in the low 80s. I told her I thought she had expressed enough rage and that it was likely she was using it to cover up something else, and that I wanted her to stop it.

I continued to point out her need to be strong, her fear of being weak, her competing with men and her resentment of them, recalled her bristly attitude, belittling remarks, attempts to make me ineffective with her "I won'ts," and that she crippled her husband by making him stay at home and be a nursemaid. She kept denying the validity of my remarks, complaining that really she was weak or she would be able to stay alone, and that all she wanted was to get over her anxiety so she could be a good wife and mother. She sobbed frequently, but each time tried to control her sobbing and became provoked at herself for being so weak. I discussed my concern over the fact that she found it so difficult to give in to her emotions and I did not know how far it was possible for her to go. Her invariable reply was that she had to get well.

Still, I had made no progress with her neck and shoulders, but in spite of this and with some misgivings I set about mobilizing her pelvis and thighs. Here she objected almost ferociously. She held her thighs tightly together and said she would stand for no such treatment. Again the explanations, the résumé of the aim of therapy, and the reminder that she could stop; again we proceeded. To my great amazement, when her thighs became soft her neck and shoulders gave spontaneously and her breathing was much easier, with the impulse going well into the pelvis. I had her strike the couch with her pelvis and try to feel the hate that was there and bring it out.

Now, she accused me of being a sexual beast. She said that all I thought of was sex and that I was trying to make her feel the same. With much embarrassment and a great deal of reproach, she admitted beginning to feel sexually excited on the couch. We discussed her sexual life in detail. She resented her puritan upbringing, felt that she should have had more sexual experience, resented her husband's being so devout, and having had to force birth control on him against his religion. She dared not look at other men, although she found them attractive and interesting to speculate about. Genital feelings began to develop for the first time since the birth of her oldest child.

I suggested that her fears of being alone or of going out at night might be fears of immorality, and that she needed her husband to protect her from herself. On a deeper level, she was afraid to surrender. She lost the suspicion in her eyes and gradually developed a strong attraction to me. Her lips began to quiver and I had her give in to the urge with reaching and longing. She admitted that she was in love with me but made sure that I did not get the idea that she wanted an affair. She felt much better, became comfortable, could remain alone in the house, and go to town by herself. Genital contact with her husband became pleasurable and she even reported an occasional climax—something she had never experienced before.

However, after a short respite of a few weeks, her anxiety returned. Her fears of insanity became acute; summer was coming and her old fear of lightning returned. I told her it was a fear of her own streamings and she remembered having the same fear as a child. Her mother, too, was afraid of lightning. She could no longer go out, feared sudden death, and developed an intense fear of falling. Even when walking on the level floor she had to hang on to chairs. She dared not go out on the street and climbing stairs was a real problem. She could not go up to the second floor unless her husband was with her. I explained her orgasm anxiety and encouraged her to give in during the sexual embrace; she noticed that as sensation increased she would stiffen and hold her breath. During the embrace, she was afraid of making noises —that would be insanity. I held her head back and encouraged her to surrender to her body; she struggled as one drowning for a moment but finally breathed fully and the reflex appeared. The panic disappeared from her face and she was radiant and soft. I relaxed and sighed a deep sigh; therapy to that point had required ninety bitterly fought hours.

This state lasted for two days, during which she felt very alive and well, full of confidence, and without anxiety. Suddenly her former state reappeared and I never achieved as much again. She had touched the door of health but could not maintain it. On looking back, it seemed that I had essentially forced each step on her, and that with each one she seemed equally unprepared. She had entered into nothing willingly, even though she persisted in continuing, and she never seemed to have any real contact with what was happening. Her anxiety reappeared together with her suspicion, the murderous look in her face, the bristly belittling attitude, and the stiff neck. There was nothing to do, even though genital feelings remained, but to start all over again, particularly keeping in mind the necessity of establishing real contact. She had never felt her suspicions nor overcome her embarrassment. Repeated explanations, discussion, and her own experience in therapy never shortened the bitter fight necessary for each new step. Simply, she had gone through ninety sessions without accepting anything.

I concentrated on her suspicion and her stiff-necked, unyielding attitude, and discussed in greater detail her sexual life, her thoughts, and her fantasies. I learned nothing new; she loved her husband, there was not a thing against him, he was ideal, certainly she would leave him if she did not love him, her religion would not stand in her way, nor would she keep the home together just because of the four children. She wanted to get well; in fact, she had to and she was sick of being so miserable.

I turned then to discussions of her father. She loved to talk about him, but these discussions were equally unproductive. He was the most admired person in her life; in fact she married her husband because he was in many ways like her father—he was kind and understanding and she felt safe with him as she did with her father. She recalled many wonderful days when she went on trips with her father, many delightful evenings talking with him; she resented her mother, who seemed jealous of their companionship. When the father died suddenly, she was very broken up. Although he had been an alcoholic, she rather remarkably recalled no unpleasant experiences because of the condition and consistently minimized the habit. She could recall no sexual thoughts or feeling toward him, just admiration and a feeling of contact. In fact, she remembered no genital urge prior to falling in love with her husband. She could fantasy genital contact with her father without disgust but at the same time without feeling, and she insisted she had never had any such urge and didn't then.

While we were in the midst of this discussion, her mother-in-law made plans to visit them for a month. As the time for the visit drew closer, she became increasingly angry, brought out many bitter things against her husband's whole family, and finally against her husband. She remained angry until the mother-in-law left, complained bitterly that her husband was spineless, that he seemed more concerned about his mother's feeling than hers, that he wasn't man enough to send his mother away when he found how the visit upset her, that he insisted on taking his mother to church every Sunday, and that she had to be dragged along to avoid family scenes. Finally, she decided she would leave him, at last she knew that she had never loved him but had put up with him because he resembled her father. Emotionally, she felt much better. She could again remain alone—in fact much preferred solitude to being with her mother-in-law.

She went out at every opportunity to escape the woman she hated so much, and even came to therapy without her husband, which was something really new for her. She looked admiringly at other men, and one man in particular excited her sexually. She began to lose genital feeling for her husband but her desire was there and continued unfulfilled; there was no desire to masturbate but she denied any feelings against it. For about six weeks she was thus comparatively comfortable but sexually unfulfilled.

Finally her mother-in-law left, and gradually she began to see her husband once more in a better light, and even began to deny the hatred she had expressed for him. She was sure she loved him and that he was the only man she had ever loved. However, she rapidly lost genital sensation and in the end became as anaesthetic as before. The anxiety returned with increasing intensity; the stiff neck and suspiciousness remained fixed. I persisted in following up her suspicion and her stiff neck, repeatedly pointing out her righteousness, her perfectionism, her need to be strong, and her fear of leaving her husband in spite of her resentment toward him. She began to turn on me; I was trying to break up her home, I was just a sexual beast, I did not adequately handle her transference for me but skipped over it too quickly because I had not understood it properly and would not let her talk about it enough. In fact, all I was interested in was making an animal out of her.

The issue of her transference came up many times and I felt she must be right, that I had not handled it properly; but I could find no more clues about what I had done wrong. (I suspect that it was not so much how I handled it but that she could not accept her failure to win me.) Becoming quite concerned about her condition, I suggested a consultation with Wilhelm Reich. She consistently refused until Reich had left for Maine—and then she agreed to see him, later using this repeatedly to plague me because I had not arranged a consultation. I frankly told her my concern and suggested that she go to another therapist who might see what I had missed, but she turned down each suggestion. At the same time, she kept taunting me to do something.

I discussed her situation and said I did not know if she could get well, whether she could stand health and full genitality. Yet I hesitated simply to discharge her because of her acute anxiety and her distressing symptoms. Instead of easing, as I had hoped, the symptoms became more intense as the days passed; she feared imminent death, felt she was going to explode, was certain she was going violently insane, and developed a severe dizziness. I kept reassuring her and explaining her orgasm anxiety, and she maintained that she loved her husband. I finally told her that she would simply have to understand what was happening and give in, surrender to her feelings as she had once done, and make up her mind to face her daily living in spite of her anxiety.

With this, I lengthened the time between sessions, at first to twice a month and then to once a month. This situation continued for a whole year and, to my surprise, she adjusted fairly well, reporting each time that she had not been too miserable until a day or two before she was due to return. Therefore I suggested that she go on her own and call me only if she really needed me.

In the next six months I saw her twice. Then she called for an appointment, came in and sat down and said she did not want to be on the couch, but wanted to know what I intended to do for her since she had been coming a long time and was no better. I told her I could promise her nothing, had never promised her anything, and suggested she see someone else. She wanted to know if she could see Reich and I told her I would arrange it if she were willing to make the trip to Maine. She asked for an appointment the following week, and that time she got on the couch. Her neck was as spastic as ever, she had considerable stasis, and her spite muscles were hard and tender; I pointed out her suspicious attitude and her hostility and was able to release her spite and dissolve much of the spasm in her neck. In fact, her neck became quite soft and she felt much better after the session.

I heard nothing after that until I received a call from her husband two months later. He told me that his wife was very miserable, that he had to stay home with her, that he could not stay away from his work indefinitely, that she had had a great deal of confidence in me and had come to me a long time without benefit. Now they found it necessary, he added, to take her to a good psychiatrist and pay fifteen or twenty dollars a session, which he could scarcely afford, so that he felt they had gotten a "raw deal." He told me that I had asked her once if she wanted her money back and that now she did. I asked him if she had told him the rest of the story—that once when she made a slurring remark about therapy I had asked her if she wanted to have her money back and stop coming to me, but that she had refused and continued to come. Then he asked what suggestions I had, since I did not feel the offer still held good, and I told him he would have to decide for himself because I was not in a very good position to make suggestions. An appointment was made for the two of them to see me to discuss the situation.

At that interview it was quite apparent that she was the dominant partner; he sat meekly and said nothing except to support her when she asked him to. Her eyes were wide open, suspicious, and her face was filled with hate as she told me what a "raw deal" she had gotten from me. She said that at one time I had been a respected analyst, recommended by the physicians in the county, and that she had come full of confidence, expecting that I would analyze her but instead had experimented on her with orgone therapy. I had wasted her time and money and had not helped her; the least I could do was to return her money. Now she was forced to go to a psychiatrist who would analyze her. He had told her it would take a year and if I would not return her money I should at least pay his fees. I reminded her that I had never promised a cure, that she had not paid for a cure but rather for my time and experience, that I had charged her only half of the regular fee, had given her longer than the usual sessions, and had contributed my best ability. Further, I explained that I did not feel obligated to her in any way, although I was sincerely sorry that I had been unable to help her. I told her I did not pretend to help everyone. She replied by saying she would take the matter to court, and I told her that was her privilege. I have heard nothing more about this.

We have seen here a case of a very alive woman with a high charge and an insuperable pelvic block who was driven by therapy closer and closer to a genitality she could not tolerate. She had no course but to turn on the one who drove her to such misery and attempt to destroy him. There was much that was right in her attack on me; quite probably she would have been better off if I had refused to treat her. I feel that if I had been less successful therapeutically I would be in better grace with her today, and I hesitate to think what might have happened if I had been more successful. At first I did not realize it, but as time went on I became more and more aware of the gravity of the problem—we know that the organism is justified when it refuses to break down its defenses.

My first impression of her was that she was the usual phallic whose defenses were beginning to weaken, but the problem was not that simple. Most of the signs that Reich has pointed out as reasons to discontinue therapy were present, particularly the tenacious persistence of blocks. I knew in the course of her therapy that I should heed them, but her misery and her determination and pleading kept me going. Besides, it was difficult to admit defeat. There have been few patients I wanted more to help; and I may add that difficult as she was, I personally liked and respected her.

I understand that she has been treated by at least two other psychiatrists since she left me.

A Case of Bradycardia

Bradycardia is often caused by organic heart disease, especially pathology in the Bundle of His. In this case, heart studies were normal except for the slow beat. According to the history this condition had existed since a diptheretic infection in childhood. It was the first case of bradycardia I treated and I had no opinion as to whether or not it would respond to therapy. Therefore, I consulted Reich. He studied the history and physical findings, including a biophysical examination, and concluded that bradycardia in this case was biopathic; that is, due to armoring, and that it would respond to therapy.

He believed that the bradycardia itself was probably due to an inability to cry, and that swallowing the emotion of crying is carried through by a swallowing in the esophagus, by which a pressure is exerted on the organs of the chest and diaphragm through a constant pulling in of the lower organs of the mouth and throat. Since the vagus nerve, acting as a depressor nerve on the heart, runs downward from the base of the brain through the medulla oblongata and along the esophagus and the trachea, the constant pressure exerted upon these organs most likely affected the vagus indirectly and thus caused the bradycardia. For overcoming this symptom, then, the problem was to obtain full ability to cry in order to eliminate this pressure.

The patient was a twenty-seven-year-old married schoolteacher, an only child whose primary interest in the therapy was not to correct the slow heartbeat but an ambivalence in her own life.

Her father had left the family when she was twelve, and since that time she had been torn between the two parents. Actually, although she had remained with her mother, she loved her father more. Since the separation she had lived in an atmosphere in which the mother had constantly complained about the father who had deserted them. This left the girl indecisive and unhappy, with a vague feeling of dissatisfaction in life and an anger toward both of the parents.

She had been taken to a psychiatrist for brief periods when she was three, when she was six, and again when she was sixteen. She believed the first two were for temper tantrums and constipation. The last was apparently an attempt on the part of the mother to effect an emotional separation of the daughter from her father. It was not successful.

She was toilet trained very early with resulting constipation as a child. Even as an adult she suffered from constipation whenever she moved to a new home. She was married at twenty-one to a man she had known since she was seventeen; she said she loved him and that they had a very good sexual life together. She experienced a climax frequently. Her first heterosexual experience occurred at thirteen, but she had had no genital feeling until after she reached eighteen. She had frequent dreams of being stabbed in the back and had been afraid of dying.

Biophysically, she was well developed but slightly overweight. Her blood pressure was normal, *pulse 44,* temperature and respiration normal. She presented very little muscular armor but felt pain when one pressed on the notch above the sternum and pressure on the lumbar muscles was also painful. Her sterno-cleido mastoids, lower dorsal, lumbar, and thigh muscles were tense and tender. There was a spasm of the esophagus and of the diaphragm. Full breathing produced streamings very quickly throughout her body. When her lower jaw was pushed gently backward and her submental muscles pushed upward, she burst into sobs about her parents' separation. This breakthrough produced strong currents in her body which lasted long after the session ended. This was a very alive, mobile girl whose main defense was running. In therapy, this was manifested largely by going away in the eyes, talking, laughing, and vacillating about her goals and about therapy itself.

When she returned for the second session she would not breathe adequately and, although vigorous attempts to stimulate her were made, she remained more or less immobile except for a little crying held back from expression by a tight throat. The previous breakthrough had occurred because she had been taken by surprise and was unprepared. She was by that time defended against such full response. Therefore, she was asked to discuss her early history and remembered an incident from when she was three years old. She was chased down the stairs by a woman with a broom and ran into her father's arms greatly frightened. At about the same age, she remembered sitting in a bathtub with a boy, noticing the difference in their genitals, and that she wished very much to be a boy. Vaguely, she recalled her father explaining the difference.

At this point, she began to breathe freely, experiencing streamings in her thighs and genital. She suddenly stopped, put her hands over her face in embarrassment, and said she had become very sexually excited with longing in her epigastrium. She had stopped because longing belonged only to her husband and she had not been thinking of him.

During the third session she was able to breathe well, and it brought soft crying, rather marked Parkinsonism, and a feeling of constriction in her lower neck. That was her main block and it recurred whenever sensations increased beyond her tolerance. The sternocleido mastoids and upper spinal muscles were loosened and she was asked to scream. She then breathed down well and began to show sucking movements with her lips, which were ignored because they seemed premature. Instead, she was asked to make a face. She clenched her teeth and fists but felt frustrated, so she was irritated to bring out anger and asked to bite on a towel. She did so, but not enthusiastically, and began to feel longing for her father, reaching with her arms and saying that he had broad vision while everyone else, including her husband, was narrow. I suggested that her father meant freedom —outside her blocks.

This girl, with very little armor, a tendency to run, and an obvious impatience, constantly tried to reach into deeper layers prematurely.

She returned for her fourth visit very cautious; her chest was not moving and she was passively immobile. She brought the following dream, which consisted merely of the question, "Can one have intercourse with one's therapist?" I doubted that this was a dream, but was rather her tangential way of asking that question and a running away from the goal of therapy. I asked her to discuss her feelings toward me, and she said that she liked me very much and was beginning to get a transference for me. She planned her trips and wanted to come. She wandered off the subject two or three times, began sucking movements with her lips, and said she felt longing in her lips and upper chest. This was obviously an invitation to be kissed, an effort to run away from the anxiety created by therapy; an evaluation borne out by the fact that her chest was barely moving, her neck muscles were spastic, and her eyes dull and far away. She could not have had feelings behind her sucking movements.

I mobilized her chest, spinal muscles, and the muscles of her neck, and got her to move her eyes and look at me. Then I had her gag and bite a towel. She felt much freer and was very dizzy on arising. The dizziness indicated a mobilization of energy beyond her tolerance level and showed response to therapy. In discussing her attitude toward therapy, she brought out the very familiar idea that "therapy was supposed to give me an orgasm." I explained that although we hoped that therapy would render her capable of a full orgasm, it did not give her one. Treatment to this point was more or less general in mobilizing her energy, eliciting emotional response, and learning awareness of the reactions of her organism.

During the week following this visit she felt angry and irritable and when she returned again an attempt was made to reproduce this anger, but without success. She just became helpless and frustrated, showing an expression of supplication. Her inability to tolerate and express her feelings created anger, which again could not be expressed, thus resulting in frustration and helplessness. Her forehead was immobile and she could not open her eyes. Attention was paid to this segment and it was pointed out that she had a tendency to start something and go on a tangent, and that she must be aware of this. Her pulse continued in the mid-40s.

Again at home she continued angry and irritable all week and returned quite immobilized. Her chest was not moving, her teeth were clenched, and her neck was spastic. I mobilized these areas and tried to irritate her; she felt rage but could not release it. She could not open her eyes fully but improved with practice and attempts at screaming. Finally, she broke into an angry crying, then screamed loudly and opened her eyes. Her breathing was now easy and she became very dizzy. The running away was dwelt upon, and I pointed out that she ran by immobilizing her forehead and eyes. She became contrite and said, "I hate myself. I can't follow directions. I am not getting anywhere, but that is my fault." This was again a tangential criticism of my not helping her.

She returned again irritable on her next visit, and when loosened up ran away by chattering. I pointed this out to her and she assumed a helpless attitude. I asked her to look at me and she became panicky, screaming, "I can't, I can't. I bought a lot of dresses, I pretend I wear them to you; I pretend I am in love with you." My comment was, "Well, that's nice," in order to let her know that I did not take her seriously any more than she took herself seriously.

After this she began to feel more anger, and when provoked she twisted my arm timidly, hit the couch more vigorously. When given a rolled-up sheet, she used it to hit the couch, the floor, and the walls—her anger was breaking through now. After a time she became frightened and stopped, but felt relaxed and her breathing was free to the middle of her abdomen. She said she felt better; this, as usual, was only temporary. She returned the following week with a severe block in her throat, and when this was relieved by gagging with vomiting, she complained of a constriction in her lower chest. She moaned and whined, trying to push through. Irritation of her upper spinal and costal muscles freed her chest and she was greatly impressed, commenting that at last something had been accomplished. This comment surprised me as I felt there had been more obvious occasions to comment on, but apparently she was more in contact at this time.

However, the following week she found breathing difficult, fought with her husband, and found herself very watchful during the sexual embrace. Feeling alternate love and hate for her father, she said her brain was separate from her emotions. During the session she swallowed back every emotion that came up until her forehead and occipital muscles were mobilized; this brought out considerable anxiety and she screamed in terror. Then, she breathed freely, the impulse going into her pelvis with streamings to that segment. On the way home she suddenly felt very lonely and cut off all her feelings. She lost interest in everything, even in therapy, and felt sad and withdrawn.

On her return, the gag reflex was absent, her forehead was flat, and her eyes were dull. I had her move her forehead and look frightened and this produced a tic on the right side of her mouth. When she exaggerated the tic, she began a sucking movement with her lips and burst into sobs. She was aware of a peculiar feeling in her face, which she could not describe, but continued sucking with her lips and then spontaneously began to squeeze her eyes and wrinkle her face. This produced pleasant sensations through her whole body and she was very dizzy and shaky on arising.

At this time, she left on a four-week vacation with her husband and reported a wonderful time when she returned. She had visited her father, but found him too intense to stand very long, and it tired her. She kept her eyes shut during the session; when she would open them she seemed very far away and as if staring into space. She had difficulty maintaining contact. I mobilized her eyes and then suddenly grasped her throat lightly; she gasped, showing intense anxiety, and then burst into sobs. Momentarily, she said, she felt that she could never breathe again and was almost unconscious; she felt that she had left her body and withdrawn behind her eyes. She remembered occasional dreams of being choked, but mostly had dreams of being stabbed in the lumbar region.

She continued to find herself going away in the eyes all the following week, with periods of resentment and anger. In the next session, irritation of the intercostal muscles caused her to go into a typical temper tantrum, holding her breath until she turned blue. As soon as she stopped one, she started a second. I mobilized her forehead and had her simulate a frightened look—that resulted in full free breathing. Her throat, upper abdomen, and thighs became warm, but otherwise she remained cold. She said she was afraid to let go in a rage because she might burst. At the same time, she felt genitally excited; she said her marriage had to go and that she found she had nothing in common with her mother. These feelings appeared consistently whenever she reached out toward health.

During the week she felt a block in her throat, developed ocular headaches, and a tic of the left eye. She returned discouraged and bitchy and went through several more temper tantrums. She realized she got close to things in therapy and then ran away; and said she felt it strongly and wanted to increase her sessions, reporting that her husband noticed a great change in her. However, she continued bitchy and complaining, and wondered if I knew what I was doing as she was not getting anywhere. She consistently denied other evidences of resistance. With considerable provocation, she began to hit me and to hit the couch, then she started teasing me and laughing and seemed relaxed. Her breathing went to her pelvis and her pulse rose to 64. This was the first time it had risen above the forties and demonstrated the correctness of Reich's deductions.

She said she felt her husband held her back because he was so narrow and limited and she withdrew from him sexually. On the other hand, her father was domineering and difficult to get along with; her mother was uninteresting. At this point, her sexual outlet consisted largely of masturbation, with the fantasy of women masturbating each other. When she was five, she had masturbated in the bathroom, but felt the floor had eyes and felt very guilty. At seven, she and a girl friend masturbated each other; at eight, a man masturbated her—she had pretended nothing was happening but had enjoyed it. She had always been very curious about other people's sex lives.

Her throat continued blocked and she swallowed back her emotions. She continued hanging on to her husband and making a mother out of him. She admitted sexual feelings for me, which she would hold back by clamping in her pelvis. At this point, she developed acute appendicitis and was operated on. During the operation, an ovarian cyst the size of an orange was found; it had not been present three months previously when she had been thoroughly examined by a gynecologist. Energy had been streaming in to her pelvis and she blocked there, holding it in and causing the acute surgical condition. The operation she experienced as a pelvic release, with a great deal of warmth and tingling in the whole pelvic area. Waves went through with bursts of uncontrollable laughter on the evening of the first post-operative day. It hurt to laugh but she could not stop. The sensation was accompanied by a dream of riding with several children on a sled up and down through many mountains, throwing food to starving creatures until she and the children had no food left for themselves. This was falling anxiety and a feeling of giving. On the third post-operative day, she had intense sexual feelings and masturbated.

After her discharge from the hospital she had the following dream: She meets with a very strict dean of women at the college she attended. All the men leave, laughing. The dean reproaches her with a long list of things she started and never finished. Then, she is sitting next to her girl friend and it suddenly occurs to her that she would make a good mate for a young man she knows, but she thinks, "I am wrong—that would be incest; he is her brother."

Her associations were that her stepmother had come to visit her at the hospital and they were taken for sisters; she said that lately she had been longing for and loving her father very openly. She thought the strict dean in the dream was her mother, but I felt it applied to me and that the men leaving in laughter was a derision directed at me, since I was forcing her toward recognizing her incestuous desires.

She continued to say that she did not love her husband, only pitied him and did not want to hurt him. She looked very alive but somewhat anxious; I mobilized her eyes and forehead, which produced a block in her neck at the supra sternal notch and a feeling of panic. Masturbation, she reported, caused a feeling of convulsions in her head.

Following this, she went into a slump, feeling helpless and filled with doubts. Vigorous provoking caused her to feel a desire to kill, but she could not express it. She continued discouraged, helpless, and weak; her throat and lower neck remained blocked and she was afraid to fantasy love for her father.

For several sessions crying was the only emotional response she showed.

Then, she was instructed just to breathe and to cry no more, as it was felt she was using crying to run away. She fought desperately against instructions, trying to cry, feeling frustrated and abandoned when she was not allowed to. Her pulse rose to 76, her color improved, and then she was asked to vocalize, saying ahhhhhh. She felt tingling in her tongue, neck, and upper chest, which gradually spread to her legs and arms. Her pulse reached 80 temporarily, but generally remained around 72 to 76. An increase in her voice brought an immediate spasm in her throat, and she went away in her eyes with a feeling of abandonment.

During the next week her pulse remained between 60 and 72; her throat was free but her upper chest was tight and she had some cardiac pain radiating to her left arm. Her face, neck, and upper chest were flushed. I continued to have her vocalize, increasing her voice to a yell; at this point she again developed constriction in her lower neck. Her hands and feet became cold and she experienced a feeling of abandonment.

She was out of contact and restless at the next session. She felt angry but was reluctant to breathe and vocalize, and was afraid she would explode. She commenced some vocalizing and began to expand, then grew frightened and stopped. Her pulse varied from 72 to 80.

When she returned, she looked alive and well and I had her breathe and vocalize. Her organism almost gave in completely but she hid her face and clamped down. She refused to look at me and obviously felt guilty but would not discuss it. She denied fantasies of me, but reported the following dreams: (1) She was at the North Pole; a long train of dead people, piled high, was passing and her mother was one of them. (2) An older man was shot but a younger man fell dead. Here, she got rid of both her mother and her husband.

On the next visit she was cheerful and looked at me fairly easily. I had her move her eyes and try to snap my finger with her mouth; she became too embarrassed to enter into it enthusiastically, laughed, acted girlish, and said she was embarrassed about developing sexual feelings for me. Since I was her therapist, it was wrong. Also, it was wrong to have thoughts about her father. She reported that on a recent walk in the woods she had felt anxiety in the lumbar region—it reminded her of being chased downstairs and running into her father's arms. She could look and long with her eyes better, and she could reach with longing, but when anything touched her deeply she joked and laughed to run away and blocked her diaphragm. This was relieved by repeated gagging. Her pulse continued about 72.

Then, I began to mobilize her pelvis, loosening her thighs. She brought out that she remembered being punished for soiling the bed, together with a fear that she would move her bowels and bladder if she let go. She held her legs with her arms (hanging on to her mother[4]) but showed longing in her eyes and mouth, and became nauseated. At this point, she insisted that her marriage was good (again hanging on to the mother she hates). She had to hang on to those she hated and could not reach those she loved. Here was a hook between the tantrum of her father leaving the family and the earlier tantrum of bowel training. If she lets go, she will "shit" on those she hates.

We returned to vocalizing; this created a great deal of anxiety and her epigastrium became cold. She became intensely angry at me but could do nothing about it; she was afraid to express anger toward me. Anger, she said, was a new emotion to her. After this, her eyes became warm and illuminated—another new experience, which was followed directly by contraction with anxiety and cardiac and epigastric cramps.

The next session she was far away, split. Her pulse was 54. I mobilized her eyes and had her vocalize with general stimulation. She became very angry—"The most I ever felt"—but could not express it. I then proceeded to her lumbar region, which produced intense anxiety and rage; but she held in her diaphragm. She was afraid to let the anger out for fear she would soil herself. Asked to strike with her pelvis, she became immobilized, so I encouraged her to kick with her legs. Then she was made to

[4] In therapeutic cases, I have found that this gesture has meant clinging to mother, as a child clings to its mother's legs.

look at me and became warm in her pelvis, but gritted her teeth and contracted down, giving the appearance of straining at stool.

On her next visit she was again contracted, her pulse was down to 52, and she was withdrawn and very dead. She felt split and had no feelings. She insisted her marriage was good and that she loved her husband—whenever she contracted she hung on to her husband or her mother. When she felt free her feelings were all for her father. Recognizing that her husband was the holdup in her progress, she brought the following dream that explained her withdrawal: A strong man had his arm around her back and held her close to him; she felt great excitement through her whole body and awoke with her heart pounding.

First, I mobilized her, but she became faint and thought her heart would stop, going away in the eyes, which were dull and sluggish. I asked her to reach; she did so, but with an attitude of supplication and then cried bitterly. After that she felt more connected and I told her that her father was the strong man, asking her to imagine her father with his arm around her back. She quickly said, "I can't, I can't—but it is exciting. I never thought before that the anxiety in my back might be pleasure."

Following, this she kept going away for several days, had intestinal cramps, and pain over her heart; she would not let herself feel. She had contracted against the sensations brought up for her father—the common struggle to maintain the moral teachings of childhood.

I had her kick and hit with her pelvis while vocalizing and her pulse rose to 80. She said she wanted her father but was afraid of him; he was too much for her. She always fought with him when she saw him and was afraid to give in to her feelings for him. She knew that incestual feelings stood in the way, and added that it even interfered during the genital embrace with her husband. She had a very unhappy childhood, she said, and her mother never gave her much love. I asked her to let her fantasies come through and she became very anxious, and said it would be wrong, and blocked her throat.

The following week she was withdrawn and her eyes were sluggish. When her eyes and body were mobilized she felt streamings to her lower abdomen. Her body felt warm and comfortable, but as if it belonged to someone else—her "self" had become detached and contactless. She reported that the sexual act with her husband was very enjoyable but that she clamped at the climax (orgasm anxiety) and was very dizzy on arising from this session.

Feeling more in contact during the week, she experienced considerable longing; still she felt anxiety at the climax and became afraid of dying or falling apart. She planned to separate from her husband; although she resumed sexual relations with him, his narrow attitudes interfered with her feeling any love or respect for him. She was quite soft all over but when I got up to leave she looked forsaken. Remembering her father's desertion, I returned; she burst into tears and clung to me.

The following week she was again immobile and I asked her to reach with her eyes, mouth, and arms. Her pulse became weak; somehow she could never reach the emotion just around the corner. However, she began to tingle all through her body; the feeling continued after the session with strong sexual responses.

I continued to mobilize her pelvis and the reflex appeared, but she felt holding in her rectum and had no sensation in her genital. I asked her alternately to relax and contract her pelvic floor but she became embarrassed and could not let herself go because she was afraid she would pass flatus. When she did breathe through with the reflex, she developed a spasm in her throat.

She brought the following dream on her return: She was outside the world, as Aphrodite; she saw a handsome young man and longed for him intensely in her genital. He told her that she should find someone else. She said, "I realized it was my father." She had felt very well all week but held in her shoulders. Reaching brought on crying, wailing, and despair; she said she could not stand her longing. She had decided to leave her husband and felt very much alone.

The next visit she was again withdrawn, her eyes were dull and she had no feeling. It was the first day of her menses and she had considerable pain. Her thighs and pelvis were spastic, as were her shoulders and neck, while her eyes were dull and lifeless. She was contactless. I released the spasm of her shoulders and neck and mobilized her eyes. The menstrual cramps ceased and she felt elated and much improved at the end of the session. I told her to allow herself to feel her love for her father; she could remember being sexually excited once when riding on his shoulders when she was a little girl. She was, however, afraid to allow sexual feelings for him and asked what would happen if she did; I told her that I did not know but that she would have to face it or forever have to run away to her mother and her husband for protection from herself. She replied, "My feelings for my father are tremendous."

However, after the visit she dreamed she was making sport of orgonomy, and added, "I am struggling with myself." She had no feeling during the week. I mobilized her generally and she began to get pleasant sensations in her pelvic floor and became embarrassed, saying she fantasied her father's penis entering her vagina. It was painful and she felt pain in her lower back in the lumbar region. When I relieved the spasm of these muscles she became very anxious and began to wail. She did become warm all over, except for her arms, so I told her that she needed to reach for what she wanted.

The following week she felt very well, her pulse varied from 64 to 72, and she was soft and pleasant on her return. I had her reach with her arms and she felt streamings through her whole body to her toes, except for her arms. She said she had sexual feelings toward me and shouldn't; I told her that what she felt she should accept—what she did about it was something else. I then worked on her shoulders and arms and she began to tingle to her fingers. She reached without embarrassment, vigorously with sucking of her lips and tongue, until her throat contracted down and I stopped her. She said she felt her pelvis move forward and then her throat blocked, and that she felt pleasant but sad. The throat being her main block, it consistently blocked when she expanded beyond her tolerance level.

Again she ran away; her eyes were dull and seemed distant. Her forehead was flat and she said the whole crown of her head felt away; she seemed helpless. Her pulse dropped to 44 and she developed a spasm over most of her body. I mobilized her generally, had her reach and vocalize again. She said that she was away because her feelings became so intense, but she was not worried because there was too much health in her.

At this point she divorced her husband, having simply outgrown him. She became more serious, with less tendency to run. Also, she became more aware of her central weakness of "not really meaning it," the eternal ambivalence and withdrawal from fullest contact with a helplessness at bottom. She described it as a life and death struggle. At times she felt carried along in a mountain stream of movement and flow within her, and knew a great tremulousness; most of the time she felt very clearheaded, warm, happy, and very much herself with an inner strength.

I discontinued regular sessions but remained in touch with her and saw her on an occasional visit. She continued to develop and dreamed openly of incest with her father. She had several episodes of nausea and retching with breakthroughs of rage and a final yielding of her diaphragm, totally uniting the upper and lower halves of her body.

She met and fell in love with a young man whom she later married. The genital embrace was extremely pleasurable, but she began to block in her eyes, with a dull heaviness, a constricting tenseness in the eyeball, and a sense of going mad and losing reality. This did not last long and the embrace, in her own words, became involuntary, soft, a beautiful streaming into one another, deepening in cosmic intensity.

She continued well for ten years after which I lost contact with her. Her pulse remained around 70. Therapy consisted of fifty-two sessions.

A Case of Chronic Depression With a Hook

The chronic depressive is one of the most difficult problems the therapist has to face in which a cure can be expected. His early and severe repression makes adequate mobilization a serious challenge. Add to this a hook, and one is faced with real trouble. It is extremely rare that one finds a hook in chronic depressives because of the usual low energy. In this case, however, the energy level was surprisingly high and shrinking therefore was absent. The patient's depression was not obvious but had been in the past and recurred during therapy. Seriousness was present. Only ten years ago we would have considered this case beyond the reach of deep, biophysical therapy.

To review: A hook is that situation where, in the presence of a high energy, the pelvis has been freed before blocks, especially the major block higher up, have been dissolved. When these blocks are attacked, the organism cannot stand the increased charge and reacts with psychosis, suicide, or serious physical breakdown. The organism has to be allowed to adjust slowly to the rise of energy and needs adequate holding in the pelvis until it has accustomed itself to the higher level of functioning. Even then, when the pelvis is opened a jump occurs in functioning which is dangerous enough in ordinary circumstances. This particular case would have been impossible except for the patient's extraordinary understanding and cooperation.

The patient was a thirty-one-year-old, single, white male, a civil engineer who grew up in the western part of the country. He complained of sexual inadequacy which kept him from any serious relationship with women, a feeling of worthlessness and hopelessness, and a wish that he were dead so that the misery of meeting life would end. He could not concentrate or absorb knowledge. He felt that if he showed any serious interest toward a girl she would expect sexual advances and he could not bear the shame of showing his inadequacy. He could accomplish only a partial erection, and if the sexual embrace were attempted he would be premature, even ejaculating before entry. He suspected that he must have homosexual tendencies, and, as in the phallic character, sexual potency was crucial for his survival. Without it, he was nothing. On the other hand, his work was more than satisfactory and women were very attracted to him. Indeed, one of his problems was keeping them from expecting too much of him as he never wished to offend them or hurt them.

As a child he grew up in a very rigid environment; although kindly, it was cold and austere and he was expected to deport himself as a perfect gentleman. His father, a rancher and cattle breeder, developed pneumonia and died when the patient was three years old. At that time he was kept at the home of an aunt, and felt rejected by his mother. He had a brother and sister—twins seven years older than he. Although a good student at school he was constantly made aware of the superior success of his brother, especially in sports, and his father was held up to him as the acme of perfection. The father had been very successful, was a well-read man, and wrote several important papers on cattle breeding. The patient never had felt able to live up to the accomplishments of either father or brother and so always felt more or less a failure.

He did, however, excel in running and became a good shot with the rifle.

His sister supplied the only real affection and warmth in his childhood. Adding to all this, the time was filled with fears. Rattlesnakes, copperheads, and mountain lions were common in his area, and he was constantly warned about them and told stories of their dangerousness. The family lived on a ranch with an outside privy and to go out there at night was a real ordeal. Every step was filled with terror from an expected attack by either a lion or a snake. Further, he was conditioned not to breathe in the toilet for fear the odor would give him a disease. Therefore, he held his breath.

When he finished high school he joined the Air Force and served as bombardier on a flying fortress until the end of World War II. On one occasion, when he returned home on leave he was jumped and beaten about the face by a gang of sailors for no discernible reason; he arrived home quite upset and miserable and was greeted by his sister, who threw her arms around him, which frightened and repelled him. He tried to renew acquaintance with a girl he had admired for years and who had been first introduced to him by his sister, but found himself unable to make contact with her. He felt out of place, uncomfortable, and literally ran from her, thinking she could never care for him. He also found that while in the Air Force his legs had become stiff and he could not run as he had previously. His mother had had a stroke and died while he was away.

Following his discharge from the Air Force he started college, intending to take up animal husbandry and become a cattle breeder like his father, but unable to tolerate the imagined competition he switched to civil engineering. At college he had a few tentative affairs, was sexually potent but more or less conscious that girls he was interested in resembled his sister. He became very angry when they tried to do things for him, having to defend himself from serious relationships.

On one occasion during college, he was severely reprimanded by a professor for something he was not to blame for. That evening he had a date with a girl at his apartment; he was rather uneasy and upset, and following the sexual embrace he wanted her to leave. He finally took her home and on the way back became violently ill with abdominal cramps, diarrhea, headache, and a temperature. He was admitted to the hospital and remained there for two weeks. Since that time he had felt differently, more or less as described when he first came to me. It is more than probable that this series of incidents marked a regression from a fairly well-maintained phallic appearance to chronic depression.

He sought therapy and was treated by another orgonomist for several months before he came to me.

Biophysically, he was a well-developed young man, serious and immediately likable. One felt he had a thoroughly decent character and, with all his misery, he had a good sense of humor. His face was stiff and immobile, eyes fixed, jaws tight and spastic, neck bulging but held as though ballooned by inner pressure rather than muscular contraction, and the shoulders and arms were stiff. Except for the shoulder girdle, his chest was soft and moving, abdomen soft, and pelvis free of armor and freely movable. He gave the impression of intense holding from the shoulder girdle up, seemed about ready to explode holding the energy from the lower part of his body, which was soft but pale and lifeless. It was quite evident that there was a hook here, and that he was holding on for dear life. In fact he admitted he had fears of insanity, and considered himself schizophrenic. I explained his condition to him, told him therapy would have to be slow and would be extremely difficult, but that with his help we would see what could be done. The object was gradually to reduce his upper holding, hoping that the pelvis would begin to rearmor and that at the same time the organism would develop more and more tolerance to movement. One could not feel safe until he was free down to the chest, by which time it was hoped he would be armored in the lower part of his body if therapy was conducted properly. From then on, therapy would deal only with the usual problems found. But until that point, psychosis or suicide were real possibilities.

He reacted acutely to any stimulus because of his high charge and severe holding. I asked him to breathe and move his eyes around the room; he let out a cry of panic, stiffened even more, including his legs, and soon his face turned blue. I became frightened, asked him to stop and talked to him a bit to re-establish the status quo. I cautioned him to try to keep his throat open but it soon closed in spasm and his face turned blue, occasionally becoming gray and really frightening. This was accompanied by a cold perspiration; in fact, this cold perspiration appeared throughout most of therapy. Each time we reestablished calm before trying again and each time I encouraged him to allow his voice to come through more and more strongly; then I asked him to open his eyes. This again produced panic, but his voice and expression began to show rage. The rage made an opportunity to discharge some energy and I asked him to clench his fists and hit the couch. At first he hit rather mechanically, but soon could allow enough freedom to even stand up and beat the couch with all his might while making roaring sounds with his voice. However, with all his hitting, it never seemed satisfying to him.

We continued with his eyes, forehead, and occiput, mobilizing them gradually more and more, and expressing rage by pounding. He recalled that he could never look at anyone without going dead in his eyes, and also that when going to the outside privy at night he would never look from side to side, but always fixed his gaze straight ahead and awaited an attack by a lion. While in the privy he always had to hurry because he had to hold his breath; he would take a deep breath before going in and hold it until he got out in the fresh air again. Also, he was afraid snakes were down in the privy and would bite him if he sat down. Loosening in his nose was almost as important in therapy as loosening his eyes in producing sensations.

Gradually he became aware that as he opened or moved his

eyes pleasant sensations streamed down his body, but he was able to maintain them only momentarily. Many childhood memories came up, leaving home at three, the sadness and lonesomeness he felt sitting at the table with his family and uncle all cold and proper, his mother's demands that he be a good student so his father would have been proud of him, peeping at his mother and sister, his uncle beating their dog unmercifully and chopping the chicken's heads off. Frequently he cried softly, but only from his eyes. Mostly his cry was that of an angry baby demanding attention that never came.

Eventually he could tolerate movement of the eyes and could breathe without cyanosis; instead his face became pink. At that point I asked him to begin looking at me, which was difficult and filled him with guilt. He felt that I could see how worthless he was, that he should be dead and he wished he would die. He had thought a great deal that the only rational thing would be to kill himself and end it all. He would never be of any value to a woman. After all, how could I expect to cure him—he was a schizophrenic and would probably end up insane. At this point I told him he was not a schizophrenic, but that he was depressed, and feeling sorry for himself would not help. He did not believe me, but wasn't sure whether I didn't want to admit his schizophrenia or couldn't see it myself.

There was, of course, basis for his fears of insanity, but even more the fear was an expression of his fear of loss of control, in the deepest sense orgasm anxiety. He began to doubt my ability, thought I was really not so bright, and admitted being disappointed when he first saw me because I was not large and powerful as he had heard Dr. Reich was. However, he was willing to continue even though he felt I could not help him—because probably no one could. He would keep going until it was clear that only suicide was left. There were a few bright spots, in which he reported seeing things more clearly, as he had when a child; he also reported momentary glimpses of pleasant sensations in his body and of feeling alive.

He began to talk with more understanding of his therapy, which at first had been entirely mechanical. He could begin to feel the reality of energy and movement in his body. I needed these bright aspects myself as time went on and a hundred sessions found me no further than the eyes. At last, however, I felt they were quite free; they were freely movable and movements did not disturb his organism; he could make contact with me and fleeting contact with other people, but soon found himself looking down or away.

Sensations of wanting to bite began to appear, and I decided to proceed to the oral segment. I loosened his masseters and asked him to yell and scream. Again his face turned blue, his eyes became fixed, and he looked just as he had a hundred sessions before. We returned to the eyes and more mobilization and tried again; this time I asked him to bite on a sheet. He immediately started to gag, became cyanotic, and went away in the eyes. It was necessary to keep his eyes mobile or any further work would be to no avail. Therefore, each step with the jaw was started by moving or opening the eyes, moving the forehead or pressing the occipital muscles. Any movement of the jaw would result in a cry of panic, and a spontaneous raising of the arms as though protecting himself. The arms were held stiffly. I had him growl, beat the couch, and bite and twist a sheet. Although he entered into everything willingly, he would choke, turn blue, hold his breath, and fix his eyes after the initial try. At the same time, he could go dead in his jaw and nothing would happen, while any movement of his jaw with contact produced panic. I began to see that the jaw would take another year.

I mentally hoped that each segment would not take that long, but at least his eyes were mobilized and he had tolerated it. At the same time, I was glad to note that his legs became more and more tense. As time went on his arms became more active; although held stiffly they made striking movements with each cry. It was difficult to determine whether this was a restricted hitting or rather as it appeared—an effort to maintain balance as though he were falling whenever the movement of the jaw released energy. Still he could go dead in the jaw, move it freely with nothing happening. Contact with it made him feel increasingly angry. At times murderous rage would show; it frightened him and he decided he really hated everybody and wanted to kill.

He remembered shooting birds as a youngster, and recalled fantasies of twisting their necks. He remembered being told that his father had shot a mountain lion near their house; he also had many memories of the ranch, his uncle, and of how his uncle had beaten him severely for cruelty to the dog when he was three—after the beating he had followed his uncle around like a dog for weeks. On another occasion, he had bitten his uncle on the cheek and scratched him and was severely reprimanded. His uncle had great meaning to him as a youngster; he was afraid of him, but felt he was stupid as was also his mother. His father had been intelligent and intelligence was the only thing that counted. Occasionally his eyes would fill with tears and he would cry momentarily.

By this time his legs had become quite spastic and painful when touched. I began to loosen them a bit sometimes to gradually accustom the pelvic segment to movement of energy coming down from above. This worried my patient, who could not understand why I would work on it if I wanted the pelvis to armor. However, his energy level was so high I felt that the more of his organism that could absorb it and still tolerate it the better it would be. Since the legs had armored so well, it seemed safe enough. Work on the legs created great anxiety.

His jaw eventually became softer; he found himself conversing more easily with people and was even able to get angry and show it to his co-workers. He noticed the girls in his office, who had, I am sure, long been aware of him, and went out on an occasional date. He was still careful not to allow his companions to get any ideas that he was serious, telling them he had no intentions of marriage. The girls accepted this, believing they could wear him down. He was also careful not to go out too often with any one of them for fear they would expect advances and thus show him up.

We then proceeded to the neck, where there was a peculiar condition. The neck, especially above the sternum, was bulging, yet the muscles were easily softened. It seemed as though pressure inside were ballooning it out. I felt there must be a lot of screaming behind that, and had him scream and scream. His eyes became fixed and his jaw tight; it was necessary to return to them repeatedly. His arms became more active and he began to claw the air with his hands, growing angry. I suggested they looked like the talons of a bird and he said he felt like a hawk. Suddenly the arms began to flutter like the wings of a bird—something I recognized from previous cases who had grown up on farms; he was a chicken with its head cut off. When it subsided and I asked him to tell me about it, he said he had visualized his uncle chopping the chickens' heads off and became a chicken waiting for its head to be cut off. He recognized that as a castration fear, and following this, the bulge in his neck disappeared. I suggested that he start gagging every morning; this is one of the most important procedures in helping to dissolve armor and keeping the organism from rearmoring.

At this point he was basically free in the first three segments. Streamings went through to his legs with some sensations even in the penis. With each progress, armoring in these three segments recurred but was easy to dissolve.

Just as I was starting on his chest he went mountain climbing with a girl friend and broke his arm. He came to therapy even with his arm and chest in a cast, but he had accomplished a neat revenge. I could do little with his shoulder girdle—especially the arms which had always been held so tightly. Therapy was held up for six weeks. During that time he went into a severe depression; he was hopeless, he said, there was little point in looking forward to anything. He was offered a promotion at the office but refused it, saying he intended to leave. He wanted to go back to his home, he could never feel right in the East; he could never get well and was a schizophrenic after all. I reminded him that he was depressed, that his broken arm was no accident, that he had indeed tried to castrate himself and now wanted to run. I pointed out that he could run if he wanted to, and asked, "But what then?" He continued to come. I could only concentrate on consolidating the gains in the first three segments.

I think I felt better than he did when the cast was removed and we could go on again; I did not dare have him hit for a while and wondered how much the immobilization from the cast would interfere. We proceeded cautiously, although here he was more daring than I was. He began to breathe and claw the air. Suddenly it dawned on me that his stiff arms were held like the legs of an animal. I told him this and he said yes they felt like it . . . in fact he felt like an animal . . . yes, he was a cougar wanting to pounce on people. This continued for several sessions and he began to enjoy the feeling of power and aggression. His shoulder girdle became soft but the lower half of his chest was restricted and below the elbows his hands and forearms were stiff and mechanical.

I had him rotate his forearms and open and close his hands; this produced considerable anxiety and cold perspiration. The epigastrium was cold. I suspected this restriction was a "verboten" against masturbation, but we continued although he seemed less interested in this procedure and stopped it frequently to talk or do something else—he was obviously running from it. At this time he was associating more with women and became quite attracted to one, but complained that although she was lively and charming she was too young for him and so he really shouldn't get serious with her. She soon left on an extended vacation and her absence depressed him more than he wished to admit. However, he turned his attention toward another girl with whom he became more seriously involved. Still undecided though, he complained that she seemed stupid and reminded him of his sister. He began to report genital feeling and occasional masturbation. His arms were now quite free and he moved them in a different way when breathing; he began to wave them freely in the air, and said suddenly he felt like a baby waving his arms and that it was very pleasurable.

The first four segments were now free and the diaphragm, fortunately, had never armored, so that only the abdomen and the pelvis remained. This situation exactly reversed that presented when he first came. Then, the lower two segments had been free and the upper body armored. The hook was overcome. At this time I considered inducing reaching with the arms, but decided against it because of the hate I knew still remained in the pelvis. At this time, he was engaging in sexual relations with women, with satisfactory erective potency and considerable pleasure.

The abdomen was no problem. Deep, gentle pressure on the

abdominal wall started fibrillation and relaxation. He began to feel itching in the perineum.

Now I began on the pelvis, dividing it into anal and genital, with anal to be released first. When I released the spasm in the legs and buttocks he began to raise and lower his legs slightly and stiffly. I asked him to kick and he did, not too willingly at first but he reacted more and more later. His legs trembled and he began to report burning sensations in the perineum, which eventually became pleasurable. Also, he reported masturbation with anal excitation.

Sensations of falling apart over the occiput and sacrum appeared and he said that when he really looked or smelled he felt angry. He wanted to kill with his eyes and at times would protect his face, feeling that something was coming at it. Protected, he would look at the world from the safety of the peephole, and he recalled first peeping at his sister. He could at the same time kill his eyes and look and nothing would happen. He noticed that when his girl wrote endearing things he would become angry—this was standard throughout his life. When a girl did anything for him he became angry.

Gradually his jaws wanted to join with his eyes to kill, manifesting a desire to bite; also, his arms wanted to hit. He began hitting and kicking, feeling that if he really let himself go he could kill. He bit and clawed until he developed a severe pain in the pylorus. His jaw began to tremble. At this time he brought two dreams:

1. I was visiting the home of my girl friend; she was part colored and had large breasts. Her mother and her younger brother were there —the brother in the background. The mother was white and wore only a robe, which I noticed was open and exposed her pubic hair. I looked away embarrassed. At this, my girl friend, who was not exposed, made efforts to cover herself. The dream shifted and the girl friend and her brother went swimming. I was aware in the dream that I had no sexual feeling.

2. I was walking along and a large dog came running to me. It did not seem vicious but I knocked it down. It fell between the roots at the base of a tree and seemed dead. However, it soon got up again and several other dogs came and started to attack me. They were vicious and tried to bite. I pulled out two guns and held them off. A

man and a young woman came along in a donkey cart and I hailed them to escape the dogs; they gladly offered me a ride. They were sitting in the back and I got in front and found myself sitting on boxes of flower beds, so I kept myself raised up. The donkey cart became a motor cart. We came to a restaurant and the man said they would stop there and eat. He picked some of the flowers, which I thought were for the young woman, but the man said they were for his wife and went off to give them to his wife. The young girl and I went in to eat.

In the first dream, the girl friend was his sister who was forbidden to him sexually (part colored). All girl friends he liked were brunette like his sister and had large breasts. He had slept in the same room as his sister and his mother until he was six years old, and would try to peep at his sister, who was seven years older than he.

The second dream was his therapy. The dogs were his problems, which he could meet better now that he was more potent (guns). I was the driver and brought a girl with me and finally left her with him (I develop his interest in women). He is emerging from the anal stage (sitting on flowers). At first therapy was slow (donkey cart) but then went faster (motor cart).

He said that when he was young he was close to his sister and that, in fact, she was the only one with whom he had sustained contact. There was never real contact with his mother and he was afraid of his uncle. The only other person he ever felt close to was the girl his sister had introduced him to when he was in his teens. He transferred all the feeling he had for his sister to her until he ran from her when he was home on leave. He had felt she could never care for him. His mother had given him a great deal of attention but no warmth. His sister gave him warmth, and had probably taken care of him when he was young. He could not allow himself to imagine any sexual thoughts toward her; it would be wrong.

As a matter of fact sex is dirty and disgusting, he said (from anal eroticism), and he could not understand why everyone did not feel that way. Sex makes you get involved, he explained, and without sex you are independent of other people. He had imagined having his genital cut off clean; it would be a great relief. Women have their genitals cut off—they are even indented.

He had had thoughts of returning home to his sister and living with her; it would be comfortable and there would be no sex. Recently he had received a letter from her saying that she had made him guardian of her two daughters. In a sense he has children, he told me, and feels responsible for them. He was reluctant to think of sex in relation to his sister and felt dead all over. He added that he was reluctant to accept my interpretation of his dreams and did not like to have his sister brought into it. I pointed out his great reluctance as an urge to run again. Logical progression of therapy had now brought us to the very core of his problem: the incest barrier, the Oedipus situation. The sexual activity of only a few months previously was discontinued, since he had lost interest in sex.

Following this, he developed pains in his abdomen and remembered he had had them as a child and in college. His face was stiff and he felt inhibited. Everything seemed no use; he felt like a baby with no one there. He asked, "Don't I look miserable enough for anyone to come?" with his face. Mobilization of his eyes and forehead caused the pain to disappear, but he felt angry, and said, "I feel I am in a struggle to the end with Mother; I won't produce a movement no matter how much she massages my perineum." (The mother had done this to overcome constipation when he was a child.) So, since he had said, "I would like to destroy someone by shitting on them," I asked him to kick. He did and liked it and felt better.

He brought two more dreams after this:

1. I was in a room with three beds with my mother and sister as we used to sleep when I was a boy. My sister was sleeping in my mother's bed. The middle bed was not made up and I was going to sleep with my mother. Outside through a large window I noticed that the oak trees were gone and the river had become a flood flowing past the house. It was flowing the wrong way.

The window was the one he had been used to peep through at his mother and sister going to the bathroom, and listen to them urinating. It sounded different from men and they urinated quickly (flood) and flowed the wrong way. Their genitals were cut off (no oak trees).

2. I was riding with my uncle in a car. Another car whizzed ahead of us, ran off the road, and rolled over. We drove off the road to see it and I was afraid we would turn over too. The head of the man in the overturned car was bashed in as though the top of it had been cut off.

I suggested that if one is "fast" he loses his head (is castrated).

After this, my patient began to feel pleasant sensations in the pelvic floor, but only in the posterior part, not in the genital. It felt loose, as though his intestines could fall through.

Then he had the following dream:

I was at a party where there were many girls. I selected one whom I felt I could dare make advances to, but wondered if she were worth it. She moved out into the open but went near two girls, whom I recognized as my sister and teen-age girl friend. Then I could not go near her and let the two girls see me.

This dream showed that his sister was still keeping him from girls. He felt angry, began to cry angrily and reach with his arms. I told him to stop because I felt there was something missing. I had noticed that he had never brought out any real sobbing in therapy and felt that was acting as a holdup. He had always felt that if he really sobbed he could not stop and would want to die. He told me he thought he was held in the jaw and I found that the floor of his mouth and tongue were held rigid. I had him vocalize, la-la-la—and then he spontaneously began to reach with longing. His abdomen became very cold and painful and this brought out a new and rather unexpected sensation; he felt like a fish and moved his body as a fish does swimming and waved his arms gently. He said he had used to do a lot of fishing, and when the fish grabbed the hook would jerk to drive the hook through the lower jaw and the tongue—a fish tongue is stiff. He had been, it appeared, afraid of getting hooked in the mouth. He said that he used to hit the fish on the back of the head or break their necks to kill them rather than let them suffer. He began to feel pain in the back of the head and said he felt as if he were being hit there, became quite frightened and screamed in terror.

After this, his neck felt as if it had gills going in and out; he felt both as if he was being hit and that he was hitting the fish on the back of the head. He began to wave his arms and acted out both holding a fish and hitting it, and when he breathed he had the sensation of falling back from being hit on the back of the head. He said he used to compete with his uncle but after his uncle had beaten him on the buttocks and legs he could only compete in fishing and shooting—never directly. (The incident of being beaten had come out in the first therapy with the early opening of his pelvis.) He had had, then, thoughts of hitting his uncle on the back of the head or running the car into him from behind.

After about a week it suddenly occurred to him that he was not a fish and so could let air into his lungs without suffocating. He found that he would hold his neck to shut off his chest and arms; when he breathed his hands felt strong and he wanted to choke and scratch and hit. He could not let me be a person for fear of what he might do to me, but knew it was really his uncle he wanted to destroy. He added that he also wanted to be tender with his hands.

Then, he began to reach with his arms and cry like a baby. Outside of therapy he reported more social activity and was able to really enjoy himself. Then he developed sensations of falling when he lay down. He felt his head would fall off and something would fall out of him below. He had always been afraid of falling through the privy as a child at home, especially when the feces came out; he felt part of him was falling and his anus would clamp down tight and be painful and his arms would spread out to catch himself to keep from falling through. He felt he could save himself that way. The hole was deep and dark, and he said that when he felt he was falling he felt contracted (vegetative system contracts). At that point I had him begin to hit with his pelvis. He felt his pelvic floor tighten, so I stopped him and turned him on his side. The reflex appeared. He screamed and caught himself, but said it was pleasant.

After this he began to feel he wanted to sob but could not; he had been called a cry baby as a child but that was only a stifled crying, nor did he cry after he grew up or show any mourning for the deaths of his relatives. He felt that it was weak to cry, that if he sobbed he would want to die. I told him that I thought sobbing would clear up his problem of contact.

But then he felt nothing was of any use; he was no good to anyone and was out of contact. He felt that he must not cry; he could not stand contact and was quite contracted and immobilized. This state continued for two or three days and then he asked himself why he shouldn't cry. He found that when he moved his eyes or eyelids or something in his nose gave he felt like crying. He remembered being very sad when his brother left for college; although his brother was seven years older they were very good friends, but he had not remembered it before. He developed a feeling of reaching affectionately with his eyes and said he had not felt that way since he was a boy. He recognized that he kept himself stiff to hold back crying, and finally burst into a more complete sobbing than he had yet shown and felt more relaxed than he had in years.

Crying and reaching became easier and he began to feel more genuine than he had ever felt in his life. He said "I am really me" and "It is the first time I ever reached out with the expectation of touching something with my hands. Before I just reached with my eyes and floundered with my arms."

Sensations increased and he consciously held in his jaw to control them. When he loosened his jaw just a little he got sensations at the base of his penis. However, he continued to avoid accepting people as persons and only momentarily could accept me as a person—when he did he became very uneasy. To him, I was just a therapist; complete contact requires an open pelvis.

During the following week he developed sensations in his scrotum and in the base of the penis. These sensations would come and go, and when they were present his body felt free. He even felt longing in his penis for his girl (the first one described, who had been on a long vacation) and recognized the second girl as a substitute. That longing could be felt in the penis was a surprising discovery to him.

On the couch he seemed rather uneasy and anxious, and reported that the outer surface of his left thigh felt cold and tight. That was the surface toward me. I suggested that I was a threat and he recognized that he was afraid of me; I told him that he would not let me be a person not because of what he might do to me but because of what I might do to him. Asking him to flex his knees I loosened the holding in his thighs; his neck spontaneously gave and felt relaxed. His legs trembled and he began to reach, saying he did not feel passive any more but wanted to reach out for something.

He felt sensations in the base of his penis but his pelvic floor tightened in a painful contraction and he said he felt that I did not want him to feel his penis. He kept moving his feet because when he held them still the sensations were too strong in his legs and he would want to reach with his penis and would like to have an erection.

I suggested that between sessions he practice loosening and contracting his pelvic floor to accustom it to the movement of energy. Experiencing some difficulty in maintaining contact with the pelvic floor, he realized he was holding back sensations from his penis, but when he had contact with the pelvis his body felt loose. I had had him hit with the pelvis previously, and he said that he wanted to hit with it at this time. He had not wanted to when I asked him before, and he added that in hitting then he had had no contact with his genital but only with his buttocks. Then I worked on his thigh muscles, supra pubic area, and ileopsoas muscles. Following this, he developed some feeling in his penis, especially prickling sensations in the area of his circumcision. He observed that a few months before he had experienced considerable heterosexual activity with a good deal of pleasure and had only occasionally been premature.

Alternating sensations of passivity and activity now became prominent and he said he felt it very strongly. Also, he said, individual parts of his body seemed to want to reach by themselves, especially his genital, and he remarked that he was afraid he would have an erection and that I wouldn't approve. He longed for his girl friend, the lively one who was away at the time. Again, however, he hedged, saying that he was worried that if he married her he might die and leave her with small children. He had always felt he would die young like his father. And he added an interesting note: he had always considered himself of Irish descent like his mother but lately he had been thinking of himself as English. His father was of English background. Regarding marriage and dying, I suggested that in life we have to take chances and that no one knows what the future will bring. The posterior part of his pelvic floor was now fully relaxed, but the anterior part, especially at the base of the penis, continued to go into spasm after relaxing for short periods.

His hands again became central because sensations in them grew strong and they tingled, which caused anxiety. He recalled that his aunt sewed up the pockets of his pants when he was a child to keep his hands from holding his genital; she had also threatened to cut it off if he touched himself. To her, sex was very bad; she was an old maid and terrified of lightning.

He wanted to feel his pelvis and wanted me to work on it and loosen it up, which was encouraging. He had gained contact with his organism and felt his armor as foreign and restricting and wished to be free of it. He no longer worried about erective potency, nor did he have any fear of the female genital, but he had not yet obtained full pleasure in the sexual embrace and would stiffen at climax (orgasm anxiety). Pleasure could be expected to increase over the year or two after therapy ended.

After this point therapy proceeded smoothly. Remaining holding yielded; there is a sort of cleanup operation to be done on holdings that do not give until the pelvis begins to function. For example, a deeper expression of biting, in wanting to bite his girl's breast and finally his mother's breast came out. This was followed by an intense desire to suck. More and deeper sobbing appeared, accompanied by a desire to urinate. In his home urinating was spoken of as "shedding a tear." This was followed by intense urethral anxiety and eventually pleasure sensations in the urethra. He was afraid he would urinate on the couch. Periods of depression, feelings of worthlessness, and impotence also recurred.

On one occasion he came in irritable and cross, complaining that his scalp and back of his neck were tight. His head felt as though it were being pressed down on. I loosened his eyes. He raised his arms with his fists closed and held close together and made peculiar grunting sounds. He looked to me like a baby in distress and I asked him if he felt like a baby. He said no. He was going through a scene from early childhood in which he had observed his uncle castrating calves. Their forelegs were tied together as were the back legs and someone held the head while his uncle castrated them. His arms felt like the forelegs of the calf. The calves would stiffen and groan as the scrotum was cut, and grunt again when the base of the testicles were clamped off. He had been told not to watch but saw through a hole in the door of the barn. He was fascinated, but had not been able to identify with the calves before and did not now as he had when he felt he was a fish. He added, "Why do I always identify with the animal being hurt?" (On one occasion he didn't—the cougar.)

Following this he went into another depression and again wanted to return to the West. He became critical of his girl friend and expressed a great deal of hatred toward the East. He did not feel at home here and felt he would never belong. It evolved that he could not stand the freedom in the East but longed for the quieter life of his repressed home environment. He could not look and see the beauty of the East. He dared not become part of it. How fiercely the human organism, accustomed to armor, fights against its yielding to free flowing life: The East was the adolescent with his demand for life, his home the armored adult who is quiet and safe.

One day he brought the following dream:

I had a sore on my body or leg, the place was indefinite. It had a protrusion on it like a graft. This had a dressing over it. I was trying to pull the dressing off. Some of the flesh came off with it. I remarked casually that some of myself had come off. A woman was there.

It reminded him of his circumcision. He thinks, perhaps, he was circumcised when he was three years old. He recalled again a very clear memory of his aunt cutting flowers with scissors. She said she would cut off his penis if he touched it again.

I had him mobilize his eyes and loosen his face. He noticed he could stop all feeling by immobilizing his head and pulling his chin back. He became increasingly afraid, feeling more and more terror. Finally he had the thought that he was afraid he would have an erection and his penis would be cut off.

He noticed he felt his eyes move and they felt different than before. Also he was more aware of sensation in his arms. They continued to move upward when he breathed as though he were using them for balance. It suddenly occurred to him that he actually did balance himself that way when he used to peep at his sister. He had had to walk along the veranda in the dark. Many boards were rotting and he was afraid of making a noise. He would hold his breath and walk gingerly, holding up his arms for balance. He would have an erection while anticipating peeping. In the session then, he was afraid he would have an erection and I wouldn't like it. I might cut his penis off or gently masturbate it, either of which would be very frightening.

His aunt told him when he was about six years old that the punishment for peeping was to have his eyes put out. In spite of this he couldn't resist the urge to peep. This threat gradually became effective and he found it difficult to look at girls directly. Even at that time it was difficult to look at his fiancée in the nude. He was afraid his peeping would show up. When he looked at people he looked down very quickly with shame. He always felt great shame over peeping.

After he had brought this out he began to feel very young and imagined he could hear heavy breathing. He was back at his home as an infant and listening to his parents in the sexual embrace. He was afraid his breathing would get in rhythm with the breathing he heard and he would be discovered. After this he felt pleasure in his body which he had not felt for years, not even during sex. He discovered he could hold his breath by fixing his eyes.

At the next session he reported that he had experimented at home and felt intense anxiety when tiptoeing with his arms outstretched, as he had walked when peeping. During the therapy the movement of his arms became free like a baby's. He said that when he looked things seem clearer than they ever had and that he could feel excitement directly in his genital.

At the next session he complained of tightness in his occipital region and pelvic floor. I loosened the occipital muscles and had him roll his eyes. His arms began to move but rather stiffly and irregularly. I asked him just to let his arms hang loose because he was using them to hold his shoulders back. I told him to bring up his knees and allow his shoulders to come forward.

Strong impulses going to the pelvis occurred but they were irregular due to holding back. He again began to wave his arms in an erratic fashion and visualized his uncle holding their dog by the hind leg and beating it. He identified with the dog, and became afraid his left leg would be torn off. He had always been afraid of his left leg falling off at the hip. He thought the dog's leg would tear off when his uncle held it up. He had been very angry at his uncle but was afraid to say anything. At this point he got off the couch and beat it with all his might, fantasying his uncle. After this his arms felt more relaxed than he could remember.

This was followed by a short depression ending in a rage of wanting to claw and scratch. He remembered with satisfaction scratching his uncle's face and even wanted to dig his nails into his own cheeks. He continued to bring his arms forward and I noticed again that with this movement his shoulders were pulled backward. I manually brought them forward with each breath and instructed him to let his arms relax. Strong impulses flowed to the pelvis and his face became stiff. Loosening his face made him aware that he was avoiding sensations developing in his penis. Genital sensations caused intense anxiety and made him feel that he was falling through space, feet first (falling anxiety). Now all that remained was to develop tolerance to his genital sensations of full orgastic surrender. Much of this he could accomplish by himself. This process continues long after therapy is discontinued. He incidentally reported an occasion of seeing in true binocular vision.

He has kept in touch with me during the past two years and has continued to consolidate his gains. Therapy required three hundred and fifty sessions.

PART IV

CHARACTER MANAGEMENT:

The Prevention of Armoring

18 · Prenatal and Natal Care

ANYONE WHO DEALS SERIOUSLY with the problem of emotional disease, either in its cure or in its prevention, must be prepared for bitter attacks from those who represent society, because he must meet and handle the sexual problem. Broadly speaking, men can be divided into two categories: those who make social mores, and those who are crushed by them. The former, of course, have also been made sick by society, but in defending their own sexual anxiety must crush everything that excites natural feelings within them. These are the emotional plague characters discussed above. Those in the second category are made to abide by the rules of the former, but have never incorporated them into their structures. They are the simple neurotics and those few who have maintained health. It is always easier to rear a repressed child than a healthy one who asserts his independence and demands his rights. Everyone is familiar with the way Freud was plagued and ostracized. Probably few are aware that Brill, who brought psychoanalysis to America, was threatened with jail and the loss of his license by a group of narrow-minded physicians. I personally heard a well-known neurologist say at a meeting, "Dr. Brill, keep your filthy hands off our children." The attacks on Margaret Sanger are history. Reich experienced similar violent attacks. Natural sexuality is the great "do not touch it."

But if there is to be an end to the misery of the world,

natural sexuality has to be faced and accepted, especially for children and adolescents. To treat the neuroses is not enough. It is an endless and slow process for which there could never be enough therapists. Prevention can be the only successful solution, and prevention entails the acceptance of natural genital functioning.

Preparation for Delivery

Toward such prevention, about fifteen years ago, at the suggestion of Reich I started a project for pregnant mothers, preparing them for delivery and the care of the infant and, where possible, continuing to see the child at intervals through the years. I wished to see what could be done to bring up children in as natural a way as we knew. And to see how well they could meet life.

In preparing the mother for delivery, the object was to increase her ability to accept delivery and the baby, not to effect a cure of her neurosis. Preparation included sex-economic counseling, routine hygienic measures, removal of common practices which are known to harm the growth of the embryo, such as the use of tight girdles, lack of orgastic release during pregnancy, and so forth. Careful periodic examination of the bioenergetic behavior of the organism in general and the pelvis in particular was also made. Particular attention was paid to the eyes, to prevent going away and development of possible psychotic tendencies during delivery. Correct breathing and expression of emotions—screaming, crying, or rage—were also established. The pelvis was mobilized to allow a relaxed uterus for growth of the fetus and to facilitate delivery. The patient was encouraged to let out her emotions freely during delivery in order to avoid holding. Where possible, it was considered desirable to be present at the delivery to aid the patient in case difficulties should arise.

Delivery

Labor naturally should proceed smoothly with strong but not severely painful contractions. This is because the uterus contracting down on the fetus does not meet an immobility, but rather the fetus pushes on the cervix and finds that it gives with the pressure and each contraction advances the progress of delivery. Pain occurs only when the uterus contracts down on a fetus that cannot give with the contractions because of lower holding. In many primitive peoples labor is said to be very short in duration and taken rather nonchalantly. Similar cases can occur in our society.

When I was eighteen and teaching school far in the country, I was awakened in the middle of a cold February night by the husband of the family with whom I lived. He said his wife was in labor and asked me to ride horseback two miles to a phone to call the doctor. Before I arrived there, the husband caught up with me to say it was all over and not to bother with the doctor. The next morning the mother was up and cooked my breakfast as usual.

I was present as a medical orgonomist at a natural home delivery of this kind. The mother, a former patient of mine, was well prepared. My duty was to see that the mother did not suffer any acute contraction that would interfere with delivery and that she maintained contact in the eyes. Very frankly I had nothing to do except occasionally remind the mother not to hold her breath when she became too interested in what was happening and forgot to breathe. I did have a pleasant conversation with her, which may in itself have assisted the process by helping to prevent the development of any anxiety.

It is true that in both cases it was not a first child, but labor generally should be of this order. It can be expected to last somewhat longer in primiparas but the process should otherwise not be much different.

Difficulties arise in such cases only when the pelvic opening is unusually small or where the fetus shows an abnormal presentation. These are factors which should be known and prepared for prior to the onset of labor.

When the cervix is fully dilated and labor enters the second stage, unarmored mothers have reported feeling a sense of exhilaration and power with no further discomfort. This sense of exhilaration and well-being may last for several hours. It is sometimes accompanied by a feeling of floating and mild ecstasy.

Real problems arise when the mother approaches delivery with a great deal of anxiety. She may have experienced considerable discomfort during her pregnancy, such as persistent vomiting, backaches, urinary frequency, constipation, and a myriad other complaints, until she has resented the whole thing and even her husband for his part in it. Perhaps she has heard stories of the suffering of labor and the dangers to her own life. She has heard it spoken of as travail, an ominous-sounding word. She has even worried that she might give birth to a malformed or idiot child. She has known nothing of the joy of expecting a new birth, her very own child. She has perhaps not done too badly with the initial pains of labor until she finds herself in the hospital.[1] There, in an unfamiliar environment, a bare room next to the delivery room, she hears the groans and screams of other women. The nurses are businesslike and unsympathetic, too busy to bother with her fears, and her doctor is not there to offer her reassurance. In fact she is told they cannot possibly call him yet. She may see doctors coming from the delivery room in gowns covered with blood, sometimes hears rumors of a labor-room tragedy to mother or child.

Understandably, she becomes panicked and her whole organism clamps down severely. With this her pains increase to the point that she must cry out in spite of herself. Nurses admonish her to be brave and stand it and she feels ashamed and contracts more. She tightens her jaw, pulls up her shoulders, clenches her fists and holds her breath. She presses her legs together, pulls back her pelvis and contracts the pelvic floor. Pains continue to increase because the uterus is contracting against an immovable object and little progress is made toward expelling the baby, which is held high in the uterus and cannot descend. This state can go on for two and even three days until, utterly discouraged and exhausted, she feels she cannot stand another moment. Everything terrible that she had heard about delivery was true and more.

In the meantime the fetus is being squeezed unmercifully and its heart rate may go up alarmingly. The nurses who are watching the fetal heart rate become worried and anxious, which only adds to the mother's distress. Eventually narcotics are administered to give the tired and distraught mother some rest. This only adds to

---

[1] The following is not typical of the better hospitals today, but it does represent all too many.

the baby's precarious state. When she awakens the mother is given drugs again to resume the contractions and the whole picture is repeated. At last the cervix is fully dilated and delivery either occurs spontaneously or by the use of forceps or manual rotation. The mother is of course given an anesthetic to relax the muscles, but tears of the cervix and perineum are certain to occur. Even more important the baby too is anesthetized and enters the world pale, half dead, or half asphyxiated from drugs, anesthesia, a tight cord around its neck, or from contractions of the mother that have cut off circulation in the cord. What an event for the mother, when she should feel joy in the new baby and the baby should be able to respond to her. All this matters not to armored man. The baby is given oxygen or artificial respiration, mucus is sucked out of his windpipe, and then he is hurried off to the nursery with business-like efficiency. There is no understanding warmth, no emotional contact, all is done with mechanical routine. The mother, sick from anesthesia and exhausted, is rushed off to a room to recover from her experience and sob in her loneliness. She receives no evidence of empathy from her environment after the greatest emotional experience of her life. Because of all this the mother may not produce milk in her breasts for a day or two—sometimes not at all. The baby is too drugged and half asphyxiated to nurse for twelve, twenty-four, or even forty-eight hours. This is so common that it is now taken for granted and no one will believe that a really alive baby will nurse within an hour or two after birth and the mother will have the milk.

What can a medical orgonomist do in cases like this? He understands her emotional state and her contraction. This understanding can very quickly be conveyed to the mother, giving her reassurance. He first explains the situation that is preventing the progress of labor and that this is simply a result of her anxiety, her terror. He next explains what both must do about it to relieve the chaos into which she has fallen. This may accomplish a great deal in itself. At least the orgonomist hopes to obtain the mother's co-operation. Now he sets about relieving the contraction and holding back. Of first importance is the tight jaw. She is encouraged to let her jaw drop as in sleep and to breathe through her mouth. If she cannot do this herself the mouth must be manually opened. This eliminates some ability to hold and establishes a better respiration. Her shoulders are then loosened and pushed downward and the chest mobilized by pressing on the sternum or sides of the chest during expiration. She is encouraged to scream or shout, especially with the pains, and otherwise to sigh out loud. Sometimes she will give in and sob if one holds her hand and says something comforting like, "don't hold it back, it's all right." This produces relaxation. She is further encouraged to loosen her legs and bring her pelvis forward to "go with" the pain instead of bracing against it. This is easier if the mother is on her side, and in fact delivery is best accomplished in this position, although it is seldom used. Contractions of the uterus will increase, but the pain will diminish and she may feel drowsy or even become interested in the process of labor instead of fighting it. During this time her eyes must be watched carefully for loss of contact and she must be made to regain contact. One must be very insistent about this and it is often quite difficult to bring the woman back to awareness. With relaxation of the mother the precarious situation of the baby improves and its pulse will slow down and even return to normal.

All of the foregoing is illustrated very clearly by the following two case histories reported by Dr. Chester M. Raphael. Dr. Raphael writes,[2]

"In the first of the two cases I am reporting here, labor was abnormally prolonged. In the second, labor appeared to be accelerated. The assistance given both mothers was stimulated by the spontaneous appreciation of the armoring process, which, under these circumstances, represented an acute armoring in response to fear and pain—an appreciation which I have gained from orgonomy and the biopsychiatric treatment of chronically armored states.

"The first case is that of a twenty-seven-year-old primipara who had been unable to conceive during a period of four years. The studies of the reason for her sterility, including tubal insufflation, semen analysis, vaginal smear study, and endometrial biopsy disclosed no positive findings except an endocervical secretion of the type found in chronic endocervicitis. This was

[2] This is part of an article entitled, "Orgone Treatment During Labor," reprinted from *Orgone Energy Bulletin*, April, 1951, with permission.

felt to be sufficiently severe to block the upward migration of the sperm into the endometrial cavity. For this reason, intrauterine insemination of the husband's semen was attempted but the procedure was not successful. The examining physician found her to be "tense and anxious out of proportion to the situation."

"Finally, she conceived. In a letter to me she wrote: "After several attempts at artificial insemination, we decided to take a respite from doctors, thermometers, daily temperature charts, Rubin tests, and regulated intercourse. Result—conception."

"Her friends and relatives were oversolicitous because she had had such difficulty in conceiving. She was very tense and unstable during the first months of her pregnancy. She had a few severe attacks of vomiting but then her pregnancy proceeded uneventfully. There was no history of serious illness prior to her conception, and she had the reputation of being a rather stoical person.

"The expected date of delivery passed. There was talk of interference, although the mother expressed the feeling that there was no need to meddle. However, when she visited her obstetrician he recommended that labor be induced. No complications had been anticipated. Her pelvis was ample, there was no undue gain in weight, and her physical condition appeared to be good. A dose of castor oil and an enema were prescribed. Several hours after receiving the castor oil she had a few contractions and was rushed to the hospital. She herself objected that it seemed too early.

"Some comments made by the patient on her experience in the hospital throw some light on the factors which contribute so often to the fear of childbirth.

Until I was admitted to the hospital, I was in excellent spirits. I wasn't particularly afraid. I knew that I would have some pain, but I certainly felt that I would not find it intolerable. When I was taken to the labor room, however, my attitude changed with a suddenness that was startling. I was greeted with blood-curdling screams and pleas for assistance which were coldly disregarded. While I was speaking to the admitting nurses on the floor, there were two deliveries in progress, every detail of which I heard. Then while still there, I saw two doctors emerge from the delivery rooms in bloodstained uniforms. The room I was taken to was barren, two beds, a chair and a window that contained mesh wire within the panes of glass, giving the impression of a barren cell. I slowly gained the impression of being in a medieval torture chamber.

"For the first five hours she continued to have contractions and then received an intramuscular injection of demerol. She fell asleep. When she awoke a few hours later, the contractions had practically disappeared. She was examined by a resident physician and her obstetrician was notified that the cervix was not dilating. That same afternoon she was still feeling quite well, although somewhat shaken by the tortured screams all around her. That evening contractions resumed and it was suggested to her that she continue to move about to help the process of dilation. In her words: "That night I must have covered about ten miles." Toward morning of the second hospital day, following another sleepless night, the contractions became very strong. No medication was administered at this time for fear that it might again cause an interruption of labor. I should like to return to her description of the proceedings:

I had no idea that I could scream so loudly. When a pain came, I would seek something to press down on until it subsided, a radiator if I happened to be near one, or a table in the hall, anything that I could press down on with all my strength. I was ashamed of myself for screaming so loudly, and when I felt a pain coming on I would head for the bathroom, where I could scream by myself. I remember apologizing to the girl who shared my room for screaming so much. My room, by the way, was directly across the hall from a sort of supply room and laboratory, and next to the delivery room so that I could hear everything that was going on. During the night, or it must have been Saturday morning, one woman had a stillbirth and I saw the nurses carry a bundle which I presume was a baby, into a room across the hall. All the nurses gathered around and spoke in hushed voices. I was quite disturbed about this. I remember telling my obstetrician that I felt I would go slowly mad, that I couldn't take it much longer and that I had heard of a stillbirth during the night.

"At this point, she received another enema and the contractions continued to be severely painful. Then she received three injections of obstetrical pituitrin. The pain became unbearable. The obstetrician, continuing his efforts to hasten matters, ruptured the membranes. Meconium was found in the fluid and the nurses were cautioned to stand by and follow the fetal heart carefully.

"At this time I was called and heard that things were going badly. The fetal heart rate was 164 and thready. When I arrived at the hospital the patient had been in labor for more than forty hours. Her condition seemed desperate. I found her sitting up, supporting herself with her arms held rigidly against the sides of the bed, her face was ashen, her lips cyanotic, her pulse thready, her hands cold and clammy, and her shoulders acutely hunched up. With each contraction, occurring at five-minute intervals, she screamed that she could not endure it any longer and wanted to die. Between contractions, her eyes rolled up into her head and her distress was extreme with each contraction. She held her breath and her body stiffened. The picture was one of acute contraction of the entire organism.

It took considerable effort to make her lower her shoulders. "Succeeding in this, I asked her to breathe more deeply, to prolong her expiration. In less than two minutes her body grew tremulous, clonic movements appeared in the lower extremities and extended upward to her lower jaw and teeth, which began to chatter uncontrollably. She clenched her jaws, but I discouraged it immediately and helped her to let her jaw drop. The spasm in her shoulders and intercostal muscles—which were exquisitely tender—was gradually overcome. Her respiration improved. Then she herself complained of a block in the region of the diaphragm. Fibrillations appeared in her thighs and strong sensations of current appeared in her hands and fingers. The severity of the pain of uterine contractions began definitely to subside.

"The color returned to her face, her pulse grew fuller and slower, and her respiratory movements now proceeded with an involuntary rhythm. She then began to belch and with this the discomfort in the region of the diaphragm subsided. She grew quieter and began to smile. Very quickly the contractions began to occur at two-minute intervals. There appeared to be relatively little discomfort with each contraction and she was able to rest between them. Despite more than forty hours in labor, a good part of it agonizingly painful, she began to look comfortable and pleased. An important quality of her reaction to pain was a distinct withdrawal in her eyes. When she did this, she appeared to lose all contact. She did not hear me, seemed confused, and it was difficult to bring her back.

"When you arrived," [she told me later] "I remember telling you that I could not go on and that I simply could not stand much more. You told me to bend my legs and while pressing down on my chest, told me to breathe regularly and exhale all the way down. You established a rhythm of breathing while pressing down on my chest that I tried to keep, but the pains were strong and once again I cried I could not go on. But you persevered and I tried awfully hard until finally we seemed to be having some results. My extremities began to tingle and feel numb. Slowly a drowsy numbness began to envelop me, my legs felt heavy, my gaze would wander. Only when you called me back would I, with a very definite effort, bring my gaze back. It was so easy to go off that I believe you had to call me back quite often. By this time, I was tingling all over, I began to feel warm and relaxed, whereas previously I was chilled and tense. Once when you left the room the nurse who was standing by commented that she thought you had hypnotized me. The pains were certainly bearable now. You told me that they were coming more frequently although to me it did not seem that way, for in the interval between pains I was able to rest. I can't quite understand it myself. I only know that it helped me tremendously."

"I had been with her for about two hours by this time. The fetal heart rate was 179 and it was obvious that something was wrong. The obstetrician was called; he arrived a few minutes later, examined her and found the cervix to be completely dilated although the head was still high. He found the fetus to be in the right occiput posterior position. This position, coupled with the infant's distress, made him decide to deliver the infant immediately with forceps. Working quickly, the mother was now under an anesthetic, the head was rotated and then delivered, the infant exhibiting three loops of cord around its neck. It was flaccid and pallid; the throat was aspirated immediately, artificial respiration was applied and oxygen administered. The infant responded quickly and was placed immediately in an incubator. Again the mother, "When I finally realized what had happened, I had a feeling of great euphoria and exhilaration, my recuperation was very rapid, I felt well immediately and had no post-delivery despondency, which I had been told could be expected."

"The second case was that of a twenty-three year old primipara who had been studied during her pregnancy by the Orgonomic Infant Research Center of the Wilhelm Reich Foundation. The period of gestation had been entirely uneventful and she, in general, appeared to fulfill the criteria for relatively healthy functioning. In this instance the hospital situation was much more favorable. The obstetrician had agreed to refrain from routine use of medications, anesthesia, and routine episiotomy, and even the promonitory spank with which the infant is frequently greeted had been carefully discussed with him and he had agreed to refrain from it as a routine gesture. Plans for immediate contact of the infant with its mother after delivery were made. The entire hospital situation was as favorable as possible, so as to reduce to the minimum the pathological atmosphere and emotional contagion of the labor room.

"The patient experienced her first faint contractions at approximately 8:00 A.M. and continued at about twenty-minute intervals. She arrived at the hospital at 10:30 A.M. Shortly thereafter the contractions practically stopped and she was dubious that she would proceed. The occasional contraction she likened to a menstrual cramp. Her obstetrician estimated that she would not deliver before midnight.

"I arrived at the hospital at 4:45 P.M. Contractions were mild, of short duration, and approximately seven to ten minutes apart. She was calm, with a somewhat exaggerated attitude of unconcern. She complained of slight discomfort in her lower back, her face was placid, her jaws relaxed. However, the shoulders and upper chest were held somewhat and breathing was moderately restricted. She complained of some pain in the left groin. The thigh adductors were moderately spastic and while the thighs were held initially, they could be moved easily. I proceeded to help her establish fuller respiration. The almost immediate effect of this was to induce a state of sleepiness. I encouraged her to rest. About fifteen minutes elapsed when she suddenly experienced a strong and much prolonged contraction. She reacted to this with an inhibition of her breathing, for the moment, a facial grimace, a tightening of the abdominal and thigh muscles. I encouraged her and helped her reestablish fuller respiration.

The entire organism relaxed again. Within a few minutes, another contraction occurred with the same contraction of the organism in response to pain. Thereafter, the contractions occurred regularly and intensely at two- to three-minute intervals. What appeared most prominently with each contraction was a reaction of withdrawal, particularly noticeable in the eyes. This required almost constant attention until delivery. She felt disinclined to breathe deeply, complaining that it increased the pain. At first, with strong contractions, she felt dizzy and appeared restless and slightly confused. This could be mitigated to a considerable extent by insisting that she "come back" every time she showed any sign of withdrawal. At first, she was reluctant to do so, but as time went on she appreciated its advantage. The pain was less severe when she could achieve it and progress appeared more orderly and effective. Sensations of current appeared in the upper part of the body and to some extent in the lower extremities.

"At the spot in the left groin where she complained of pain, a hard, tender cord, running longitudinally, could be palpated. I was not able to overcome this in spite of my efforts. It was not until the cervix had dilated completely and the head of the fetus had passed through the birth canal to the pelvic floor that this painfully tender spot disappeared. Now she began to experience sensations of current in her abdomen and pelvis. She began to belch and finally felt much more comfortable. Then the sensations of pressure on the rectum began to increase and she grew more apprehensive and restless and slightly confused.

"She felt she wanted to have a bowel movement and wanted to walk to the bathroom, but then decided against this. Her face became flushed and she complained of a feeling of heat throughout her body. Then coldness, a clammy sweat, and marked dryness of the mouth occurred. She grew less cooperative. Her jaws and legs were held stiffly and much more effort had to be exerted to overcome this holding. I had to proceed more energetically to get her to "come back" in her eyes. The vegetative sensations were now very intense. As they began to subside, the procedure became simply one of voluntary effort with rest and at times sleepiness between contractions. The entire process became more rhythmical. Her respirations increased in amplitude and she was able to bring herself back; at times she was actually able to prevent the withdrawal.

"At 6:30 P.M. a slight bulging was observed. The membranes then appeared at the introitus and passed through without rupturing. The obstetrician was called and the patient was removed to the delivery room. At 7:15 P.M. she began to deliver the head of the infant. And now, again, an acute contraction set in. It was more marked than at any time before. I could pry her jaws apart only with the greatest effort and her breathing required considerable attention. She began to tremble, and exclaimed with an expression of terror that it felt like something terrible might happen. She later said that she had the feeling she wanted to push but was afraid she might burst. The infant was delivered at 7:20 P.M., appeared moderately cyanotic but responded immediately, cried lustily, and became healthily pink. Two and one-quarter hours appeared to be the span for really active labor. A moderate first-degree laceration of the perineum occurred in the delivery of the head and required suturing under an anesthetic.

Dr. Raphael concludes:

"I have gained the impression from both cases that with the establishment of full respiration, the dissolving of acute armoring, the overcoming and prevention of the tendency to withdraw, and the acute contraction of the total organism, the process of labor and delivery is, in general, very much accelerated. Knowledge of the orgasm reflex and the segmental arrangement of the armoring as discovered and described by Wilhelm Reich excites an immediate appreciation of the problem and technique to be used in rendering assistance during labor. Without this knowledge, the physician must view the problem with bewilderment, helplessness, and dismay. His only recourse is to drugs with attendant danger to both mother and infant; more or less ineffective persuasion to relax; calloused indifference; or meddlesome interference of one sort or another, as for example, the so-called prophylactic forceps, routine episiotomy, etc. What Reich has said concerning the bodily attitude of the armored organism and the dissolution of this attitude is readily applicable to the acutely contracted organism. Active assistance is necessary for overcoming this "holding back." It is expressed automatically and the individual is unable to comprehend or respond to exhortations to relax, or other such persuasion. The holding back process is so acutely manifest that the obstetrician cannot fail, now and then, instinctively to suggest to the patient to stop holding her breath, or to take a deep breath, but he is generally unable to help actively. His assistance is, at best, abortive. He is unable to proceed systematically or consistently. Without the knowledge of the function of pulsation and the armoring process, he is unable to formulate his therapeutic task. It goes without saying that the amount of assistance required in labor is dependent on the previous state of the organism. The prevention or effective dissolution of chronic armoring—prior to pregnancy or before delivery—would facilitate the process of labor. In a primipara, to whom childbirth is new and who approaches it with superstition and trepidation, the shock of the experience can be allayed to some extent by correct education regarding the mechanism of labor. The setting, as was apparent from the first case presented, plays a significant part.

"From this preliminary study, it would appear that there are very practical preventive and therapeutic measures, the application of which would alleviate much of the discomfort of labor and many of its dangers. The most important results of such a facilitated process would be the reduction of danger of injury to the child to the very minimum. It is this result which interests us in this study and encourages its continuation.

To Dr. Raphael's conclusions I would like to add: Delivery should occur at home in a familiar environment with loved ones near. Unfortunately few obstetricians today will consent to this. They argue that in case of emergency the hospital is a safer place to be and besides there has to be more preparation at home since the home is not set up as is the hospital for childbirth. Also it is much more convenient for the obstetrician. He has a nurse to watch the progress of labor and has to be called only at the last minute. All of this may be perfectly true, but if we are concerned only with the welfare of the mother and the baby both fare better at home except in the presence of some complication, which can usually be foreseen long in advance. Further, both are less apt to suffer subsequent infection, which can easily be incurred in the hospital.

The baby should remain with the mother after it is born so that each can be a comfort to the other. The baby is allowed to nurse as soon as it shows desire by sucking movements of its lips. Under these conditions both mother and baby respond quickly after the strange event they have experienced. One can scarcely believe the difference between babies born in this manner and the usual baby born in a hospital under the routine procedures. Stinging drops in the eyes, tight wraps, separation from the mother, and feedings that are withheld for twenty-four hours following birth are not in the best interest of the baby's development. They may contribute to many difficulties the baby will suffer in the following months and even perhaps affect his whole life.

19 · Babies

No one can adequately understand the energic concept of functioning unless he has worked with and carefully observed babies, for it is here that movement both unitary and interrupted is most clearly seen. It never ceases to be a cause of both wonder and amazement how nature in nine months can produce from one sperm and one ovum such a complex but beautifully functioning organism as the human baby. When allowed to develop in the uterus of a relaxed and loving mother and born naturally, it becomes immediately an independent and efficient functioning unit. Its breathing commences immediately, and immediately it is able to observe and contact the world.

I assisted with a natural home delivery and the father, a medical orgonomist friend, and myself observed carefully the newborn baby girl. Within a few minutes after birth she looked up at one of us and then the other and followed us with her eyes as we deliberately walked about, turning her head to keep us in view. Her eyes were open and clear. We wondered what impression she had at her first look at the world. At this time, she was allowed to lie on her mother's abdomen, both receiving warmth and enhancing the contractions of the mother's uterus through the contact. Within the hour, she nursed vigorously and, from her expression, with full pleasure. Her whole organism responded to every move, for there with her mother she could expand and be unafraid.

It is inconceivable that doctors, nurses, even mothers and fathers, can still accept the concept of separating mother and child at birth. Many mothers do, of course, object, and then they are met with the inflexible rules of hospitals concerned only with efficiency, convenience, and old erroneous medical ideas which have become dogma, never with the emotional needs of the child.

This arbitrary attitude is at times carried to the point of absurdity. An acquaintance of mine consulted me about a situation that worried him. His six-year-old daughter had to have a small subcutaneous cyst removed from her arm. The surgeon refused to operate in his office under local anesthesia, and said that it must be done in the hospital under sodium pentathol. The hospital insisted the girl must remain in the hospital overnight for observation prior to the operation. Her mother could not remain with her. This little girl had never slept away from home and the father was worried that all the elaborate preparation would be more frightening than the operation. In my earlier years, I did many minor operations under local anesthesia on small children and found them excellent little patients when everything is explained properly and truthfully to them.

So, I agreed wholeheartedly with my acquaintance and told him to try to persuade the surgeon to operate in his office; failing this, to insist on taking the girl to the hospital the morning of the operation. Too many parents and even doctors, hoping to calm children, minimize everything, only to have the child find he has been deceived. This makes him mistrust all adults. I have found that the average child can accept as much as the adult, sometimes more, if he is made aware of exactly what he is up against.

However, in this case, the surgeon refused an office treatment, so the man tried to arrange to take his daughter to the hospital in the morning. And here the surgeon added his persuasion too. To no avail. The little girl was taken to the hospital in the evening, left alone in a strange and forbidding place awaiting an unknown ordeal. She lay awake most of the night sobbing, faced her operation tired, frightened, and heartbroken. Several months later, she was still afraid to be left alone or to have her parents go out. She keeps going over the details of her experience until she comes to the point, "Now is it time I came home from the hospital?"

But, when they are not restricted in such incredible fashion, babies develop very rapidly in accomplishing movements and control.[1] Breathing in the unblocked baby affects the whole organism. The impulse can be seen going into the pelvis and ending with a soft tilting forward of that segment. The skin is warm and pink, the body a soft and plastic energy system which, out of its own resources, will make contact with its environment and begin to shape it according to its needs. The eyes are open, frank, and serious. The mouth is a remarkable and well-developed, functioning organ. One is amazed at the strength and vigor of suckling; if one allows the infant to suck on a finger one finds a strong and rhythmic reflex which soon starts streamings in the finger, which gradually extend up the arm. It is easy to understand the effect on the mother's nipple; nursing sends energy streaming through the body to the pelvis. With the mother responding to her infant, a deep feeling of love is felt with genital sensations. Where these sensations are interpreted as incestuous, the mother withdraws anxiously and loses contact with her child.

At the end of nursing one frequently observes a quivering of the lips in the infant. These quiverings spread to the face, finally ending in trembling and soft convulsive movements of the head and throat, sometimes of the whole body. The eyes turn up under

---

[1] Obstetricians frequently advise placing newborn babies on their stomachs when they are lying down. The rationalization is that if the baby should vomit or regurgitate his milk he will not drown himself by inhaling the fluid into the lungs. As a matter of fact, especially weak and sick babies are more apt to regurgitate and drown themselves in this position unless properly burped. Besides this position does force the baby to retract his pelvis and arch his back assuming a holding back attitude. Vigorous babies overcome this hindrance by drawing their knees up under them. Babies should be allowed to lie on their backs or on their sides; these positions are more natural and allow greater movement. Of perhaps even greater importance is that these positions allow more freedom in looking and following moving objects which aid in development of the eyes.

the upper lids and the baby gives himself over completely to this pleasurable surrender (the oral orgasm).

Where the mother develops anxiety and loses contact, the infant too contracts and his downward path to misery begins. He first contracts in the diaphragm and chest, both reducing sensation and separating the upper and lower parts of his body. This is easily observed in his breathing, but other signs and symptoms soon present themselves. His feet and buttocks become cold and blue, or pale; his eyes lose their sparkle, his face that open and contented look. His back becomes arched and his whole body may be rigid. He becomes restless, irritable, and his cry instead of communicating a confident demand takes on a whimpering pleading. Eating becomes upset, so do bowel functioning and sleeping habits, and he loses weight and may develop temperature, colds, or other illness.

The mother, alarmed and unable to understand what has happened and unable to correct the problem, becomes more and more anxious. Finally she resents the husband, who was responsible for the baby in the first place, and we have a chaotic situation which is a vicious circle. It is usually at this stage that the medical orgonomist is consulted.

Examination of Babies

History

For history, the therapist must know five things; First, the complaints that tell why the baby was brought to a doctor. Secondly, the general circumstances of pregnancy and delivery, including any difficulties there may have been, and whether or not the baby was wanted. Then he must know the circumstances at birth—what medication was used, whether there were difficulties in getting the baby to breathe or nurse.

Fourth, he must find out something about the baby's behavior since birth, in nursing, sleeping, bowel movements, creeping[2]

2 Robert J. Doman, et al, The Doman Delacato Institute for the Achievement of Human Potential, Philadelphia. These researchers have shown the importance of crawling, creeping, walking, and other movements for the

and so forth. He must find out if the cry is full or whining, if he is generally content or cross, if he is too thin or too fat, whether he can cuddle. Inability to cuddle is serious and indicates an autistic baby. Finally, the therapist must know if a male child has been circumcised.

The fifth point of the history concerns the mother's attitude. The therapist must know what her feelings have been toward her child since birth, if the situation is chaotic, and whether the mother had developed genital anxiety.

Examination

The following six points cover the general questions the therapist must ask himself as he examines the baby.

1) General appearance: Is the baby crying, happy, or struggling? Does he cuddle to his mother and how does the mother handle him? Does the baby appear frightened, angry, or sad?

2) Eyes: Are the eyes open, frank, serious, friendly, and able to flirt, or are they suspicious, sad, frightened, and kept partially closed?

3) Skin: Is it warm and pink or cold and blue, especially about the legs and buttocks?

4) Position: Is the back arched with the pelvis held or can the baby give forward? If one holds up hands and feet, does the baby still hold rigidly or does he give anteriorly?

5) Throat and jaw: Are the throat and jaw open or held? This is determined most easily by fullness of cry. When the baby's mouth is held open and he cries, does he get angry and really assert himself?

6) Pelvis: Is the pelvis movable or held? This is easily determined by raising both feet.

Blocks are very easy to release in babies. They are very fragile, though, and must be worked with tenderly. Even if he hurts the baby in the process, the therapist will be rewarded with a smile of appreciation and friendship when he is successful.

---

adequate development of coordination and integration. Even reading disabilities improved when the individuals were put through the process of crawling and creeping which they had not done during their development. The side to side movements of the head during crawling and creeping seem to be very important for the development of the eye segment.

Convulsive Seizures in a Baby

The following case history is one of the clearest illustrations of the possibilities of this therapy. The patient was a well-developed, handsome boy of seventeen months.

His parents stated that, since the age of three months, he had experienced periods of blanking out which the pediatrician diagnosed as petit mal. (See the discussion of epilepsy, p. 147.) When he was nine months old, these blanking-out periods changed into grand mal seizures occurring several times a month. The seizures had persisted until the time I saw him. When he was brought to me, he had been on medication (phenobarbital and Dilantin) for five weeks, but was still having an occasional seizure. Each attack started as a temper tantrum during which he would hold his breath, turn blue, and end by going into a convulsive seizure. Except for these attacks, he had been an exceptionally good baby. He almost never cried or got angry, was quiet and well behaved, and showed evidence of high intelligence —all this in spite of the fact that he could only say two or three words, and those very indistinctly. At ten and a half months he started to walk and would lead his parents toward what he wanted and indicate what he wanted them to do about it. The father reported that the baby behaved better with him than with his mother; the temper tantrums occurred when he was with his mother.

After the convulsions began he was studied by several physicians and was finally hospitalized in a large neuropsychiatric institute for complete study. The general physical examination gave normal results. Blood examinations, including blood calcium and phosphorus estimations, were also normal. One specialist thought there was a beginning atrophy of the retina in the left eye, but two others said the fundi were both normal. Electroencephalograms showed abnormal brain waves; therefore epilepsy and early brain tumor were suspected. Repeat examinations were recommended when he reached eighteen months. The interim diagnosis was "instability of the cortex." He was placed on a regimen of phenobarbital and Dilantin with the statement that after four or five years medication might be discontinued with a hope that the convulsions would not return.

He was a wanted child, the first, and to that time, the only one. He was born normally after nine hours' labor with no instruments used in delivery. The mother suffered from hyperemesis gravidarum, and for the first six weeks after delivery found nursing a trial because the baby demanded feeding every one and a half or two hours. Either he was not getting enough to eat, or he was demanding nursing because he could not get adequate contact from the mother. However, his nursing was vigorous, and at ten and a half months he voluntarily stopped and accepted a bottle. (He started to walk at the same time.) No specific information could be obtained from the parents to account for his condition.

The father seemed to be quiet, permissive, and gentle; he apparently had good rapport with the baby. Overtly, the mother's relationship was not as good, but she seemed to be genuinely interested in the baby's welfare. She tried to be a good mother and religiously tried to follow a book on child care. Of course, following a book indicated that she was unable to follow or trust any natural maternal instincts. She was quite contactless and had a great deal of buried hostility; sexually she was frigid. The father stated that prior to and during the first three months of marriage before the pregnancy she had been quite free sexually and had adjusted well. Since then, she had gradually withdrawn from sexual activity and when I saw them had no interest in it. Her lack of interest was accentuated by a vaginal infection. One could guess that when she nursed her nipples were cold; she reported no pleasure in nursing.

For the first visit, both parents came with the baby and remained in the room while I examined him. The father took charge of the baby, undressing him and putting him on the couch. The baby whimpered a bit and I talked to him, trying to make some contact. Suddenly, he stood up, ran to me, and threw his arms around my neck, holding me tight. I held him, continuing to talk to him and explaining that I wanted to examine him and see if I could help him feel less miserable. Then I laid him on the couch. He was a beautiful child, but I have never seen one so badly damaged biophysically at that age. His jaws were held rigidly tight, and his throat was so constricted that he gasped for breath with his head shaking every time he inhaled. His chest did not move in breathing and his spinal muscles felt like iron bands. The occipital muscles were extremely contracted and the pelvis was held rigid. His eyes were only partly open and his expression was one of a determined holding back at all costs. The submental area was rigid and pushed down by pressure from the tongue—indicating held back crying. It was not difficult to see that he was holding back at least two emotions, rage and crying.

All the time I was examining him, the baby was very cooperative. I explained the holding to the parents and demonstrated it, letting the father feel the rigid muscles. I told them the baby needed to let out rage and crying, and that if that were successfully accomplished the pressures and tensions would be relieved, as well as, I hoped, his symptoms. What I would have to do to relieve the muscle spasms would be unpleasant and even painful for the baby, but I felt it would be worth while. On their part, the parents would have to learn to accept the child's aggression.

At that first session, I worked on the baby's sternocleido mastoid muscles, softening them somewhat, then turning to the masseters. They were tremendously rigid and gave very little; I did not dare use very great pressure. Turning him over, I worked on the spinal muscles, releasing the right side fairly easily but making no impression on the left side, which was rocklike. However, the occipital muscles gave fairly easily and the eye segment was relieved; I hoped the epileptic seizures would not recur so long as the occipital area could be kept mobile and the eyes therefore free. Returning him to his back, after releasing the occiput, I manually opened his eyes wide and tried to open his mouth. Up to this point the baby had made little fuss and I had felt he understood I was trying to help. However, he resisted my attempt to open his mouth with all his might; whenever I got his jaws apart he kept his lips tightly closed. As well as possible I held his mouth open and pressed up on the floor of the mouth, hoping he would breathe and cry more freely. He squirmed and got very angry, occasionally letting out a cry. Continuing to hold his mouth open with one hand, I pressed on his chest with the other and succeeded in getting about every third breath through as a fairly open cry. I was also pleased to see the amount of rage he expressed, both in his face and in trying to fight me off.

At that point I told him that would be all, both because I did not want him to overreach himself and because I did not want to subject him to too long and unpleasant experience. He jumped up and went to his father and, to my great pleasure, looked back at me with his eyes wide open and smiled. Then he went about the room exploring; both parents remarked that he seemed more relaxed and open.

I told them that since we did not definitely know the diagnosis, we could not know what I would be able to accomplish. My impression, I explained, was that his severe holding could account for his symptoms; I cautioned them to think over whether or not they wanted me to work with him. I was only able to promise my best efforts, but if they did want me to treat him, I told them, one of the first things I would do would be to cut down the medication so that in three weeks he would be given none at all. I suggested that they call me in a week.

When the father called, he reported that the baby had shown a great change—noticed not only by himself and his wife but also by their neighbors. The baby was using several new words, had started hitting the mother, and would pick up dirt and throw it at other children (peculiarly, only at blond children). He had never been able to express this sort of aggression before and the father seemed to understand its importance. At times, the baby had cried quite freely and had had a temper tantrum that did not lead into a convulsion. The parents had voluntarily cut the medication in half after I saw them, and wanted me to continue working with the baby. I agreed to see the baby once a week.

The mother brought him alone and remained with him during each session. At the second session, I was wearing a patch over one infected eye, and when he saw it the baby became frightened and started to cry quite freely. I talked to him, explaining my patch, and he ran to me and again threw his arms around my neck. I held him for a while and then put him on the couch.

Again I was amazed at how readily babies respond to therapy —his eyes remained open and he cried quite freely, only occasionally gasping and shaking his head as he breathed. The occipital muscles had stayed soft and his mouth was not so difficult to open as it had been before. After ten minutes I stopped work and turned him over to his mother. His left spinal muscles were still rigid. I told the mother to stop the Dilantin completely.

At the third session, the mother reported the baby had been hitting her a great deal and hitting other children, too. She wanted to know what she should do if he picked on very little children; I suggested that she tell him not to hit them but to hit her instead. The baby had also had a temper tantrum during which he had cried without holding his breath or turning blue at all. He cried a lot, struggled, and got very angry at me during this session, finally showing sucking movements of the lips. When I gave him a bottle he took it eagerly and smiled at me. Turning him over to his mother again, I told her to stop all medication and was informed that it had been practically stopped because the child had refused to take any of it.

When he arrived for the fourth session, he had been completely off medication for a week. There had been one temper tantrum —he had held his breath and turned blue but had not gone into a seizure. The aggressiveness and belligerence had been maintained; he had been hitting and fighting and even taking on three- and four-year-olds. He was really fighting for his life. The mother reported that he had not attacked any children smaller than himself when he had come in contact with them. But he was making a new demand on her. She used a stroller for long excursions as a usual thing, but now he was refusing the stroller and insisting she carry him. He wanted contact.

He did not like this session at all; he kicked and bit vigorously, crying angrily the whole time. For the first time his spinal muscles relaxed well, however, and his jaws, throat, and chest were much better. Only rarely would his throat tighten and his head shake as he breathed, and his color remained good. As soon as the session was over he quieted, smiled, and waved good-by when he left me.

At the fifth session, the mother reported that he continued to fight with other children, but that over the weekend he had become very quiet and good, and that she had worried that he had regressed. They had gone to visit her father and stepmother over the weekend; she didn't like them and thought the baby disliked them too. The baby had indeed regressed; his eyes were dull, far away, held half closed, his occipital and spinal muscles were spastic, his throat was tight. When he breathed he turned blue and swallowed his tongue. After I loosened his spinal and occipital muscles, he opened his eyes wide and began to cry. I held his mouth open, pressing on the floor of his mouth until he could cry quite freely, then turned him over to his mother. Safe with her, he looked back with his eyes fully open and bright, smiling.

After this session the father reported that the baby bit him once mildly and had drawn blood when he bit his mother. He had begun to cling to the mother, and the father had noticed she was unconsciously drawing away from the child, although consciously she was trying very hard to accept him and help him to express himself. The father also felt that he himself had recently been drawing away from the baby. Apparently, both parents liked the quiet baby and wanted him relieved of his seizures but not otherwise changed. I explained that their desires were not realizable. The baby had the convulsions because of the way he was, and could only grow away from the seizures as he grew away from his former behavior. Tactfully, I hinted at the fact that parents mold children to their own needs, which sometimes conflict with the child's needs. The father brought up the question of whether or not both parents should have therapy, and I told him I thought it would be wise, particularly for the mother, if any permanent good were to be done to the baby. During that week, the baby had had some very good days; there had been one temper tantrum, but no convulsion, and his cry had usually been free.

At the sixth session, the baby cried hard, tried to get to his mother, and showed very marked *arc du cercle*. The spinal muscles were quite spastic but easily softened. The throat was tight and he swallowed his tongue, interfering with his breathing.

This condition was alleviated by pressure in the submental region. The occipital muscles were also spastic and had to be relieved before the eyes lost their dullness. He kicked and fought, looked very angry, and cried angrily. When I let him go he ran quickly to his mother and clung to her, but then looked back with wide open eyes to smile and wave. Quite spontaneously, the mother brought up the question of therapy for herself. She was guilt-laden over her performance as a mother, and added that she was pregnant again and didn't want to do the same things to another baby. I told her I thought therapy was advisable and referred her to another orgonomist.

At the seventh session, the mother reported that the baby had not held his breath at all that week, although he had continued to fight and bite her and to fight three- and four-year-olds, who seemed unable to stand up against him. There had been two days when he was very good and loving. His eyes were quite bright and wide open, and during the session he kicked and fought and cried loudly. His throat caught only for a moment and he swallowed his tongue. His armor was easily reduced, but he still pulled backward in an *arc du cercle* instead of giving anteriorly. As soon as the session was over he ran to his mother and asked for a bottle, and did not forget to smile to show he had no hard feelings.

The mother reported, during the eighth session, that he had held his breath on one occasion and turned blue or even grayish, and that he had seemed more subdued and had even gone to sleep in the waiting room. He clung tenaciously to his mother. During the session his eyes were dull, although he cried quite freely, and he seemed less vigorous in his movements. Toward the close of the session he swallowed his tongue and choked a good deal. I was able to improve his eyes by work on the occipital muscles, but his bodily attitude continued to be a great holding back. The total impression was one of general withdrawal; I did not quite understand why he presented such a picture and could get no reason from the mother.

At the ninth session the mother reported that he had been quieter but had seemed cheerful and cooperative. He was still clinging to his mother; and, as soon as I took him, he went "dead," and lifeless. The muscles were quite relaxed and he struggled very little and would not cry vigorously. Since I did not understand his reactions I did no work but merely observed him. As soon as I said we were finished he jumped up and ran to his mother, quite alive at once. He reminded me of a opossum.

At the tenth session the mother reported that he had been quite good. He had not held his breath at all and there was very little to report. When he saw me he cried and clung to his mother; as soon as I took him he again went "dead." He did not struggle at all; his eyes were bright and clear but he dulled them somewhat during the session. On the whole, he was relaxed and seemed to be playing opossum. When I said, "That is all," he jumped up full of life again and went to his mother, smiling back at me and waving good-by.

During the eleventh session the mother said he had been very aggressive, fighting with his friends and biting his parents all week. He had started to refuse the bottle, did not want to go to bed at night, and seemed afraid. Once at breakfast he had seemed to be "away" for a few seconds. On the couch he stayed very quiet and still, holding his breath, not struggling against any work I did. His neck and left spinal muscles were spastic but his pelvis had become movable spontaneously.

On a trip myself, I left him with a student for the next month. The student was a young woman who has very good contact with children and she had sat in on my sessions with him. He continued to be aggressive, hitting and biting his parents. There were three temper tantrums during the month; in one he went stiff and in the other two he turned blue, but he had no convulsions.

When I saw him for a twelfth session, his eyes were well opened and he appeared to be quite alive. However, as soon as he was on the couch he closed his eyes and offered no resistance. The spinal muscles were tense and he cried when I worked on them; otherwise he remained still. Once again he was full of life when I had finished. This boy was outsmarting me—he withdrew contact as soon as he got on the couch.

He continued to be aggressive and to fight. The day after the session, he was jumping on his bed when he fell and hit his mother's face with his head. She screamed and frightened him. After she had pacified him he wanted her to sit in the little chair he had lately been given for Christmas. She said she would stay where she was and suggested he sit in his chair, and he responded with a temper tantrum. He held his breath, and one arm and the opposite leg twitched. There were no aftereffects from the tantrum. When I asked the mother why she had refused his overtures, she said that she had not understood the offer of the chair.

Again during the thirteenth session he was passively cooperative. The spinal muscles were very spastic and the baby cried when I freed them. He was still refusing to go to bed early, but was sleeping late in the morning instead. It became apparent that the day following each session was the baby's low point in the week *and* the mother's. Each session brought up her own guilt, and she admitted that she had been very angry at the baby and felt very guilty about his condition. Obviously, the mother found it difficult to tolerate the changes taking place in the baby and was unconsciously sabotaging therapy; at least some of her guilt was because of this.

He ignored me completely at the fourteenth session. He was entirely passive and had a disgusted expression on his face. However, he came to life quickly when I released him.

At the fifteenth session the mother reported that he had had a temper tantrum a few hours before the session, during which he had gone stiff but had not developed convulsions. She said the father could not stand the baby's aggression. During the session he expressed crying more fully but still showed a passive attitude. There was some evidence of constriction in his throat.

His passivity on the couch was becoming a problem; such attitudes are quite common in adults but I had never before seen this attitude so marked or so consistent in such a young baby. In adults, this contactlessness can be attacked by reverting to character analysis, pointing out what is happening, mimicing them, having them describe their sensations or even lack of sensation. Sometimes the contactlessness can be broken through by acting out the emotion in exaggerated form. None of these methods are possible with a baby. What we knew was that the contactlessness was a defense against strong feeling, and since he seemed at this point to have little difficulty in expressing rage and very little more trouble in crying, it seemed that what he had not had was love and the opportunity to express love. The mother was unable to give him this love. Therefore I felt such expression was the current problem and played with him a bit and talked to him. He, however, remained unconcerned.

My student had grown to love him, and I discussed with her the possibility that she take him over and just love and play with him. She was delighted. I was concerned, however, with his habit of holding his breath when he had a temper tantrum, and wanted to clear that up if possible before turning the treatment over to her.

At his sixteenth session the mother reported that he had had three temper tantrums. He had held his breath but there had been no twitching or convulsion. His spinal muscles were spastic again and his throat was tight. He continued to be passive. I freed the spasms and got him to cry freely.

The mother reported, at the seventeenth session, that he had had one temper tantrum, during which he cried and breathed freely. However, he had become passive with his playmates. It seemed definite that he was withdrawing because his parents could not tolerate him in any other way; and he had learned to hold back very well, but not to live and express himself. On the couch he was still passive and contactless, but he was quite free of muscular armor. I felt he was ready to be turned over to my student and the mother seemed pleased at the idea.

After this session he cried freely with no tendency to hold his breath, and was taken over by my student from this point on. She reported that at the first session he seemed timid, clung to his mother. Therefore she tried only to make contact with him, holding him, talking to him, nuzzling him. When she put her face against his, he broke into pitiful sobbing and drew away as though he could not stand the feeling. He did not hold his breath and his contactlessness was dissolving. At the second session he was more active, engaging in play and eventually becoming rough, hitting and kicking but able to accept fondling.

Gradually he responded more and more, coming to enjoy the relationship and growing very loving. He had no more temper tantrums.

The baby four months later is still under observation and care at this writing, but I feel he has gone far enough to safely say that he has been saved from the life of an epileptic. He had no convulsive seizures after the time of the first session, even though medication was discontinued. He has had no temper tantrums for some time, and for a longer period has not held his breath nor shown any difficulty in breathing.

The mother is in therapy, trying to solve some of her problems, and the father at least has some understanding of the trauma caused by both of them. We do not, of course, know what the child's response to the new baby will be, but I believe the outlook for the child should be quite hopeful.[3]

If the process of the therapy should seem severe for a young child, it should be recalled that he was suffering most severely before the therapy and would have continued to suffer all the difficulties an epileptic must face. The mother reported that on several occasions the child asked to come to therapy, and he never showed any sign of confusing the momentary pain inflicted during treatment with ill will on my part. He was always friendly and trusting off the couch, no matter how anxious he was to get away from it. He knew I was helping him, in the same way one knows one is being helped even though it hurts when a bone is set or an abscess lanced.

[3] This boy, three years later, has continued to develop into a healthy and alive youngster with none of his former symptoms. He accepted his young sister very well.

20 · Care of the Infant

ABOUT TEN DAYS TO TWO WEEKS following delivery, difficulties may confront the mother in her handling of and relationship to her baby because she develops genital anxiety. This anxiety comes from the increase in energy and excitation of the pregnancy and nursing, together with the opening of the pelvis by the softening during pregnancy and the full opening during delivery.

Reich has shown how vital the contact between mother and infant is for healthy development of the baby.[1] Loss of contact creates anxiety (a contraction) in the infant, primarily at the diaphragm, and results in respiratory blocking. A continuation of this state may be expected to result in extension of the armoring upward and downward, laying the foundation for future biopathies.

Here, in the following case report, are some of the problems encountered when contact was lost because of genital anxiety in the mother.

The baby, in this case, had been planned with the expectation of letting "only the interests of the child determine the course of events, and if at all possible, nothing else." Many features in the setting were favorable for such a project. The mother, aged

[1] Besides Reich, Anna Freud, René Spitz and others have shown the importance for the child of contact with the mother. Harry B. Harlow at the University of Michigan, working with baby monkeys, demonstrated this clearly.

twenty-eight, had essentially completed psychiatric orgone therapy. The father, a year older than she, was patient, understanding, and kind; he had solved most of his problems by the same means. The grandmother, with whom the parents were closely associated, was in therapy; and a sister of the mother and one of the father had each been in treatment. All were intelligent, well educated, had read orgonomic literature extensively, and were well acquainted and in complete agreement with the principles of sex-economic self-regulation. All were warm, likable people.

There was one child, a boy four years old, who, although born prior to the parents' acquaintance with orgonomy, was nearly healthy with good sexual expression and evidence of only fleeting, occasional armoring. I saw him a few times for minor difficulties. He had been circumcised at one month and his birth had been easy and uncomplicated.

Although the mother was freed of armor, and the orgasm reflex had been established, she continued to be somewhat anxious and flighty and chattered in a repetitious manner with endless, anxious questions. She had never been able consistently to accept her genital feelings, and when they were particularly strong she would control their intensity by holding her breath. She enjoyed the genital embrace, experienced real pleasure, but could never let herself go completely. At the acme, she would usually hold her breath and either lie still or retract her pelvis, all of this with a conscious feeling of anxiety. She was quite aware of the genital anxiety which she could not solve, and survived by occasional therapeutic sessions. She had been quite eager to become pregnant for some time and she wanted another baby. However, in view of her continuing anxiety, I repeatedly suggested waiting until she had had more opportunity to attain genital potency. She was so determined that she eventually proceeded in spite of my objections.

I observed her throughout her pregnancy and saw her every two weeks. The pregnancy presented no problems and was free of nausea and other symptoms, except for continuing anxiety. She frequently held back in her upper chest whenever genital feelings became too strong. It was always very simple to get her to move and breathe through, taking but a few minutes.

She was willing and eager to be accepted as a research project and was determined to bring the baby up according to the concept of sex-economic self-regulation. Arrangements were made with an orgonomically oriented obstetrician and nurse, and rooming-in was arranged at the hospital.

She felt life at a little under four months, and the baby's movements were always vigorous and active but never violent. Three weeks before the expected date of delivery she awoke at two o'clock in the morning with some mild cramps and show; the pains rapidly increased in severity and frequency and she went to the hospital. At 3:30 A.M. she delivered a five pound, five and a half ounce girl without anesthesia. Labor was uneventful and uncomplicated and she breathed down throughout. At the point of delivery she became frightened, but remembered not to hold her breath and screamed in order to breathe.

The baby was born with the cord around its neck and the face was blue, but it became pink in a few seconds after the cord was removed. No artificial respiration or resuscitative methods were necessary. No silver nitrate or other solution was placed in the baby's eyes and no mucus was noted in her throat. Because the weigh was below five pounds, eight ounces, the baby was placed in an incubator. This was a hospital rule. However, the hospital (which had never had rooming-in before) allowed the incubator to be placed in the room with the mother and the special nurse. The mother could have the baby whenever she wished. No interference on the part of the hospital was met.

Shortly after birth the baby was placed at the breast, when sucking movements were noticed. She suckled vigorously but the mother did not believe there was any milk. I saw the baby at 1:00 P.M., the time of the second nursing. At this time the mother and baby both looked very well.

The mother reported she had felt pleasurable streamings through her body and thighs during labor, but had developed considerable anxiety at the point of delivery. Up to the time of the second nursing she had felt no streamings in her breasts; this appeared shortly after, accompanied by a profuse flow of milk, which oozed out of her nipples. Streamings were felt in the uterus, pelvis, and thighs. The uterus, was well contracted, but not as hard and spastic as one is accustomed to feeling in obstetric wards.

The baby was rosy pink and warm throughout, with full breathing showing the reflex. Her cry when hungry was full and angry. She showed strong sucking movements and smacking of the lips, and nursed vigorously. I observed an oral orgasm during nursing at this time. The hospital shirt which the baby wore had the ends of the sleeves sewed up to prevent the babies from scratching their faces. Since this hampered the movements of hands, I asked the nurse to cut the sleeves and it was done. The baby was lively, alert, and reacted to touch. One felt that she focused momentarily when looking at people. On my second visit, I was convinced that she did focus. No evidence of cyanosis or trauma from the cord could be found; her neck was soft, chest free, breathing full, abdomen soft and warm, and her feet and hands were warm. She could move about freely, turning from side to side, and by the third day she could turn completely over.

Two days later I saw her for the second time, together with another orgonomist trained in infant research. The mother was up and about and had been so after the first twenty-four hours; the mother had streamings in her breasts and uterus when nursing, with pain at times when sensations became too strong. There was much flow of milk.

The baby, still in the incubator, now weighed five pounds, five and a quarter ounces, which was only a quarter ounce below the birth weight—a contrast to the usual marked loss of weight. It is probable that under ideal conditions there would be no loss or even progressive gain. She was warm all over, nursed vigorously, and had a strong cry when she was hungry. However, she seldom cried and was an amazement to the nurses on the ward as the only baby who never seemed to cry. She definitely focused her eyes and followed persons about her. She could turn over quite freely. While nursing, she was seen to have an oral orgasm again, and the mother reported she had noticed others. The other orgonomist suggested removing the beads from the baby's neck, especially in view of the cord having been around her neck and it was done. He felt there was a slight catch in her throat in breathing but the impulse went through to the pelvis with the reflex. The mother and baby returned home on the fifth day.

On the fifth and seventh days the baby was seen by our orgonomic social worker. She reported that the abdomen appeared distended and hard on both days. The baby had regurgitated slightly and appeared uncomfortable. The social worker had also reported that the stools were watery and forceful. After a while the baby vomited and seemed relieved.

I saw the baby again eight days after birth, together with the second orgonomist. No evidence was found at this time of distension of the abdomen. One stool was somewhat watery but mostly well formed. Oral orgasms continued; the baby was warm, breathed well, and no blocks could be seen. She was sleeping peacefully when first seen, awoke gradually and pleasantly, and nursed. She was very alive and one was drawn to her spontaneously. She was able to hold her head up very well.

At this time I examined the mother, who showed no armor and felt well. The uterus could not be palpated abdominally. She reported having several exciting sexual dreams.

I do not believe that in her first ten days this baby had any serious traumatizing experience.

I continued to keep in touch by telephone with the mother, who reported that the baby had shown no problems. However, on the twenty-second day, while I was away, the baby developed a marked regurgitation and diarrhea; her stools were greenish in color and twelve to fourteen a day. The mother became quite concerned, tried to locate me, and finally called the second orgonomist; she remained under his care until I returned. I saw the baby on her twenty-fifth day; she had continued very fretful, crying almost constantly, slept very little at night, and would be only momentarily relieved after nursing. Her chest was not moving, her breathing was abdominal, and crying was not full. On questioning the mother I found that she herself had been very anxious previously, having felt strong genital sensations which she had been unable to tolerate or fulfill. She found herself withdrawing from the baby, could not stand to be near her, held her stiffly, and even felt hostile toward her older child. She was angry at herself for this attitude; she felt that such behavior was not acceptable from the standpoint of being a "healthy mother" and presented considerable guilt. I spent quite some time explaining the mechanism of her feelings, which had arisen out of genital anxiety, and helped free the baby from her blocks.

The baby appeared in distress, miserable and pale. I mobilized her chest and she began to cry and it was an angry crying, although still inhibited in her throat. After making her gag and stimulating the muscles in the back of her neck, I heard her voice become more free. Her face flushed, she looked angry, and cried a free angry cry. Immediately after this, she went to sleep and rested peacefully with her chest moving.

I saw the baby next on her twenty-eighth day. The mother reported that the baby had continued free for two days following the last treatment. She had slept well at night and seemed satisfied after eating, although the mother herself had continued anxious, guilty, and without contact with the baby. When I examined the baby, her chest was pale, the abdomen and legs were bluish, there was a slight discharge from the left eye, and some lack of contact in the eyes. Her chest, again, was not moving. Diarrhea was still present but to a lesser degree. Again I mobilized the chest; the baby cried angrily and her body became a bright pink down to the middle of her abdomen. Afterward she seemed more alert and restful. I also examined the mother, who presented some stasis. I succeeded in mobilizing her energy, discussed in some detail her resentment about her lack of sexual fulfillment, her resentment toward the baby because of this, and the resulting lack of contact.

On her thirty-second day, the baby was definitely better; her cry was lusty, her chest was moving though not freely, and a general tendency 'toward holding back was seen. Her spinal muscles and the back of her neck were quite spastic. The abdomen and legs still had a bluish tinge. She had continued to cry and the mother had developed a habit of nursing her more and more frequently in the hope of quieting her. I explained that the baby accepted nursing so frequently because of anxiety and not hunger, that the anxiety was an outcome of lack of contact, and that the mother found it impossible to supply the contact the baby needed, so she should let the grandmother or father attempt to supply it. She had noticed that the baby was much better when being taken care of by either of them. I again released the spastic muscles and the baby seemed much better. Diarrhea had practically subsided.

Five days later, her color was good, all the blueness had disappeared. Her body was warm, chest moving though not fully, but the spinal muscles were spastic again. Her abdomen was quite tense and she had had no movement in twenty-four hours. I again freed her chest.

On the forty-sixth day, when I next saw the baby, the mother reported that the baby had been crying almost constantly, did not sleep at night, demanded half-hourly nursing, and had irregular bowel movements. During the first few days of the past two weeks the mother said she had enjoyed the sexual embrace, with initial full pleasure resulting in anxiety at the acme. Following this period she had developed "terrific anxiety and became sexually disinterested." Quite obviously, she had run from genitality to the tedious care of constant attention to the baby.

At the time of my examination, the baby presented a surprisingly healthy picture. Her chest was moving, she was warm, was not crying, and her body was quite soft. I decided that certainly now the difficulty was not with the baby but entirely with the mother. I explained that she had set up too much of an ideal which she had been unable to follow and that from now on she was going to be an ordinary mother. I explained also that she would put the baby on a feeding schedule during which she would not feed her more often than every two or three hours, that she was not going to walk the floor all night because the baby cried, and that after investigating and finding that the baby was not suffering she would simply let her cry. I made these suggestions to release the mother of the burden she had made of the baby and hoped she would thus regain contact.

She called me two days later, saying that although the baby had cried a great deal the first night that by the second day she had been content to nurse every four hours and slept the majority of the night. The mother felt quite relieved.

When I next saw her on the baby's fifty-third day, the mother reported the baby had continued very well during most of the week, but that on the last day or two she had lost contact with the baby, did not know what the baby wanted when she cried, and that the baby had started crying again. However, during my examination she was smiling, her body, including the abdomen, was soft, and her chest was moving freely. I found nothing that required working on the baby.

For three weeks she continued very well; the mother said the baby had been happy, awoke smiling, ate regularly every four hours, and slept through the night. The mother herself felt happy and relaxed.

Then, a month elapsed during which I kept in touch by telephone but did not see either mother or child. During this interval the family bought and moved into their own home. In the period of readjustment the mother developed considerable anxiety and became afraid to stay at home alone with the children. The baby also reacted with anxiety, crying, and some disturbances in sleeping and eating habits.

When I next saw them, the mother reported that, although the baby had not been crying, she would sleep for only short intervals, sucked her thumb a great deal when she woke up at night, and had not been gaining any weight until recently when she had been given a bottle. She accepted the bottle avidly. She had two to three bowel movements a day, was not constipated but tended to strain at stool. Her color was quite good and she looked well nourished and she was warm, but presented a rather shocking picture of very typical and almost total holding back. Her chest was high, moved only slightly, she held her arms, and the only noticeable movement was a rather vigorous kicking of the legs. Her shoulders were pulled back, her thighs and spinal muscles quite spastic. Mobilization was a problem and I did not succeed in completely freeing her shoulders. Her cry, which had been markedly restricted, became fairly full but with a still noticeable block in her throat. I planned on seeing her again the following week but she developed an illness, diagnosed by her physician as rose fever, with which she had a high temperature for two days, then broke out in bright red blotches over her body.

Her temperature fell but she showed a marked irritability. Two weeks elapsed before I saw her again.

When I did see her again, the mother had this to report: During the past week she had had to stop nursing the baby because she could not stand the sensations in her breasts and wanted to cry. However, these sensations had continued in spite of her action. She had consistently avoided the genital embrace, had withdrawn from her husband and her son, and had developed "a love for her baby which was more than she could stand."[2]

The baby had accepted the bottle very well, suckled vigorously, and seemed to have a strong oral need. She would grab everything and put it into her mouth eagerly. She seldom cried but continued to wake frequently at night and suck her thumb. No evidence of genital play had been observed. She enjoyed her bath immensely and loved being lifted and allowed to fall with the mother's arms, but the mother frequently felt too much anxiety in this play to do her part. The mother noticed that the baby's bowel movements depended almost entirely on her own anxiety.

The mother's anxiety was almost constant, with occasional short periods of feeling very well and alive. These periods would last perhaps an hour or two. Her anxiety usually disappeared when holding the baby, but at times increased, "because," the mother said, "I was afraid of my love—it was so strong." I expected to find in the baby a picture similar to that of my last visit. I must say I was very much surprised. The baby looked very well, she was smiling, and although a slight gurgle in her throat was noticeable, her chest movements were quite full with the impulse going well down into the pelvis. She had an occasional tilting forward of the pelvis at the end of expiration. There was none of the holding back seen on the last occasion. The baby was quite alive and happy and weighed fifteen pounds.

Somehow the mother seemed to have established some contact in spite of her anxiety—but, we may add, at the cost of complete rejection of her own genitality. (After this visit, the mother's genital feeling returned and she accepted the genital embrace, but continued to react with anxiety at the climax.)

[2] This was a reaction formation. Actually she hated the baby for the disruption it caused in her life.

During the period that I observed this baby, I found it necessary to treat the husband and the older child, both at their own request. The husband had developed considerable stasis, had almost lost his proverbial patience, and had become thoroughly disappointed and disillusioned in the situation with regard to his wife. The four-year-old had become a problem. He was mean, destructive, constantly whining, fighting his little heart out to regain some of his lost recognition.

The mother was entirely aware of this tragedy but eased the heartbreak by her devotion to the cause of becoming an ideal mother, a result of the mystical connotation of being selected in a research project.

This case supports Reich's findings and illustrates the disastrous effects on the infant when contact with the mother is lost. It also shows the ability of the infant, its surprising ability to recuperate before chronic armoring is met, providing contact with the mother can be reestablished. I feel that somehow the rose fever represented an emotional breakthrough with marked relief to the child.

During the first two weeks following the birth of the baby, the mother was apparently able to accept her streamings better than she could after this period. At first she was the center of attention, at the start of a new and exciting experience. When the genital embrace was not feasible because of her condition, she blamed the baby for her lack of sexual expression; when this was no longer rational she withdrew from sexuality. We thus see the important place genital sexuality can play in producing loss of contact between mother and infant and its resultant effect on the whole family.

I am in part at fault in this case, for I feel that much of the effects of anxiety could have been prevented by more vigorous and consistent work on the mother, from the very beginning. I had wondered, though, ever since her own therapy whether she would ever be capable of accepting full genitality.

This project is scarcely started. A dozen or more years lie ahead before we can see whether or not this infant can be saved from chronic armoring and what unfortunate effects can be avoided in the family as a whole.

21 · Conclusions

So far the best that we have been able to do is to remove blocks when they develop.[1] None has escaped occasional blocking, but by preventing armoring in the children affected by the project described in the last chapter, we have enabled them to grow up with considerable independence, self-assurance, and ability to enjoy living. By the age of three, the little girl of the case reported above would tell her mother when she needed to come to me, would come into the office alone and prepared for the session, dressing and undressing herself. At five, she told me what to do for her. The saucy look of the healthy young animal was perfectly charming. There is great hope in this little experiment but the children have to fight large odds in society and the final answer is still not reached. Individuals can survive and function; we do not know if masses can remain free of armor. Even these children would have developed armor had they not been under constant supervision. They still must be observed through adolescence to see how well they meet that period.

During the past twenty years, since I have been familiar with biophysical functioning, I have had occasion to examine one adult whom I would unhesitatingly consider healthy. She came

[1] We are watching one baby (now over three years old) who has so far required no therapeutic help and has remained free of blocks.

from a home one would consider antithetical to health, with neurotic parents, one of whom was alcoholic, and a neurotic sister. She could not tell me how she had survived, except that her parents' teaching went in one ear and out the other. She was considered a black sheep by her rigid, tyrannical parents. She had left home at the age of sixteen, at which time she experienced her first heterosexual contact with a boy she loved; afterward she continued to have a sexual outlet. She was sex-positive but selective and had experienced streamings in the genital, loved children, and had married at twenty-one. At the time I saw her she had that enviable charm of health, self-assurance, natural poise and was beautiful in expression, body, and character. Although she had never read or even heard of Reich, her ideas could have been copied from his writing. If we knew exactly how she had maintained health it might add much to the solution of our task. I suspect there is a developmental capacity for health or predilection for the various character types. I hope healthy people are not as rare as my experience indicates. We must remember that it is not usual for a healthy person to wander into a psychiatrist's office and ask for an examination just as they might go to their family doctor for a checkup—which is what this young lady did.

The genital character is defenseless against the armored individual until he learns how to meet him. This young woman was glad to hear that her ideas and feelings were natural because she had been made to feel different by society. She was different, of course, but to her credit. The incredible part is that she had survived and had followed her feelings without knowing she was right, knowing only that she was decent and devoid of hate. Such people are usually crushed in adolescence.

Adolescents need assurance that their feelings and urges are natural, and knowledge and guidance in meeting society's anti-sexual attitude are needed, too. Adults have become frightened of natural feelings through their own necessity to armor, and they look upon such natural functioning as something to be controlled. Besides, they cannot distinguish between primary and secondary drives and try to repress both. Secondary drives are antisocial and need to be handled, but primary drives can be trusted to lead to good judgment and avoidance of difficulties. The healthy adolescent, it is true, would demand his sexual rights but would shun sex without love—not to mention promiscuity, rape, perversion, or brutality. There would be no prostitution. Natural feelings are more moral than the feelings of armored society but show some important differences. For example, continued marriage without love would be unthinkable, whereas armored society refuses to allow "merely" this as adequate reason for divorce.

An individual with natural functioning would not expect church on Sunday to absolve his sins of the week, nor do those who function naturally persecute those who do not follow their own beliefs. Our society is built out of armored terror. Its laws are made and enforced by that terror. And so it is society's laws that we must follow, irrational as they may be, and so we will continue to stifle our children and crush our adolescents to destroy their "animal" nature and so "civilize" them. Our culture has known only how to repress and quell rebellion. It cannot understand and support life. For some thousands of years man has been trying to get out of this trap but has always fallen back into it, because he has not known what trapped him or how. Now, we know that he is trapped by his own muscular armoring, which binds his orgasm anxiety and inhibits free and natural functioning.

Can man gradually make use of this knowledge to save himself before he brings about his own destruction? Reich believed he could and worked all his life toward that end.

Selected Bibliography

Books by Wilhelm Reich

The following books by Reich are listed in chronological order with English translations listed parenthetically where the original publication was in German.

1927—*Die Funktion des Orgasamus*, Vienna (Int. Psychonal Verlag). *The Function of the Orgasm*, New York (Orgone Institute Press), 1942.

1933—*Character Analysis*, Sexpolverlag. Translation, New York (Orgone Institute Press), 1949.

1933—*The Mass Psychology of Fascism*, Sexpolverlag. Translation, New York (Orgone Institute Press), 1946.

1936—*The Sexual Revolution*, Sexpolverlag. Translation, New York (Orgone Institute Press), 1945.

1938—*Die Bione*, Sexpolverlag.

1939—*Bion Experiments on the Cancer Problem*, Sexpolverlag.

1941—*The Emotional Plague of Mankind*, Sexpolverlag. Translated in two volumes: *The Murder of Christ* and *People in Trouble*, New York (Orgone Institute Press), 1953.

1948—*The Cancer Biopathy*, New York (Orgone Institute Press).

1948—*Listen, Little Man*, New York (Orgone Institute Press).

1951—*Ether, God and Devil*, New York (Orgone Institute Press).

1951—*Cosmic Superimposition*, New York (Orgone Institute Press).

1951—*The Oranur Experiment*, New York (Orgone Institute Press).

1951—*The Orgone Energy Accumulator: Its Scientific and Medical Use*, New York (Orgone Institute Press).

1957—*Contact with Space*, New York (Core Pilot Press).

1960—*Selected Writings of Wilhelm Reich*, New York (Farrar, Strauss, and Cudahy).

Orgonomic Journals

International Journal of Sex Economy and Orgone Research, New York (Orgone Institute Press), 1942–45.

Annals of the Orgone Institute, New York (Orgone Institute Press), 1942–49.

Orgone Energy Bulletin, New York (Orgone Institute Press), 1949–53.

Core, New York (Core Pilot Press), 1954–55.

Orgonomic Medicine, New York (Tenney Press), 1955–56.

Articles

Of the thousand-odd articles and references published, only the more important for the purposes of this volume are listed below. The first section contains the original articles by Reich; the second lists articles *in English* by his co-workers. Periodicals are identified by initials as follows:

Zeitschrift fur Sexualwissenschraft (Journal for Sexology) *ZSW*.

Zeitschrift fur Psychoanalyse Pedagogik (Journal for Psychoanalytic Pedogogy) *ZPP*.

Internationale Zeitschrift fur Psychoanalyse (International Journal of Psychoanalysis) *IZP*.

Zeitschrift fur Aerzticke Psychotherapie (Journal for Medical Psychotherapy) *ZAP*.

Zeitschrift fur Politische und Sexualoekonomie (Journal for Political Psychology and Sex-Economy) *ZPS*.

International Journal for Sex Economy and Orgone Research IJSO.

Orgone Energy Bulletin OEB.

Annals of the Orgone Institute AOI.

Orgonomic Medicine OM.

Original Articles in Orgonomy by
Wilhelm Reich

"Ueber einen Fall von Durchbruch der Inzestschranke," *ZSW*, vii, 1920.

"Triebegriffe von Forel bis Jung," *ZSW*, 1921.

"Der Koitus und die Geschlechten," *ZSW*, 1921.

"Ueber Spezifitact Der Onanieformen," *IZP*, viii, 1922.

"Zur Triebenergetik," *ZSW*, 1923.

"Kindliche Tagtraeume einer spaeteren Zwanganeurose," *IZP*, 1923.

"Ueber Genitalitaet," *IZP*, ix, 1923.

"Der Tic als Onanieequivalent," *ZSW*, 1924.

"Die Therapeutische Badeutung der Genitallibido," *IZP*, x, 1924.

"Die Rolle der Genitalitaet in der Neurosentherapie," *ZAP*, 1925.

"Weitere Bemurkungen Ueber die Therapeutische Bedeutung der Genitallibido," *IZP*, xii, 1926.

"The Sources of Neurotic Anxiety, *IZP* (London), vii, 1926.

"Ueber die chronische hypochrondische Neurasthenie mit Genitalen Asthenie," *IZP*, xii, 1926.

"Eltern als Erzieher," *ZPP*, Heft 3, 1926.

"Eltern als Erzieher," continued, *ZPP*, Heft 7, 8, 9, 1927.

"Hysterical Psychoses in Statu Nascendi," *IZP*, (London), p. 159–173, viii, 1927.

"Ueber den epileptischen Anfall," *IZP*, xvii, 1931.

"Der Orgasmus als elektrophysiologische Entladung," *ZPS*, p. 29–43, i, 1934.

"Der Urgegensatz des vegetativen Lebens," *ZPS*, p. 125–142 and 207–225, i, 1934.

"Zur Anwendung der Psychoanalyse in der Geschicktsforschung," *ZPS*, p. 4–16, i, 1934.

"Ein Widerspruch der Freud schen verdraengungslehre," *ZPS*, p. 115–125, i, 1934.

Roheim's "Psychoanalyse primitiven Kulturen," *ZPS*, p. 169–195, i, 1934.

"Was is Klassenbewusstsein," *ZPS*, p. 16–29, 90–107, and 226–255, i, 1934.

"Ueberblick ueber das Forschungagebeit der Sexualoekonomie," *ZPS*, p. 5–13, ii, 1935.

"Zur massenpsychologischen Wirkung des Kriegsfilmo," *ZPS*, p. 26–31, ii, 1935.

"Die Funktion der Objektiven Wertwelt," *ZPS*, p. 32–43, ii, 1935.

"Fortpflanzung—eine Funktion der Sexualitaet," *ZPS*, p. 24–31, iii, 1936.

"Einige aktualle Fragen der Zweiter Front," *ZPS*, p. 1–12, iv, 1937.

"Character and Society," *IJSO*, i, 1942.

"Biophysical Functionalism and Mechanistic Natural Science," *IJSO*, i, 1942.

"Orgone Biophysics, Mechanistic Science, and 'Atomic Energy,'" *IJSO*, iv, 1945.

"About Genital Self-Gratification in Children," *OEB*, ii, 2, 1950.

"Orgonomic Functionalism," Part 11, *OEB*, ii, i, 1950; continued *OEB* ii, 2, 1950; continued, *OEB*, ii, 3, 1950.

"Orgonomic and Chemical Cancer Research," *OEB*, ii, 3, 1950.

"Orgonomy," 1935–50, *OEB*, ii, 3, 1950.

"Children of the Future," *OEB*, ii, 4, 1950.

"Cancer Cells in Experiment XX," *OEB*, iii, 1, 1951.

"The Leukemia Problem; Approach," *OEB*, iii, 2, 1951.

"Armoring in a Newborn Infant," *OEB*, iii, 3, 1951.

"Wilhelm Reich on the Road to Biogenesis (1935–39)," *OEB*, iii, 3, 1951.

"Orgonomic Thinking in Medicine," *OEB*, iv, i, 1952.

"Orgonomic Functionalism," Part II continued, *OEB*, iv, 4, 1952.

"Early Diagnosis of Uterine Cancer," *Core*, vii, 1–2, 1955.

"The Medical Dor-Buster," *Core*, vii, 3–4, 1955.

"The Energetics of Drives," *OM*, i, i, 1955.

"The Source of the Human 'No,'" *OM*, i, 2, 1955.

"Re-Emergence of Freud's 'Death Instinct' as 'DOR' Energy," *OM*, ii, 1, April 1956.

"Orgonomic Therapy of the Ocular Segment," *OM*, ii, 1, 1956.

Articles in Orgonomy by Co-Workers of Reich, in Chronological Order

Raknes, Ola, Ph.D. (Carl Arnold), "The Treatment of a Depression," *IJSO*, i, 1942.

Havrewold, Odd, M.D. (Walter Frank), "Vegetotherapy," *IJSO*, i, 1942.

Philipson, Tage, M.D. (Paul Martin), "Sex-Economic 'Upbringing,'" *IJSO*, i, 1942.

Wolfe, Theodore P., M.D., "The Sex-Economic Concept of Psychosomatic Identity and Antithesis," *IJSO*, i, 1942.

    "A Sex-Economic Note on Academic Sexology," *IJSO*, i, 1942.

"Misconceptions of Sex-Economy as Evidenced in Book Reviews," *IJSO*, ii, 1943.

Raknes, Ola, Ph.D., "Sex-Economy: A Theory of Living Functioning," *IJSO*, iii, 1944.

Wolfe, Theodore P., M.D., "The Stumbling Block in Medicine and Psychiatry," *IJSO*, iii, 1944.

Neill, A. S., "Coeducation and Sex," *IJSO*, iv, 1945.

Hoppe, Walter, M.D., "Sex-Economy and Orgone Research in Palestine," *AOI*, i, 1947.

Ollendorff, Ilse, "About Self-Regulation in a Healthy Child," *AOI*, i, 1947.

Baker, Elsworth F., M.D., "The Concept of Self-Regulation," *OEB*, i, 4, 1949.

Raknes, Ola, Ph.D., "A Short Treatment with Orgone Therapy," *OEB*, ii, 1, 1950.

Sobey, Victor, M.D., "Six Clinical Cases," *OEB*, ii, 1, 1950.

Anderston, William, A., M.D., "Orgone Therapy in Rheumatic Fever," *OEB*, ii, 2, 1950.

Oller, Charles, I., M.D., "Orgone Therapy of Frigidity; A Case History," *OEB*, ii, 4, 1950.

Levine, Emanuel, M.D., "Treatment of a Hypertensive Biopathy with the Orgone Energy Accumulator," *OEB*, iii, 1, 1951.

Raknes, Ola, Ph.D., "Orgonomic Work in Scandinavia," *OEB*, iii, 1, 1951.

Raphael, Chester M., M.D., "Orgone Treatment During Labor," *OEB*, iii, 2, 1951.

Wevrick, N., M.D., "Physical Orgone Treatment in Diabetes," *OEB*, iii, 2, 1951.

Cott, A. Allan, M.D., "Orgonomic Treatment of Ichthyosis," *OEB*, iii, 3, 1951.

Gold, Philip, M.D., "Orgonotic Functions in a Manic-Depressive Case," *OEB*, 3, 1951.

Raknes, Ola, Ph.D., "From Libido Theory to Orgonomy," *OEB*, iv, 1, 1952.

Baker, Elsworth F., M.D., "Genital Anxiety in Nursing Mothers," *OEB*, iv, 1, 1952.

Levine, Emanuel, M.D., "Observations on a Case of Coronary Occlusion," *OEB*, iv, 1, 1952.

Baker, Elsworth F., M.D., "A Grave Therapeutic Problem," *OEB*, v, 1 & 2, 1953.

Raphael, Chester M., M.D., "Dor Sickness, A Review of Reich's Findings," *Core*, vii, 1 & 2, 1955.

Willie, James A., M.D., "The Schizophrenic Biopathy" (Part I), *OM*, i, 1, 1955.

Silvert, Michael, M.D., "Orgonomic Practices in Obstetrics," *OM*, i, 1, 1955.

"Adolescent Genital Misery from High School Classrooms in New York and Maine," *OM*, i, 1, 1955.

Raknes, Ola, Ph.D., "The Orgonomic Concept of Health and Its Social Consequences," *OM*, i, 2, 1955.

Sobey, Victor M., M.D., "Treatment of Pulmonary Tuberculosis with Orgone Energy," *OM*, i, 2, 1955.

Hoppe, Walter, M.D., "Orgone versus Radium Therapy in Skin Cancer," *OM*, i, 2, 1955.

Sandel, Francine, "Adolescents and Babies in Trouble," *OM*, ii, 1, 1956.

Sobey, Victor M., M.D., "A Case of Rheumatoid Arthritis Treated with Orgone Energy," *OM*, ii, 1, 1956.

Index